Dental Ethics At Chairside:

PROFESSIONAL PRINCIPLES AND PRACTICAL APPLICATIONS

Dental Ethics At Chairside:

PROFESSIONAL PRINCIPLES
AND PRACTICAL APPLICATIONS

David T. Ozar, Ph.D.

Professor of Philosophy
Codirector of Graduate Studies in Health Care Ethics
Loyola University of Chicago;
Formerly, Clinical Professor of Professional Ethics
Loyola School of Dentistry
Chicago, Illinois

David J. Sokol, D.D.S., J.D., F.A.G.D.

In Private Practice of General Dentistry and Health Law
Newburgh, New York
Formerly, Associate Attending Dentist
Section Chief, Prosthodontic Section
Jewish Memorial Hospital
New York, New York

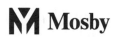 Mosby

St. Louis Baltimore Berlin Boston Carlsbad Chicago London Madrid
Naples New York Philadelphia Sydney Tokyo Toronto

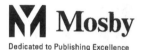

Mosby
Dedicated to Publishing Excellence

Executive Editor: Linda L. Duncan
Developmental Editor: Melba Steube
Project Manager: Mark Spann
Production Editor: Elizabeth Fathman
Designer: Dave Zielinski
Manufacturing Manager: Kathy Grone

Printed in the United States of America
Composition by University Graphics, Inc.
Printing/binding by Maple-Vail Binghamton

Mosby–Year Book, Inc.
11830 Westline Industrial Drive
St. Louis, Missouri 63146

Library of Congress Cataloging in Publication Data
Ozar, David T.
    Dental ethics at chairside : professional principles and practical
applications / David T. Ozar, David J. Sokol. — 1st ed.
        p.   cm.
    Includes bibliographical references.
    ISBN 0-8016-7400-X
    1. Dental ethics.   I. Sokol, David J.   II. Title.
    [DNLM: 1. Ethics, Dental.   WU 500 099d 1994]
    RK52.7.096 1994
    174′.2—dc20
    DNLM/DLC
    for Library of Congress   94-184
                                                                CIP

94 95 96 97 98 / 9 8 7 6 5 4 3 2 1

PREFACE

Most people still trust the health professionals who serve them, surveys show, even in this cynical age, and dentists are still among the most trusted of professionals. It is important for a dentist to keep this fact in mind and to reflect often on its implications, especially when dental practice seems to be changing so much under the influence of the malpractice crisis, the changing economic scene, the changing regulatory environment, and so on. The most important implication of this fact is that in the minds of the large majority of dentistry's patients, the principal realities of dental practice are still what they have long been: that dentists have the knowledge and skills needed to serve their patients' oral health needs and that dentists are professionally committed to acting by a certain set of standards to use this expertise properly.

The vast majority of dentists also consider professional expertise and professional commitment as the principal realities of dental practice and are concerned, in spite of the challenges of our age, to maintain both of them at the highest possible level. Maintaining one's professional expertise is a continuing challenge as dental scientists advance scientific understanding of the oral cavity and develop new techniques, materials, and technologies. But at least the resources for maintaining expertise are readily available through the journals, professional organizations, continuing education programs, and peer support that takes many concrete forms.

But resources to assist the practicing dentist in maintaining the commitment to practice ethically as well as expertly are not as much in evidence. There is much encouragement for ethical conduct within the dental profession, but relatively little assistance for judging what conduct is ethically best in the concrete situation. Few dentists have had extensive training in professional ethics, in dental school or elsewhere, and continuing education programs on ethical concerns in dental practice are few and far between. Most dentists' personal resources for professional-ethical reflection are considerable, and many have thoughtful peers, spouses, and friends to whom they can turn when particularly pressed. But few would deny that they often choose a course of professional action without a sense that they have given the matter all the ethical reflection it deserved and that they frequently do so because they have run out of ideas about how to consider it. Most dentists, we believe, would appreciate the chance to examine some additional ideas and well-developed intellectual tools to use in reflecting on the professional judgments and choices they must make.

This book is written for the sake of such dentists and for the sake of dental students who aspire to be like them. It is also written in the hope that some members of the nondental community would care to understand what professional-ethical reflection in dental practice is about. But in one respect it is written first of all for the sake of dentistry's patients who—for the most part—

still trust their dentists to be not only competent, but ethically adept in their professional practice as well. If this book can contribute to the continued fulfillment of their trust by contributing to dentists' fulfillment of their professional-ethical commitments, it will have accomplished its principal goal.

This book could not have been written without the encouragement, support, and valuable insights of our families and of many colleagues. We are particularly grateful to the members of the Professional Ethics in Dentistry Network, especially Tom Hasegawa, Don Patthoff, Pat Odom, Mickey Bebeau, John Gilbert, Mary Ellen Waithe, Al Rosenblum, and Bruce Weinstein. We are also grateful to Loyola University of Chicago for a research leave that made the timely completion of this book possible and to Professors James Sandrik, Donald Doemling, James Koelbl, and Dean Aidan Stephens, all formerly of Loyola University School of Dentisty, for their continuing support.

David T. Ozar
David J. Sokol

CONTENTS

PART ONE

THE DENTAL PROFESSION
AND PROFESSIONAL ETHICS

CHAPTER 1

Introduction

ETHICAL ISSUES IN DENTAL PRACTICE

To an unprecedented degree, dentists today are facing difficult ethical questions with far-reaching consequences. Of course, dentists have been facing ethical dilemmas in their professional practice for as long as dentistry has existed. But in recent years, the complexity of the ethical issues faced by dentists has increased, and difficult ethical judgments seem to arise much more frequently. That is why a lot of talk among dentists today, both at professional meetings and in social gatherings, concerns how they ought to respond to ethically difficult situations. In the minds of many dentists today, dental professionals need to increase the level of attention and reflection directed to these problems.

Consider this sampling of ethical decisions that almost every dentist faces regularly:

1. When examining a new patient, a dentist finds evidence of poor dental work. What should the dentist say to the patient? Should the dentist contact the previous dentist to discuss the matter? Should the dentist contact the local dental society?
2. May a dentist ethically advertise that his or her practice will produce "happy smiles" as well as quality dental care?
3. May a dentist tell a patient that his or her teeth are unattractive, with a view to recommending aesthetic treatment, when the patient has not asked for this opinion and has indicated no displeasure with their appearance?
4. Can a dentist justify manipulating data on an insurance form to secure a better kind of therapy or more timely therapy for a patient who could otherwise not afford it? May a dentist ethically refrain from recommending a superior kind of therapy to a patient in a capitation health plan and recommend instead a clinically acceptable but minimal form of therapy because the dentist knows that the payment the dentist receives for that patient will cover only the minimal therapy, and the patient may need still more care during this payment period?
5. May a dentist ethically decline to treat a patient with a highly infectious disease? May a dentist decline to treat such a patient unless the patient's charges include a surcharge for additional infection precautions? What

obligations does the dentist have regarding the information that this patient is a carrier of infection?

6. How ought a dentist deal with an adult patient who cannot fully partici- pate in deciding about care? Does this depend on the reason for the patient's inability? What ought a dentist do when the guardian of a minor or of an incompetent adult patient refuses to approve the best kind of therapy for the patient?

7. What may a dentist do to obtain cooperative behavior from a young patient who needs dental care but is uncontrollable in the chair?

8. Do dentists have an obligation to warn their patients, even when patients don't want to hear it, about the dangers of smoking or other substance dependencies?

9. What obligations does a dentist have, and to whom, when the dentist learns that another dentist is substance dependent in a manner that likely affects the care he or she is providing?

10. What may dentists require of other dentists who are their employees? What may they require of the dental hygienists and dental assistants whom they employ? What are the obligations of dentist-employers toward these groups?

This is a representative list of ethical questions that dentists regularly ask. It is hardly an exhaustive list of such questions; there are many more. This book will aim to provide dentists with a systematic account of professional ethics in dental practice to help them understand and judge wisely about issues like these. The first part of the book will offer an account of the nature of a profession, of several important categories of professional obligation that apply to dental practice, and of the elements of an ethical decision-making process. The second part will examine a variety of ethical issues that dentists face and show how the themes developed in the first part can assist in reflect- ing on them. The objective of the book is that its readers come to reflect more clearly and articulately on the ethics of dental practice.

ETHICAL QUESTIONS AND LEGAL QUESTIONS

Many of the ethical questions listed above also have legal ramifications. A number of books, journal articles, and continuing education programs are available to help dentists act within the law and protect themselves from suits and other legal risks. But questions of ethics are different from questions of law. They have a different basis, and they approach matters in a different way. In addition, ethical questions often concern matters about which law has no opinion.

In fact, ethics is more fundamental than law. That is, laws can be either ethical or unethical, but the converse is not true. Thus the clear-thinking per- son will ask the ethical question first and the legal question only later; and one of the first questions that a thoughtful person will ask about a law that applies to his or her situation is whether it is an ethical law or not, both in what it requires in general and in how it applies to the particular case. If it is not, then being ethical may require a person to work to change that law, or possibly, if the matter is important enough, even to conscientiously violate that law or to engage in civil disobedience to change it. These facts about law and ethics do not mean that law is unimportant, but only that ethical ques- tions are different from and are more important than legal questions.

courage such discussion and thus foster the development of a dental
munity much more reflective and articulate on ethical issues. Then the
l community can formulate codes and contribute to committees' delib-
ions in ways that will enable both structures to offer still better guidance
thical practice.

S

A little reflection makes it clear that most of the actions we perform in life
are not the product of careful, self-conscious deliberation about our alternatives. Most of our actions are, as we might say, "just done." That is, they are
done without careful reflection at the time. But this does not mean that most
of our actions are irrational. Rather they are done from habit. <u>Probably 95%</u>
<u>or more of our actions are the product of various habits of acting, perceiving,</u>
<u>valuing,</u> and so on. Indeed, it seems clear that we could not function psycho-
logically if most of our actions were not the products of our habits.

The reason that these actions, though they are not carefully reflected upon
one at the time, cannot be simply described as irrational is that the habits
these actions come from are, for the most part, available for careful reflection
and subject to thoughtful choice. That is, if we choose, we can usually identify the habits that are most formative of a particular action, and we can then
examine these habits, compare them with alternative ways of acting, perceiving, and valuing, and then make a judgment about whether this is a habit that
we want to keep or whether we should try to change it <u>so that our actions are</u>
<u>based on habits more suited to what we judge best for that set of circum-</u>
<u>stances.</u>

Some habits are difficult to "break," whether this means changing the habit
or eliminating it completely. In some cases, a person can only change or eliminate a habitual pattern of acting, perceiving, or valuing with professional
assistance. But except in the most extreme cases—which we justifiably think
of as instances of mental or emotional illness—our habits are subject to our
choices and, a step before that, to our judgments about what habits we do
and do not want to have. So doing something from habit is not necessarily
irrational.

This point about habits is particularly important in a book about ethics.
Because so many of our actions are not the products of self-conscious ethical
thinking, but rather, as has been said, the product of habits, any discussion of
ethics must therefore be as much a discussion of ethical habits as a discussion of individual ethical actions.

Given how many of our actions are the product of habits, it might seem
that discussions of ethics are actually pointless. Won't we ordinarily do what
we are in the habit of doing, the objector might say, whether that is what is
ethical or not? What this objection overlooks, however, is our limited but real
ability, just discussed, <u>to judge and choose our habits</u>. If we judge that acting
in a certain way under certain circumstances is the ethical thing to do, then
we should work to support our habits if they are in the right direction, and to
change our habits if they are not, so that we habitually do precisely that
which we would judge best if we were to stop and deliberate carefully about
it.

Talk of "virtues" may seem a bit old fashioned today. But <u>a virtue is noth-</u>
<u>ing but a good habit,</u> a habit of acting, perceiving, and valuing in the best way

The focus of this book is on ethical o·
although an occasional comment a!
nates the ethical issue involved. Ot
specific questions, a good lawyer shou
law (in each particular jurisdiction) requ
from legal risk.

CHOOSING TO BE ETHICAL

This book will examine many of the ethical is:
tice and will offer a set of guidelines to assist den:
cal in the particular issues that arise for them. But ,
anyone that they should be ethical.

This is not because there are no carefully reasoned ;
made in support of being ethical. It is for two other reaso
ments, when they are well constructed, are complex and ,
are well beyond the scope of this book. Secondly, most peopl·
ily choose to become ethical or to continue being ethical whe
sacrifice and risk simply because someone has offered them a ,
soned argument about being ethical (although such arguments d·
important reasons that are involved in such choices). They do so ,
more complex reflections about the sort of person they want to be, th
ties of the persons in their lives whom they admire, the communities
which they want to be identified, and the efficacy of various courses of ac,
and patterns of life in relation to these matters. In fact, one who chooses
pay little or no attention to ethical questions may very possibly be just as dis-
interested in arguments that show such a stance to be irrational.

This book does not pretend to be able to replace reflections of this sort,
although it may contribute to such reflections for some people by articulating
the values and ideals to which individual dentists and the dental community
as a whole are committed as professionals. This book's task is rather to offer a
careful account, for consideration by all concerned, of what counts as ethical
practice in dentistry.

PUBLISHED CODES OF CONDUCT AND ETHICS COMMITTEES

Most dental organizations, such as the American Dental Association, the
Canadian Dental Association, regional and local associations, and the various
specialty organizations, have published codes of ethical conduct to guide dentists in ethical practice. Many also have ethics committees that offer formal
opinions or informal advice to dentists on difficult ethical questions.

This book is not offered as a commentary on these codes or on the work of
these committees, much less as a competitor to them. It tries to accomplish a
different, and in some ways more basic function. Those who draft, approve,
and interpret these codes and opinions have conceptions of the nature of the
dental profession and its goals, values, and ideals, upon which these codes
and opinions are based. But the codes and opinions do not—and, in practice,
cannot—articulate these underlying conceptions in a systematic way so that
they can be discussed and enriched by the experience of the dental community at large. Therefore a book like this, which offers a systematic account of
the nature of the dental profession, of its goals, values, and ideals, and of the
implications of these for ethical practice, can be very useful. It can facilitate

possible for the situation. It is therefore accurate to say that this book is as much about professional virtue as it is about professional ethics or professions' and professionals' obligations.

Throughout the book, cases and examples will be used to help explain types of ethical issues and characteristics and other aspects of professional ethics in dentistry. In each instance, the reader should reflect not just on the individual case described, but on the habits of acting, perceiving, and valuing of which the case is an instance. It is these habits, more than the particular actions involved in the case, that are the real subject matter of this book. To keep the language of the book simpler, however, the cases and examples will be discussed directly, without continually referring to the habits—or virtues— they embody.

THE TERMS *MORAL* AND *ETHICAL*

Some people use the term *moral* to mean one thing and the term *ethical* to mean something slightly, or even quite a bit, different. But people who use these terms differently often do not explain the difference, and in any case there is no pattern of differentiating their meanings that is widely and consistently employed, much less commonly understood. As a result, serious misunderstandings frequently result from people's differing use of these terms. So it is important to explain how the terms *ethical* and *moral* will be used in these pages. In this book these two terms will be treated as synonyms, and they will be used to mean only that the issue, question, reflection, or judgment to which they apply concerns what ought or ought not to be done or what is a matter of someone's obligation. More detailed or more complicated distinctions within this general arena of discussion—for example, the kinds of obligations there are and their relevance to some situation at hand—will be explicitly made when they are needed.

In the same way, the word *obligation* will be used in a very general way in these pages. To say someone has an obligation will simply mean that there is something that the person ought or ought not do. More detailed or more complicated distinctions among obligations will be explicitly made as needed.

DO ETHICAL QUESTIONS HAVE ANSWERS?

There is a view widespread within our society that there are no correct answers to moral or ethical questions or, what amounts to the same thing, that one answer to a moral or ethical question is just as good as every other answer. There is no time to examine this fundamental issue carefully in this book. Instead, it will be most productive for our purposes to simply say that the matter is at least an open question.

That is, on the one hand, no one who has tried to has yet succeeded in demonstrating that there are no correct answers to moral questions, although we know that people have differing views on many of these questions. In point of fact, of course, we know that in some situations people have differing views because some of the people's views, all but one, or sometimes even all of the people's views are in fact mistaken. On the other hand, there are some moral or ethical questions on which the level of agreement, even among people from very diverse backgrounds, is quite impressive. Yet so far no one has demonstrated to every one else's satisfaction that one particular ethical system provides all the correct answers to ethical questions.

We hope, of course, that pursuing this inquiry, looking for answers, and developing our resources for answering ethical questions about dentistry will prove valuable. But at the very minimum, as a starting position, we can confidently assert that there is no good reason to believe that the project represents a waste of effort. This is what is implied when we say, on the question whether there are correct answers to ethical questions, that the matter is at least an open question.

SOURCES OF ETHICAL VIEWS AND CONVICTIONS

People's ethical views and convictions have many sources. People learn various aspects of their ethical views and convictions from their family and other important figures in their upbringing, from their formal education, from informal life contacts, both prior to maturity and afterward, from the culture of the society at large as well as of specific social and occupational groups, from religious upbringing during their youth and from their religious commitments as adults, and from personal reflection throughout life.

For the purposes of this book, because of the likely diversity of backgrounds and views of those who read it, all of these sources will be considered valuable as sources of ethical views and convictions, and all will be considered limited and incomplete in this role. That is, none of them will be viewed as a privileged source of ethical answers, as having the last word, or as authoritative in its own right. The answers that this book seeks will ideally be answers that resonate with people's experience generally, either experiences that every inquirer actually has had or others' experiences that each inquirer can nevertheless understand because of similarities to their own. So everyone's experience is data for ethical reflection and no one's experience is authoritative for others unless it actually resonates with their own experience.

WHO WRITES A BOOK ON DENTAL ETHICS?

It might seem that to write a book on ethics, an author would have to think he or she has the answers to people's questions about how they ought and they ought not act. But most people, probably including most readers of this book, are quite suspicious of those who would tell them how they ought and ought not act. Even if correct answers to ethical questions are possible, most of us doubt that there are experts, in the usual sense, in ethics or morality. So what kind of person writes a book on dental ethics?

As the authors of this book, we do not claim to be experts about what people ought and ought not do. We believe that objectivity (the move away from subjectivity) in ethical judgments, as in all judgments, is increasingly achieved as one's judgments are grounded in a broader and broader base of human experience—both one's own experience and the experience of others. The experience that is relevant to the discussion of ethical issues is not exclusive to any particular group; all humans can learn from each other on these matters. In this sense, while there are no "experts" (in the usual sense) on ethical matters, every person who reflects carefully on his or her experience has expertise to share with others.

As the authors of this book, then, we view ourselves as fellow-inquirers with all those who are concerned to understand ethical issues both in the dental profession specifically, and in other areas of human life. We have had the benefit of a number of years of study in this field and of contact with many of the other thinkers who have studied these issues closely. This book is an effort both to distill what we have learned so far and to share it with others who are interested in order to assist them in reflecting carefully and in broadening the range of experience on which their reflections are based, and to widen the circle of inquirers who share a common base of experience and reflection on these issues.

In other words, we have written this book because dental ethics raises important questions whose answers require far more collective wisdom than is available if only our two heads are put together. The goal is to broaden and deepen the dialogue, within the dental community and in the community at large, on the important professional ethical issues that arise in dental practice.

CHAPTER 2

_____

Profession and Professional Obligation

Case: Grind It Out!

Jack Williamson, a fourth-year dental student, has just returned from an interview with a prospective employer, Dr. Edward Prentice. Dr. Prentice runs three dental offices and plans to open a fourth office in the summer. He has been interviewing a large number of senior students from dental schools in the state in order to hire a group of young dentists to staff his new office.

Like many dental students today, Jack Williamson will graduate with large debts, so the chances that a bank will give him an additional loan to start up his own practice are slim even if the urban market were not already flooded with dentists. But Jack's wife's job and their desire to remain near his ailing parents make a move away from the city unacceptable at present. So Jack has been looking for a job in the area. He has just returned from visiting Dr. Prentice's main office to take a look at the practice and to be interviewed.

As soon as Jack walked into the students' common room, everyone knew he had been out on an interview. "Very nice suit, Jack! Are you trying to upgrade the clinic? Too much boring white?" The speaker was Len Billings, another fourth-year student. "How did it go?" he asked.

"It was a little weird. You know where I was? Prentice's Smile Centers."

"I've seen the ads. What was it like?"

"Very cushy. The new place is going to look like the Taj Mahal. All the latest equipment is going in there, too. That part was pretty interesting."

"What wasn't so interesting?" asked Becky Lissen, another of Jack's classmates.

"The part about taking care of patients," said Jack. "I spent about an hour and a half at the place on Oakville Boulevard; that was Prentice's second office, and it's where he has his own executive office. There were a huge number of patients being taken care of and waiting for treatment, a huge number; and it looked to me like 'Grind it out' was the motto."

"What do you mean?" said Robert Teng, another fourth-year student.

"The dentists—four men and two women, pretty much like us, all just out of school—working as fast as they could. The latest technology and lots of assistants, but all in the interest of speed and volume. They might as well have had 'Grind it out' tattooed on their foreheads."

"You mean Prentice pushes them hard?" asked Len. "What do you expect? If we can't afford our own practices, then we have to take what we can get.

But you could handle that, Jack; any of us in our group could. We all know how to work hard, and we're pretty fast, too. . . I mean, unless Prentice is some sort of jerk. That would be a problem."

"He doesn't strike me as a jerk, Len, and hard work doesn't bother me either," said Jack. "I've worked for plenty of bosses who pushed you on the job, not to mention the pressure on students in this place. No, it's the quotas that got me, Len. They have target numbers, a certain amount of billable work per patient, per hour, per day, and so on, that they are judged by. Prentice is apparently very clear about it; that is simply what is expected. One time, while Prentice was on the phone, I saw that one of the guys was between patients, so I went into his operatory and asked him if there was a lot of pressure to get patients in and out, or to pressure them to buy a lot of care. He looked first to see who could hear him and then said, 'Grind it out or get your butt out of here; that's the story.'"

"So I said to him, 'Prentice doesn't seem like a bad guy,' and the guy said, 'He's not nasty about it. He's a very friendly sort of guy, in fact, but that doesn't change the expectations. He doesn't have to be nasty; he's in charge. He hires and he fires. If someone doesn't perform, they get the boot.'"

"Does he force them to do unnecessary care?" asked Becky. "Are his dentists supposed to trick patients into thinking they need something when they don't? They can't do treatments without getting the patients' consent, can they?"

"I asked Prentice about it later," Jack answered, "about whether the high volume of treatment that I observed involved pressuring the patients or putting extra pressure on the dentists."

"What did he say?"

"'First of all,' he said, 'clear expectations make for good relationships with your employees. Suppose you came to work for me,' he said, 'and you wanted to know where you stood; you could figure it out yourself just by comparing your work to the target numbers. That makes things very clear between us. As for the patients, Jack, of course they have to give consent before they are treated. That's the law, and I certainly don't want my employees violating the law; I tell them that very clearly.'"

"What about pressuring the patients?" asked Becky.

"He said, 'Patients know very little about dentistry. They depend on the dentist to tell them what they need, and that's how we create our volume of work. A dentist shouldn't tell patients they need things that would harm healthy teeth; that's a given. But that still leaves us a lot of leeway. If an amalgam is showing signs of wear, we recommend that it be replaced. We don't recommend restoring a tooth with a second or third amalgam, or even a large first amalgam, when a crown will certainly last longer, and so on. Discoloration, other esthetic things, many things can be proposed as needing work without lying to a patient, much less violating their right to accept or reject our recommendations.'"

"What about patient education," asked Robert. "If they were really educating the patients, the patients would be told that some of these things are not serious reasons for treatment, at least for most people, and there are often less expensive options than a crown, too."

"I asked if patient education was a priority," said Jack. "What Prentice said was: 'Patient education is important. But it takes a lot of time, and most patients won't sit still for it when they know the meter is running. They come here to get their teeth fixed, and we fix them; that is what they are interested in and that is what we are interested in. One of the reasons they like us so much is that they can come in, get the work done, and get out. Like our ad says: 'Quick appointments when you need care; short waits when you get there.'"

"Then these patients don't really know what they are consenting to," said Becky."

"What Prentice said," said Jack, "was that if a patient asks for education, his dentists gladly provide it, but with the meter running. 'We have to be realistic here, Jack,' said Jack, imitating Prentice's slightly pompous manner. 'The rule of the marketplace is *caveat emptor:* Let the buyer beware. We never lie to patients, we only make recommendations. But if the recommendations are well made, carefully made, they can work very effectively to sell treatments that will keep our numbers high. That's what we expect of everyone in my offices, myself included. If we all follow through on that, we all make a good living out of it. Anyone who isn't interested should work someplace else.'"

"I couldn't work in a place like that," said Becky.

"It bothers me, too," said Jack. "But a dentist has to make a living, like anybody else."

"Lots of dentists make a good living without doing it that way," said Robert. "Did anyone there even mention doing what is best for the patient? That's what we've been taught, that the patient comes first. But it doesn't sound like the patients come first there; it's their wallets that come first."

"Did you ask Prentice about that?" asked Becky, "I mean that it seems unethical to practice that way?"

"Not exactly, but he could tell I was having a problem. Before I left he said, 'It looks to me like you've still got that idealism about dentistry that so many students have before they have to practice in the real world. I understand it; I was idealistic, too, when I was in school. But remember, when the patients in your school's clinic don't pay, it doesn't come out of your pocket. When it's your pocket that's involved, you find out that things don't look the way they did in school. No one is out there saying, "Dentists are good people and do a lot of good, so let's make sure they get their fair share and earn a good living." Instead, you find out very quickly that you have to make your own way. We all do. I've found a way to do that and to practice technically good dentistry at the same time. I don't hire bad dentists; I don't even interview bad dentists, Jack, only dentists in the top half of their class, because bad dentistry is bad business. But if you don't see that dentistry is a business, if you keep that idealism, Jack, then you're going to be living in a dream world. You're welcome to try it if you want, but I think you'll find out very quickly that it won't hold up.'"

"That's sure a long way from what I've been taught," said Becky, "and from the dentists I've really admired. I think it's unethical to practice like that."

"Maybe it isn't ideal," said Len, "but maybe it's realistic. It's a different world out there from what it was fifteen or twenty years ago, when the dentists that we admired as kids were starting up. They could graduate without huge debts, get a loan from a bank, and set up a lucrative practice. But that's not true any more, not for most of us anyway. They could afford to be idealistic and still make it. And maybe some of us will be lucky enough to end up in practices that are still like that. But you sure can't count on it."

"I'm not competing with Jack for a job," Len continued. "I'm going back to Minnesota. So I can hope Jack gets lots of offers so he can stay here in town. But suppose that Prentice likes Jack and makes him an offer, and suppose Jack doesn't get any other offers to choose from. He's a good dentist and a good guy and all that; he just doesn't get any other offers. Are you saying, Becky, that Jack shouldn't take Prentice's job? Maybe Prentice is a little extreme with the ads and the marketing and everything. But he doesn't practice bad dentistry; he doesn't harm people, and they still have to consent to every treatment he does for them. Are you saying that it would be unethical for Jack, or any of us, to work for a guy like Prentice if the alternative is worse, like maybe not practicing dentistry at all?"

"It may mean some hard choices," said Robert, "but if you stand for something, then you have to draw the line somewhere."

"Yes," said Jack, "you do have to draw the some somewhere. But where?"

DENTISTRY AS A PROFESSION

Dentistry has long prided itself on being a profession, and dentists routinely describe themselves as professionals. Among the most common characteristics of professions and professionals, there are several that dentists can clearly claim for themselves: (1) Dentists possess a distinctive expertise that consists of both theoretical knowledge and skills for applying it in practice, (2) dentists' expertise is a source of important benefits for those who seek their assistance, and (3) because of their expertise, dentists are accorded, both individually and collectively, extensive autonomy in matters pertaining to it.

But there is a fourth widely accepted charateristic of a profession that requires careful examination here. Many people, both inside and outside of professions, hold that professions and professionals have special obligations and consider this to be a central feature of their being professions and professionals. When a group becomes a profession, this view holds, it is precisely in doing so that it undertakes certain obligations. Similarly, when an individual becomes a professional—a member of a profession—precisely in doing this he or she undertakes certain obligations.

Is this true of dentistry and of dentists? Many people would say, "Of course it is." But others have challenged this view, claiming that it is an incorrect description of dentists and dentistry. Therefore it is important to ask, before going any further, whether it is true that dentistry as a whole, as well as each individual dentist, has special *professional* obligations. If not, then a study of "Professional Ethics in Dentistry" can be very brief, for it need only be long enough to demonstrate that there is no such thing. But if the dental community and individual dentists do have specifically *professional* obligations, if Jack, Becky, and Robert are right in thinking that they will have special obligations because they are dentists, then it is important to understand why this is so, even before asking more specifically what these obligations are.

To this end, it will be useful to contrast two fundamentally different pictures of dentistry. The Normative Picture holds that dentistry and dentists do have obligations precisely because they are professionals. The Commercial Picture denies this and sees dentistry as no different in principle from any other activity in the marketplace in which some people produce a product and other people purchase it from them. The following two sections will contrast these two pictures of dentistry in some detail.

DENTISTRY: THE COMMERCIAL PICTURE

The Commercial Picture, as indicated, takes dental practice to be no different in principle from the activity of anyone who produces and sells his or her wares in the marketplace. The dentist has a product to sell and makes such arrangements with interested purchasers as the two parties are willing to make. Depending on one's view of the marketplace, there may be some fundamental obligations that all participants in the marketplace have toward all other participants, for example, obligations not to coerce, cheat, or defraud other participants in the marketplace. If there are such obligations, they would be exclusively obligations to *refrain* from acting in these various ways, to refrain from coercing, cheating, or defrauding others. These and similar examples are specifications of a fundamental obligation not to violate the liberty of other participants. But according to this Commercial Picture of dentistry, no one in the marketplace has any obligations to *act* in one way rather than another (as contrasted with *refraining* from certain kinds of acts) toward anyone, except insofar as he or she voluntarily undertakes such obligations toward specific individuals or groups.

Consequently, according to this picture of dentistry, the fact of being a dentist and a member of the dental profession has no moral import of its own. The fundamental obligation, not to violate others' liberty, is had by all capable humans, and all other obligations that a dentist might have will come from specific voluntary arrangements between dentists and other participants in the marketplace, for example, the dentists' patients. So dentists have no obligations to their patients, nor to anyone else, simply because they are dentists and members of a profession.

According to the Commercial Picture, then, a dentist's expertise and the application of it to the lives of patients is a commodity that dentists sell and patients buy, analogous to any other commodity bought and sold in the marketplace. The dentist is a producer; the client is a consumer. Their entire relationship consists of communications about the commodity and its price, some agreement regarding an exchange (if an agreement is achieved), and the actual exchange of the agreed-upon commodity for the agreed-upon price.

Because from the Commercial point of view the dentist and the patient are self-interested participants in the marketplace, in their principal relationship they are, first and foremost, competitors. That is, each is trying to obtain from the other the greatest amount of what is needed or desired while giving up as little as possible of what is being offered in exchange. As a consequence, the proper criterion by which the dentist determines what sort of services to provide to the patient is not necessarily whatever will best meet the patient's need or best serve the patient's well-being. Instead the dentist quite properly determines what services to provide on the basis of whatever services the patient is willing to pay for and, among these, whichever ones will give the dentist the greatest return for the least cost to the dentist in terms of time, effort, money, satisfaction, and so on.

In fact, in the Commercial Picture, the patient's needs and improved well-being play only a secondary role in the dentist's judgments about which services to offer a patient. Of course, patients' needs and well-being do frequently function as motivators for patients to part with their money in return for a dentist's services. So dentists quite reasonably attend to patients' needs and well-being when doing so is useful in this way. But the patient's needs and well-being have no other significance for a dentist or for dentistry in the Commercial Picture. They certainly are not something about which a dentist or the dental profession has obligations, except insofar as these obligations are the product of explicit contractual arrangements with individual patients or other parties (e.g., insurance companies).

Of course, the dentist ordinarily communicates judgments to patients regarding their need for professional services. But any such judgments must be viewed, in the Commercial Picture, principally as efforts of good salesmanship, efforts by the dentist to motivate patients to purchase services. The case might be made that sellers are obligated to refrain from outright lies to potential buyers, to the extent that these violate, if they do, the liberty of participants in the marketplace. But it is still the case that a dentist's recommendations for services are in principle identical, according to the Commercial Picture, to any other salesperson's encouragements to buy. A dentist's recommendation that the upper left first molar needs a two-surface amalgam restoration is no different in principle, according to the Commercial Picture, from a shoe salesperson's comment that the customer looks good in a particular pair of shoes.

In addition, in the Commercial Picture, the members of any occupational group are first and foremost competitors, all striving for business from the same pool of clients. Nevertheless, members of the same occupation often have interests in common as they deal with various centers of power in the larger community, especially with the government. They will often therefore have sound, self-interested reasons for forming trade associations to perform such functions as lobbying and public relations on behalf of their common concerns. Any group that we would describe as a "professional organization" is, in the Commercial Picture, a trade association of precisely this sort. (On this view, the term "profession" is simply a collective noun, referring to the whole collection of individuals who happen to practice the same expert occupation. There is no reason to think of this group of practitioners as a community or a unified entity in any other sense.)

What about the codes of conduct that such organizations frequently publish? According to the Commercial Picture, these are, of course, simply marketing devices. They are aimed at bringing increased numbers of patients to the groups' members. The organizations' efforts to certify members' knowledge and skills, whether directly or indirectly, for example, by the certification of dental schools, and also their efforts to prevent admittance to practice by persons not so certified, are marketing techniques aimed at bolstering potential patients' confidence in the quality of the group's product, and at the same time they are a means of limiting the number of competitors their members must face. Like individual dentists, dental organizations have no particular obligations to their members' patients, nor to the larger community as a whole, nor to anyone else, simply because they are called "professional" groups and their members are "professionals." (The leaders of these organizations will, of course, have certain contractual commitments to their members, depending on how the duties of the leaders' offices have been defined and agreed upon, but these are not obligations to present or future patients of the members, nor to the community at large.)

How professional schools are viewed is also a strong indicator of how professions and professionals are viewed. According to the Commercial Picture of dentistry, the dental school is itself simply a marketplace where experienced practitioners sell their knowledge and skills to consumers—the students—who aspire to eventually resell this expertise to the public. Here again, the relationship between the parties involved is essentially a competitive one, although the exclusive possession of dental expertise by those who are already dentists puts the consumers (i.e., the students) at some disadvantage in bargaining. As above, neither the experienced dentist as teacher, nor the student as present learner and future dentist, has any particular obligation toward anyone, whether present or future patients or the larger community, simply because of their standing as present and future professionals.

DENTISTRY: THE NORMATIVE PICTURE

These implications of the Commercial Picture are easy to describe, and it is possible to find examples of conduct conforming to the Commercial Picture on the part of individual dentists and patients and certain other individuals and groups within our society. Nevertheless, it is a premise of this book that the Commercial Picture does not provide an accurate account of the dental profession in our society today. For the vast majority of dental professionals and the vast majority of the community at large do not accept the Commercial Picture of the dental profession any more than they accept it for any of the health professions. Instead they accept an alternative picture of the dental profession, which will here be called the Normative Picture.

According to the Normative Picture, the dentist, like every health professional, has joined a group of persons who have made, both individually and collectively, a set of commitments to the community at large, commitments that entail important obligations for each dentist and for the dental profession as a whole. The basis of these obligations lies in a relationship between the profession as a whole, the individual professional, and the community at large. Therefore, a brief examination of this relationship is in order.

One of the most characteristic features of a profession, as has already been noted, is expertise in a matter of great importance to the community at large. In our case it is dental care. Moreover, the kind of expertise that we ordinarily associate with a profession is exclusive in two ways. It is not only exclusive in the sense that within the division of labors that enables a society to function efficiently, only certain persons will perform, and hence become familiar with and efficient at performing, this set of activities. Effective dental care also involves both knowledge and experience sufficiently esoteric that extensive education is required as a prerequisite to providing such care, and neither this knowledge nor this experience can be gained effectively except under the direction of someone who is already expert in them. Consequently, only those who are already expert are able to train others in their expertise; only those who are expert are able both to recognize if another person has become expert or not and give dependable and timely (i.e., before irreparable damage has been done) judgments regarding the quality of particular instances of the profession's practice.

Because the larger community depends on such experts for effective dental care, but at the same time values it greatly, the members of the community can see that it is in their interest, both individually and collectively, to place dental care decisions to a significant extent into the hands of these experts. But to do so is to grant a great deal of power to these experts. Nevertheless, in the case of the dental profession, as of the health care professions generally, the community not only grants to these experts a great deal of decision-making power over people's well-being, but <u>also entrusts to them the task of supervising how they themselves use this power</u>.

Compare the power granted to the dental profession with, for example, the power granted to politicians in government. The community grants politicians power over people's well-being without a sense of trust regarding its use, and it does not trust them at all to supervise their own exercise of the power granted them. Instead, the community supports a complex and inefficient system of checks and balances within government, the institution of periodic reelection, an aggressive, prying free press, and other costly structures to maintain close supervision on the politicians' performance. But for the dental profession, <u>there is little or no such close outside supervision,</u> and there is little persistent distrust either.

Why does the community at large *trust* the members of the dental profession? What assurance does the community at large have that so much power will not be abused by dentists? The answer is the institution of a *profession*, as it is understood in the Normative Picture. That is, each profession and each individual professional is committed to using this power according to norms mutually acceptable to the community at large and to the expert group—norms that, when conformed to, assure the community that the experts will use the power in such a way as to secure the well-being of the people whom they serve rather than placing their own personal well-being ahead of that of their patients.

According to the Normative Picture of dentistry, when a person becomes a dental professional, <u>he or she makes a commitment to act in accordance with certain norms,</u> and therefore has corresponding obligations as he or she carries out the practice of dental care. A person entering the dental profession cannot legitimately say: "Dentistry may have an obligation of such-and-such a sort, but *I* don't have that obligation because I didn't accept it." The relationship between the dental community and the larger community predates the entry of the individual student into dentistry, and acceptance of that relationship is a condition of entry. In fact, it is only the continuing pattern of acceptance of this relationship by each new dentist that makes it reasonable for the larger community both to continue to trust dentists to use the power of their expertise properly and to permit them so much autonomy, both in decision-making about their patients' well-being and also in supervising themselves in how they use this power.

The accuracy of the Normative Picture of dentistry is, as indicated earlier, a premise of this book. Evidence in support of this premise can be found in each area of dental practice that was just described from the perspective of the Commercial Picture. For each area, the dominant way in which dentists conduct themselves and in which the larger community understands and expects them to conduct themselves conforms to the Normative Picture rather than the Commercial Picture.

First of all, it is widely taken for granted that dentists *do* have obligations to their patients besides the market-place obligations of not coercing or defrauding. Dentists have a positive obligation to work for the patient's well-being by properly meeting his or her needs for dental care. Merely refraining from wrong-doing is not sufficient.

Secondly, dental care is not viewed simply as a commodity to be sold and bought solely on the basis of people's desire to buy it. Dental care is taken to have objective value, to be important to people's well-being, whether a given individual happens to value it or not. It pertains to people's ability to function in a proper and healthy way and to minimizing their pain and discomfort, neither of which is ordinarily considered merely a matter of consumer preference. This is also why the dentist has a positive responsibility to practice competently because something of genuine value for the patient is at stake. *Caveat emptor,* let the buyer beware, is simply not considered as adequate account of the relationship between dentist and patient.

Thirdly, although each has interests at stake, the relationship between dentist and patient is not a competitive one. On the one hand, the dentist has obligations to the patient to act for his or her well-being in relation to oral health and function, rather than solely to maximize the dentist's own situation. In addition, at least ideally it seems that the patient and the dentist will need to work together, rather than as competitors, in achieving the goal of maximal oral function for the patient. A more detailed examination of the proper relationship between dental professional and patient will be undertaken in the next chapter. But the point for now is that this relationship is certainly not well described as one of competing self-interests.

As a consequence, there is also a sharp contrast between the way a patient hears a dentist's recommendations for treatment and a shoe salesperson's evaluation of a particular pair of shoes on his or her feet. The dentist's recommendations are not only considered to be founded on expertise, but are also trusted to be offered principally for the sake of the patient's greater well-being, rather than principally for the salesperson's.

Fourth, one important role of professional organizations within dentistry, although they may share certain characteristics with trade organizations, is to articulate, interpret, and supervise dentists' conduct in relation to the obligations that they have undertaken. In addition, the interest of such organizations in testing and approving various procedures and agents for use in dental practice, and in certifying educational programs in dental schools and elsewhere, is at least as much to secure proper dental care for patients as it is to protect the well-being of dentists themselves.

Finally, within the dental schools, dental expertise is not handed over to students as if it were a simple commodity. It is handed over only in the context of the student's understanding and undertaking the professional commitments that are its context. The relationship between dental faculty and dental students is determined by the relationship between the dental profession and the larger community, and the student's most important task is to gradually enter into that relationship and make it his or her own.

In each of these areas, as more detailed study of each of them would demonstrate further, it is the Normative Picture that describes the general situation of dentistry and of individual dentists, both in their own understanding of their role and in the larger community's understanding of it. Each of these areas could be subjected to careful sociological analysis to test more formally whether the Normative Picture accurately describes the situation of dentistry in contemporary American society. But this book will proceed on the premise that in this matter, formal sociological study would only serve to confirm what is clear to any ordinary observer, namely, that the Normative Picture of dentistry is accurate and that dentistry and dentists have special obligations precisely because they are professionals.

THE CONTENT OF PROFESSIONAL OBLIGATIONS

When a person becomes a dentist, then, he or she takes on a commitment to act in accordance with certain obligations in his or her practice of dentistry. But what determines the content of these obligations? It might appear that their content is principally determined by the published codes of ethics of the various dental organizations. But in fact the process is much more subtle than this.

The obligations of individual professionals arise because of the relationship, discussed above, between the profession as a whole and the larger community. Hence the content of these obligations must be viewed as the product of an ongoing dialogue between the profession as a group and the larger community that the profession serves. This dialogue between the dental profession and the larger community is, to be sure, subtle and complex. It is ongoing in time, probably always somewhat incomplete, and rather slow to react to new circumstances. It is also rarely explicit or formal. But this dialogue is nevertheless the source of the content of dentists' obligations specifically as professionals.

What role do dental organizations' published codes play? In each instance, these codes should be considered to be, first, very important efforts to articulate certain elements of the content of dentists' professional obligations, and second, important teaching documents to assist in the education and formation of new dentists about the obligations of the profession.

The codes certainly do not legislate dentists' professional obligations because the dental organizations do not have the authority to speak for both sides of the ongoing dialogue with the larger community. In fact, none of these organizations even includes all members of the dental profession. But these codes are still important statements of the contents of a dentist's obligations because they are the work of thoughtful and active contributors to that dialogue who frequently examine the contents of a range of views before offering an opinion. For the same reason, and also because active participation in organized dentistry is itself a commendable professional activity and may be fostered thereby, these organizational codes are also important teaching documents for young dentists. In using them for this purpose, however, it is important to view them as limited expressions, hopefully accurate but possibly flawed, of the contents of the ongoing dialogue between dentistry and the larger community, so the students return to that ongoing dialogue as the original source of this content.

Thus a dental care provider can never adequately determine what his or her professional obligations are simply by asking what he or she thinks would be best for dentists or the community, nor only what the dental community says about a situation or what its principal organizations say about it. The dental professional and the dental professions must also ask what is the larger community's current understanding of what dental care providers are committed to. This may seem a vague and often frustrating test of one's professional obligations. But if these obligations are the fruit of an ongoing dialogue with the larger community, as has been proposed here, then this is a test that may not be set aside.

What about the dental practice acts legislated by the various states? Can they be considered authoritative statements of the contents of the dialogue between the dental profession as a whole and the larger community about the content of dentists' professional obligations? In one sense, they cannot because it is unlikely that the contents of this dialogue would vary greatly from state to state, as the contents of dental practice acts could conceivably do. That is, it is not automatically the case that the products of a more localized political process will articulate the contents of this dialogue.

On the other hand, the political process that leads to such legislation ordinarily includes participation by representatives of both the dental profession and the larger community, so a part of the larger dialogue is actually a component of this process. Moreover when state practice acts are compared, there are significant similarities. These patterns, it seems reasonable to say, do express contents of the larger dialogue, and in this respect the state practice acts can be taken as authoritative statements of that dialogue insofar as they are alike. But, finally, these patterns of similarity cover only the bare minimum of standards of professional practice and are for the most part procedural. Little substantive guidance about the positive contents of dentists' professional obligations can actually be gleaned from them.

Dentists, and those studying to be dentists, are therefore obligated to reflect carefully on dental practice and to identify those aspects of conduct on which they can discern a broad consensus on the part of both the dental community and the community at large. On many matters this consensus will be obvious, although the application to the case at hand of what is widely accepted and agreed upon may be more difficult to discern. On other matters the larger community and the dental community will not reach an obvious consensus, even after careful reflection and discussion. Whereas it is impossible to make this process any simpler, it is equally both impossible and undesirable to remove the need for thoughtful, conscientious judgment about professional conduct from the dentist's professional practice. Nor does either community want to transform living, conscientious, if fallible, professionals into morally correct automatons—as if automatons were capable of moral judgment and free choice in the first place Health care is too precious and the human beings who need it too uniquely situated for it to be placed in the hands of automatons. Only living, conscientious, fallible, but committed professionals will do.

This is why it is so important that committed professionals reflect carefully on the contents of their professional obligations. But these obligations are not simple, and it is best to follow both of the two most obvious paths in order to study them carefully, looking at them both in terms of general principles and in terms of particular sorts of ethical problems.

Therefore, in the next four chapters, dentists' professional obligations will be examined from the point of view of the general principles they embody and the most important kinds of questions that need to be asked to address them. Throughout these four chapters, however, cases and other examples will keep the discussion in touch with what happens at chairside.

In Part Two of the book, the focus will shift to specific sets of ethical problems that dentists encounter in practice, examined under such headings as "Patients With Compromised Capacity," "Education and Cooperation," "HIV and AIDS in Patients," and so on. The general principles and key questions examined in Part One cannot function like little machines to compute simple answers to ethical problems. Hence the discussions of specific kinds of ethical problems in Part Two will often be messy. Professional life is like that. But the general principles and sets of important questions from Part One can still help to structure and guide ethical reflection, and that is the reason for looking at them first.

THE INTRODUCTORY CASES

Each of the remaining chapters in this book will begin, as this one did, with a case, a story about someone who (1) must make a choice about how to act in some situation, and who therefore (2) must come to a judgment about how he or she *ought* to act in that situation, and who (3) must consider his or her professional obligations as a dentist to arrive at that judgment.

The purpose of these cases is not to inform the reader of the morally correct action in each of these situations, so the reader might then act accordingly when such situations happen to arise. That would not only exceed the authors' abilities and contradict our goals in writing this book, but it would also be foolish because 14 cases cannot possibly contain all the important ethical issues that arise in dental practice. Rather the first purpose of each of these cases is to prompt readers to ask themselves what sorts of questions they have to answer in order to determine what ought to be done in a case like this. Some of these questions, as well as various possible answers to them, will then be examined in the text of each chapter. Secondly, these cases are included to assist readers in applying what is proposed in the book to their chairside experience in the hopes that any learning achieved from reading this book will not be only at the level of theory and generality, but will connect effectively with actual practice.

Consistent with these goals, there will not be a concerted effort to exhaustively analyze each case, much less to resolve any of the cases finally. In each chapter, we will only discuss certain themes from the case, namely those that accord with the subject matter of the chapter. But the *reader* should try to think through the case to a conclusion, in other words, to a judgment about what course of action the actor in the case ought to take and why. Eventually this will require the reader to consider all of the categories of professional obligation to be described in Chapter Three, and possibly other moral categories as well. But even early in the book, when very few topics have been examined in detail, the reader should still make a point of going back to the case before reading the authors' concluding commentary in order to form his or her own judgment about the ethical issues in the case. That is, we hope the reader will stop and personally do his or her *own* thinking about each chapter's case *before* reading our commentary.

Finally, as was mentioned in Chapter One, there is an important oversimplification at work whenever a particular case is presented and examined. In actual life situations, especially when there is a patient waiting in the chair, few of us are likely to take time out to engage in a meticulous weighing of professional—or any other—obligations. Instead, most of our actions, professional and otherwise, are the product of trusted habits that we have formed and reinforced over the years.

But such habits can be subjected to reasoned examination as surely as the apparently spontaneous actions that they prompt. The skills needed for such reasoned examination of our habits are the same skills needed to examine specific alternative responses to a particular concrete situation. The principal focus of this book is the development of these skills, whether for application to our habits or application to individual actions. Therefore even when the focus of discussion is on a particular case, with its specific details determining much of our reflection, the questions that must nevertheless be asked about it can in each instance be reformulated to also read: Should a dental professional have a *habit* of acting in this way or that? In other words, reflecting on particular cases like those proposed in this book is a valuable way to examine and reshape our habits so we will act ethically in all those situations when we cannot or do not stop to reflect carefully.

THINKING ABOUT THE CASE

The case presented in this chapter clearly raises many important questions about dental professional ethics. One of these questions is whether Dr. Prentice views himself and his dentist employees according to the Normative Picture of professions or whether he frankly sees dentistry as nothing but a commercial enterprise.

In posing this question, it is important to observe that the information given in the case about Dr. Prentice is quite limited. We have Jack's own observations of large numbers of patients and of dentists working hard and quickly, as well as his feeling that there is a lot of pressure on the dentist employees. We have the words of one of Dr. Prentice's employed dentists, whose comments are suggestive of a very commercially oriented operation, but who actually describes only Dr. Prentice's firmness in enforcing his expectations as an employer (in the form of "the target numbers") on his employees. This raises important questions about the proper relations between professionals when they are employer and employee, but such questions arise under the Normative Picture of dentistry as well as the Commercial and therefore don't themselves resolve the issue of Dr. Prentice's acceptance of a Normative Picture of dentistry.

Finally, we have Dr. Prentice's answers to Jack's questions. Does Dr. Prentice say anything that implies a rejection of the Normative Picture of dentistry? Are any of his answers inconsistent with the view that becoming a dentist entails accepting a set of significant obligations toward one's patients and the community at large?

On the one hand, Prentice clearly indicates that the dentists he employs are judged, and no doubt paid and retained, on the basis of the amount of income they produce for the firm. This suggests that they feel considerable pressure to do more work for each patient rather than less, which could lead to work being done that is positively harmful or that is not necessary. But Prentice explicitly rejects doing harm to healthy teeth, and the examples he gives of the kind of work that his dentists are expected to recommend in order keep "the numbers high" could be defended as being still within the range of what is clinically acceptable, though optional and obviously not urgent, care. Prentice also stresses his unwillingness to employ dentists who are not technically capable; presumably this means not just minimally capable, but able to perform technically competent dentistry quickly and with a high volume of patients.

To be sure, other dentists might not do or recommend or even mention replacing a slightly worn amalgam and might not initiate a conversation about esthetic interventions unless the patient mentioned esthetics first. But the question can at least be asked whether that more conservative "philosophy" of dentistry, which prefers to intervene in the least possible way that is effective for the patient's oral health, is professionally *required*. If it is not professionally required, then the kinds of recommendations that Dr. Prentice requires of his employees, which produce greater income for the firm than a more conservative philosophy would yield, might be professionally acceptable. Determining this would require more data about how Prentice's dentists are required to function than has been provided in the case. But in the real world, asking this question and obtaining the data necessary to answer it would be extremely important.

In fact, there seems to be a range of dental "philosophies," from more conservative to more aggressive, that are acceptable guides to ethical dental practice. Therefore another way to consider Dr. Prentice's approach is whether it is within that range or not. But answering this question carefully, it seems clear, will require answers to a number of other question, for example, about the hierarchy of values in Prentice's practice and about the relative priority of the patient's well-being, as compared with profit, in his offices. So determining how Dr. Prentice stacks up against the Normative Picture of dentistry is, from this perspective, a task that will take considerably more study.

Another tack is suggested by Becky's question about patients' consent. Could it be argued that Dr. Prentice's kind of practice is professionally defective because it deprives patients of the opportunity to give informed consent for the treatment they receive? Dr. Prentice claims that no treatments are given unless patients consent to them, but that answer does not tell us how well they understand the options available to them. However the simple phrase "informed consent" is not a clear enough standard to help us answer this question. We need to explore the relationship between dentist and patient much more carefully, especially in regard to decisions about treatment, before a clear judgment can be made about the professional adequacy or inadequacy of the kind of decision-making process that Dr. Prentice counts on.

Third, there is the question of motivation. Dr. Prentice seems to Jack, Becky, and Robert to be motivated by the wrong reasons, practicing dentistry principally for the sake of money rather than the good of patients. But, as Len and Dr. Prentice both observe, a person cannot practice dentistry in American society without also being involved in a business, and if that business fails economically, the practice of dentistry and the good of patients it produces go with it. Are Dr. Prentice and Len to be credited with being genuinely "realistic," or are their values somehow inappropriate from the perspective of the Normative Picture of dentistry?

Does the Normative Picture require everyone who becomes a dentist have the same reasons for doing so, the same values that they hope to achieve? This seems most unlikely. The Normative Picture stresses that every member of the profession undertakes a certain set of obligations, whose content is the product of an ongoing dialogue between the profession as a whole and the larger community. But it does not seem to specify the reasons why a person would undertake these obligations. So why should Dr. Prentice's emphasis on making a good living strike Jack, Becky, and Robert as professionally inappropriate, provided that he and his dentist employees are committed to fulfilling their professional obligations to their patients and the community?

The reason is that fulfilling one's professional obligations will sometimes require sacrifice of other things for the sake of one's patients; Dr. Prentice's way of speaking about dental practice may seem to imply that no such sacrifice is required, or that it may justifiably be avoided, or even that sacrificing one's own interests, for patients or anyone else, ought to be avoided. That is, even though people become dentists for a variety of reasons, the well-being of patients must be among these reasons for the person's acceptance of the Normative Picture of the dental profession to be plausible or coherent.

In fact, we don't have enough information to judge Dr. Prentice conclusively on this matter. It would surely be unwise of Jack to join Dr. Prentice's practice without getting more information first. But what is clear is that judging whether a particular dentist is practicing in a manner consistent with the Normative Picture of the dental profession requires a careful and detailed understanding of the obligations that, according to this view, dentists undertake. Most dentists practice in a professionally ethical manner without being able to fully articulate the professional obligations that they habitually fulfill. But when a set of harder questions arises, like Jack's questions about Dr. Prentice, it is important to be able to articulate the standards that ought to be applied Facilitating reflection on the professional obligations of dentists, and aiding in their more complete articulation, is the aim of this book.

CHAPTER 3

The Questions of Professional Ethics

Case: When Everything Works Right

George Anderson was a new patient, a 38-year-old plumber who had been instructed by his physician to see a dentist. Mr. Anderson had <u>had diabetes for 7 years</u>. He told Dr. Orasony that he had pain off and on in many of his teeth and that he was told by his physician that this could be related to his diabetes. He therefore asked Dr. Orasony to take out all of his teeth and replace them with full dentures because there was nothing he could do about the diabetes. He reported that he had not seen a dentist since his wisdom teeth were extracted by an oral surgeon, on referral from his childhood dentist, when he was in his early twenties. Dr. Orasony also learned that Mr. Anderson has found it very difficult to follow the strict diet that his physician had prescribed in response to his diabetes.

"Dr. Gannett is always bawling me out," he said. "So I don't go to see him, and then he bawls me out for that, or for not testing my blood sugar often enough, or for something else." But Mr. Anderson had been faithful to the requirement of a daily injection of insulin, which he administered to himself. "I've got to take that shot," he said, "or it will kill me."

An examination revealed that Mr. Anderson had carious lesions in several teeth, including one molar that was a likely candidate for endodontic therapy. He also manifested significant periodontal effects of his diabetes, exacerbated by poor oral hygiene. When Dr. Orasony asked him about this, he answered that he brushed his teeth "a few times a week, when I think about it" and that he didn't floss because "it takes a lot of time and doesn't do any good."

"Proper flossing is important for the health of the gums for anyone," said Dr. Orasony. "But for a person with diabetes, it is absolutely essential. The tiny blood vessels in the gums are very susceptible to being damaged because of diabetes' effects on blood flow. From my first look, before I take x-rays to confirm it, I'd say most of the pain in your teeth is probably from damage to the gum tissue. It is really essential that you floss properly to control the build-up of plaque where the blood flow may be compromised. Has a dentist or a dental hygienist ever given you careful instructions about how to floss and why it is so important?"

"My old dentist talked about all that when I was a kid. But when he figured out that my wisdom teeth were the problem, and then they were taken out and I felt fine again, well, I didn't go back to see him, and then he died."

"So you haven't seen a dentist since you first learned you had diabetes?"

"No. Like I said, after my wisdom teeth were pulled, my teeth felt fine," said Mr. Anderson.

"Well, your diabetes really changes things, and the pain you are having is a sign of that. It's essential that you see a dentist regularly from now on, and you have to begin to take good care of your mouth, or you will have a lot more problems than you have now. Your gums have already been affected, although the damage is at a point, I think, where it can still be corrected without a major surgical procedure. But you have to change the way you take care of your mouth."

"Yeah, but it's hard to do stuff like that, a lot harder than just taking a shot," he said. "It's like the diet. I wish they just had a shot for that, too."

"It is hard," said Dr. Orasony. "Diabetes is a real burden on those who are afflicted with it. So you really do have my sympathy."

"Well, what about just taking the teeth out and giving me dentures, like I said first off," said Mr. Anderson. "Wouldn't that solve the problem and save us both a lot of grief?"

Dr. Orasony carefully explained the long-term risks of this path and the reasons for preserving and maintaining natural dentition for as long as possible. He would support such a drastic action, he said, only in an extreme case, especially in a man as young as Mr. Anderson.

"Your situation is a hard one," he said to Mr. Anderson, "but it is not out of your control. If you are willing to work at it with the proper diet and proper oral hygiene, which we will teach you, you really can minimize the effects of the diabetes on your mouth. We will work with you every step of the way."

"I'm not so sure," said Mr. Anderson. "I haven't done very well at the diet and the other stuff so far, only the shot because it's simple and I know I need it."

"Well, why don't we try to begin now," said Dr. Orasony, "because you need these other things, too. I hate to be so blunt, but an improper diet will kill you just as surely as missing your shot; it just takes longer. And you need to develop a habit of good oral hygiene, or your mouth will give you immense amounts of trouble, and eventually develop into even worse problems."

"What should I do?" asked Mr. Anderson.

"To start on the right path, you will need several appointments to get your teeth properly cleaned and to begin the healing process for your gums. It doesn't look like surgical repair of the gum tissue will be necessary, although that is a possibility that I have to mention in case less aggressive measures aren't successful. You also have a number of teeth with cavities that will need attention once we have your gum situation under control. It may be necessary to remove the vital pulp tissue of one of the molars in order to save that tooth; that's what some people call a root canal. But I will need to take some x-rays before I can tell you precisely what work is needed there. The rest will be instruction for you so you can brush and floss properly each day to keep your mouth healthy. Is there anything I've said so far that isn't clear to you?"

"I'm not surprised that you need to do some things. I mean it is hurting and all. My union health insurance is pretty good for dental work, so I'd say go ahead. Since I'm already here, can you do some of the work today?"

"I would very much like to. The first step is to have the dental hygienist begin cleaning your teeth. She will take some diagnostic x-rays first, and then she'll start removing the largest deposits of tartar on your teeth, especially at the gum line where they do the most damage. Then we would give your gums a week or two to heal, and you would get started on a daily routine of flossing and brushing. Miss Williams will give you careful instructions on how to do that before you leave today. Then, at a second appointment, she will finish the cleaning and we can focus on the damaged gum tissue that needs assistance in healing. Once that process is under way, then I can begin working on the teeth with cavities. But as I mentioned, if your gums do not respond to less aggressive treatments, then we will need to make a judgment about gum surgery, which may mean referring you to a specialist for that work. There are several periodontists whom I respect here in town, but that is a bridge that we don't have to cross for now. Is this plan acceptable to you?"

"It's fine. But I'm just not sure I can do my part of it," said Mr. Anderson. "I wish you could take care of all of it. It's like the diet. Like I said, I wish they just had a shot you could take instead of all that."

"When Miss Williams is explaining the flossing and brushing to you," said Dr. Orasony, "you tell her about your hesitations. She is very understanding about helping people fit good oral hygiene into the rest of their lives. I think you'll find that you can take control of this aspect of your life, and more easily than you expect."

Dr. Orasony also asked Mr. Anderson for permission to call his physician so they could keep each other informed of his progress. After Sarah Williams had completed the first round of cleaning and oral hygiene education, Mr. Anderson was scheduled for an appointment 2 weeks later.

In the interim, Dr. Orasony called Mr. Anderson's physician, Dr. Gannett. Not surprisingly, Dr. Gannett was very frustrated at Mr. Anderson's inability to change his living patterns to match his medical condition. The two doctors agreed to support each others' efforts to persuade him to change. Dr. Orasony suggested that Gannett contact a nutritionist at a local hospital and set up an appointment with her for Mr. Anderson and his wife. "This woman is a very good educator," Dr. Orasony told Dr. Gannett. "I was on a community education panel with her, and after her talk, half a dozen people came up to her with questions about how to adjust their diet and fit their dietary requirements into their daily life. I was very impressed."

At the second appointment, Sarah Williams finished the initial prophylaxis. In the process, she asked a few questions to see how much Mr. Anderson had retained from his initial instruction in oral hygiene, and then she continued the educational process. Dr. Orasony explained the x-rays to Mr. Anderson and confirmed the treatment plan. He began his initial periodontal scaling and root planing in order to treat the diseased gingival tissue, which responded well to his efforts over several weeks. Both Williams and Orasony could see the effects of Mr. Anderson's flossing and brushing, and they encouraged him strongly about it. Anderson also informed them about the planned meeting with the nutritionist.

Mr. Anderson appeared faithfully for a third, fourth, and fifth appointment. Restorative treatment, including endodontic therapy for one of his molars, was instituted and nearly completed by the fifth appointment. He had also established a model daily routine of oral hygiene. Dr. Gannett called Dr. Orasony to thank him for recommending the nutritionist, who had now helped three more of Dr. Gannett's diabetic patients get their diets under control. At his sixth appointment, Mr. Anderson asked if Dr. Orasony would bring Miss Williams into the operatory for a moment before he began the last of Anderson's restorative work.

"Dr. Orasony says that this will be the last appointment for now, and from now on I'll just be coming in for checkups. So I wanted to thank the two of you for everything you've done for me. It was the two of you, and Elizabeth Collins, the nutritionist, who got me on the right track, and I just want you to know how grateful I am for what you've done."

WHY THIS KIND OF CASE?

Some readers may be puzzled to find a case like this in a book on professional ethics. There is a mistaken notion around that the only cases that are useful for learning about ethics are either cases that exemplify some form of unethical or otherwise improper conduct, or cases in which the ethical issue is complex and difficult to sort out. Why then have a case in which, as the title of this one says, "everything works right"?

There are two reasons for giving this kind of case a prominent place in this book. The first reason is as reminder that it is not from examples of unethical conduct that professionals or anyone else chiefly learn how they ought to act, and neither is it from situations in which the right course of action is difficult to determine. The first and most important source of moral learning, in any area of life, will always be examples of right conduct.

Those who wish to learn more about ethical conduct in the dental profession must attend carefully to the examples of ethically correct conduct that are all around them. It is too easy to overlook this resource for ethical growth because the vast majority of actions by the members of any profession do ordinarily conform to the profession's ethical standards. What is so common may well seem to be of little instructional value. But what is uncommon is thoughtful analysis of the specific characteristics of professionals' common ethical conduct that make their conduct ethical. One aim of this chapter is to provide an example of a kind of thinking and questioning that dentists ought to engage in regularly, asking of a case in which, from an ethical point of view, everything went very well, just what features of the dentist's conduct made that conduct ethical.

Examining instances of ethical conduct in this way will quickly reveal that ethical conduct is not something simple. It is not the case that a few narrowly definable traits make a dentist's actions professionally correct. Just as numerous elements of both knowledge and skill must come together properly for a dentist's actions in a given case to be technically correct, so for their ethical correctness as well. The difference is that specialized training by dental school faculty and by dental researchers in the subfields that make up dental science have differentiated for us the various elements that constitute technical proficiency in dental practice so we can then identify them and judge them in practice one by one.

But there has been little comparable effort to identify the components of ethical conduct. Ethical conduct is still most often judged and viewed globally, or at best in terms of vague and general directives to serve the patient, secure informed consent, seek patient participation in decisions, and so on.

Therefore one aim of this book is to identify and articulate important components of ethical conduct in dentistry. One way to achieve this is by examining, especially in Part Two, a number of ethically perplexing areas of dental practice, for example, patients who cannot participate in decision-making, patients who are uncooperative, issues about HIV-positive patients and dentists, among others. But the assumption of Part Two is that the reader will already be bringing to those discussions the fruits of careful reflection on cases that are not so perplexing, cases from their own experience in which the right thing to do is fairly clear and straightforward. The case of George Anderson, where "everything works right," is of this sort. As has already been mentioned, however, the reader should be sure to stop and think through this case, asking what about it makes it right, before reading the commentary on it.

A second reason for giving prominence to a case in which "everything works right" is to use it to develop a conceptual tool to assist ethical reflection in dentistry. This conceptual tool is a list of eight categories of professional obligations in dentistry. Or, to put it another way, <u>it consists of eight sets of questions to be asked about dentists' professional obligations</u>.

As the case of George Anderson is examined, a number of questions will come to light as being central to any discussion of ethical conduct in dentistry, whether the final judgment is that a particular course of action is professionally ethical or that it is lacking in some way. In the final section of this chapter, these central questions will be organized under eight categories of <u>professional obligation, eight sets of questions about ethical standards that can, in</u> fact, <u>be asked of any professional in any profession.</u> The claim will even be made that any professional who cannot answer these questions about ethical practice in his or her profession does not really know what, ethically, he or she is doing.

Briefly stated, in the form of the "master" questions for each category, the eight categories of questions about professional obligation to be discussed are <u>(1)</u> Who is (are) this profession's *chief client(s)?* <u>(2)</u> What is the *ideal relationship* between a member of this profession and the *client?* <u>(3)</u> What are the *central values* of this profession? <u>(4)</u> What are the norms of *competence* of this profession? <u>(5)</u> In what respects do the obligations of this profession take *priority* over other morally relevant considerations affecting its members and what sorts of sacrifices do they require? <u>(6)</u> What is the *ideal relationship* between the members of this profession and *coprofessionals?* <u>(7)</u> What is the *ideal relationship* between the members of this profession and the *larger community?* <u>(8)</u> What are the members of this profession obligated to do to preserve the *integrity* of their commitment to its values and to *educate* others about them?

But before beginning to examine the case and see these questions at work in the judgment that "everything worked right" in it, a few words are needed about the term *obligation,* which will be used often in what follows.

OBLIGATION

Throughout this book, the *ought's* that apply to dentists' conduct by reason of their being professionals (where *profession* is understood according to the Normative Picture explained in Chapter 2) will be expressed by calling them *obligations.* Some people consider the term obligation to be too strong for the oughts of professional conduct or to have other connotations that are not appropriate for the present discussion. But like the terms moral and ethical, the term obligation is used in so many different ways with so many different connotations that it is impossible to claim that one particular set of connotations constitutes the word's only *true* meaning, so that all the other uses of it are defective. Nor can it be presumed that all those who read the word obligation in these pages will understand it as it is intended unless its meaning for the purposes of this book is clearly indicated.

In this book, then, to say that something is or someone has an obligation is to say three things: (1) someone ought to act, or refrain from acting, in some way, (2) there are defensible reasons to support the claim that he, she, or they ought to act or refrain in that way, and (3) these reasons make such acting or refraining relatively important in comparison with other possible actions in the situation. Because professional practice concerns things that are important to people, as was explained in Chapter 2, the specifically professional oughts of professions will always be, in a significant sense, *important*. Consequently, it is appropriate to call them, without further qualification, obligations.

Note, however, that this element of the importance of obligations does not exclude the possibility of someone having competing obligations in a given situation. Several actions or omissions might be obligatory and important at the same time. Indeed, resolving conflicts between competing obligations is one of the principal tasks of moral reflection. Because this book is principally about *professional* obligations, however, the other kinds of reasons why an ought might be important—and hence might be properly termed an obligation—will not receive much detailed attention here. But the relative priority of professional obligations when they compete with such obligations arising from other sources will be considered in Chapter 6 and in several chapters in Part Two.

COMMENTARY ON THE CASE

Most practitioners have experienced cases that were like the one in this chapter except that they did not work out as well as this one did. One important reason is the patient. In this case, although the patient apparently did not exhibit these traits before meeting the dentist, he eventually interacts with Dr. Orasony as a reasonable, balanced, communicative man who values the assistance that a dental professional can provide, respects the efforts of the dentist and the hygienist to provide it, and is grateful besides. Though he may have lacked it before, during the time covered in the case, he acquires the courage and self-discipline he needs to respond in the best way to his situation.

Most dentists are delighted to treat patients with these traits. But a dentist is obligated to act ethically whether the patient is ideal or not. So it is the characteristics of the dentist's actions in this case, not the characteristics of the patient, that most concern us. What makes Dr. Orasony's conduct in this case ethically appropriate?

One thing, surely, is his relationship with Mr. Anderson. Dr. Orasony clearly meets the standards of informed consent, explaining the patient's needs and the various treatment options available, as well as the risks of not treating. But he does more than this. He tries to enhance the patient's own control over his situation, which necessarily involves letting go of some control that he, the dentist, might retain. He works to help the patient choose on the basis of his own values, rather than attempting to frighten him or coerce him into doing what is best. Mr. Anderson is treated with respect by both dentist and hygienist, who communicate to him their confidence that he can control his life, and he learns from this and grows more able to respect himself and trust his own powers as well as theirs.

In patients less reasonable or less communicative, for example, the steps taken by the dentist to establish a constructive relationship with the patient may be different. But the point is clear that one key standard of professional conduct concerns the relationship between dentist and patient. This is one important category of professional obligation. It will be examined in greater detail in Chapter 4 and Chapter 7.

Another feature of this case that makes it right is the match between what the dentist tries to achieve for the patient and what dentistry stands for. It is surely correct that Dr. Orasony attends to Mr. Anderson's overall health, and not the health of his oral cavity alone. It is surely correct as well that he works to strengthen Mr. Anderson's self-discipline and his ability to take control of his own life. These are all important values for dentists to foster along with the value of oral health itself.

In fact, in this particular case, with its unusually happy outcome, it seems that all manner of values are fostered for the patient, and that the often-repeated goal of benefiting the whole patient has been achieved to an unusually high degree. But is dentistry really obligated to further every kind of well-being for its patient, or only certain kinds that are connected in some important way with the profession's expertise? If the latter is the case, we must learn which values are central to dental practice and should take priority when many possibly conflicting values are at stake in a given instance of professional judgment. We must also ask whether, if dentistry is committed to furthering more than one central value, there is some ranking or hierarchy among these values.

These sorts of questions about the values that are to guide dentists' decisions for their patient, are another category of professional obligation. They will be discussed in greater detail in Chapter 5, and they will recur frequently throughout the book.

Dr. Orasony is also admirable in the extent of his commitment to Mr Anderson. He does not just hurry through the motions of giving information and receiving consent. Instead he puts himself out, calling the patient's physician, drawing on experience in other situations, and so on. It may not be that Dr. Orasony had to make significant sacrifices of time or effort to treat Mr. Anderson as he did, but he communicated to Mr. Anderson that his well-being took priority over personal concerns and many other matters for Dr. Orasony.

This theme directs us to another category of questions that must be asked about professional obligations. How much priority must the patient's general health, oral health, and other considerations be given in comparison with other values and commitments that the dentist has? The dentist is a person, too, with needs, goals, and desires. The dentist also has a family, friends, and other sorts of commitments. How much priority must be given to the patient's well-being when these other interests conflict with it in practice? This question will be a central topic of Chapter 6 and will be raised again many times in Part Two.

In addition, there is another question that, in many professions and possibly in dentistry as well, must be carefully asked even before the preceding one can be asked. Whose well-being and whose oral health and general health is the dentist professionally committed to serving. Is it the class of all persons needing dental care? Or the class of all persons who can pay for it? Is it only the person in the chair at this moment, or all a dentist's patients of record, of everyone in the land? Would Dr. Orasony have been acting in a professionally ethical manner if he had taken less time to assist Mr. Anderson in order to spend more time with other patients in the other operatories or to see more patients by scheduling more patients each day? This is another category of questions about professional obligations that dentists need to ask.

The obligation to practice in a technically competent manner, according to the profession's accepted standards for practice in each kind of clinical situation, is surely the most obvious professional obligation that a dentist has. It is most unlikely that the happy outcome of this case could have been achieved apart from competent practice on the part of the dentist and the hygienist, as well as the physician and the nutritionist who were also involved. Unless specified otherwise, the cases in this book will presuppose technically competent practice on the part of the professionals described since detailed examination of the technical aspects of the cases would take these discussions far away from their intended focus.

But there is another set of ethical questions about competence that must be raised, namely the practitioner's need to judge whether he or she is personally competent to handle a particular form of needed therapy, as in this case if periodontal surgery proved necessary. The judgment about whether to treat a condition oneself or to refer to a more skilled specialist, or even to refrain from treating if no specialist is available, is an ethical question, not merely a practical one. The delicate topic of incompetent dental work will be discussed in Chapter 9.

Dr. Orasony seems to have an excellent working relation with Sarah Williams, the hygienist. The result is that the patient views the expertise of the hygienist and the assistance she offers with respect, and benefits accordingly. In a similar way, Dr. Orasony interacts effectively with the patient's physician and works to get a professional nutritionist involved in the case, whose chief challenge is Mr. Anderson's self-discipline in relation to diet.

The relationships between dentists and coprofessionals, especially professionals who are attending to the same patient, are often overlooked in discussions of the ethics of dentistry. But fostering them properly is obviously an important component of a dentist's ethical conduct in practice. So this is another category of questions to ask about ethical dental practice. It will receive special attention in Chapter 10.

There are also other people besides patients with whom dentists interact. As a profession, dentistry is involved with the larger community in many ways, but every dentist has relationships beyond those with people who are in need of dental care that may be professionally significant. In the case at hand, for example, we know that Dr. Orasony has spoken at a public education event. We also know that access to his practice on the part of patients needing dental care depends in part upon a complex system of economic, legal, and social structures, and in part on his likely willingness and ability to practice in some ways independently of those structures, for example, by providing some amount of care free or at cost.

These points suggest that there is another category of questions to ask, namely, about what makes a dentist's professional acts ethical in relation to the larger community, both collectively and in regard to individuals who are not the dentist's patients. Chapters 13 through 15 will pay special attention to these issues.

Finally, it is important to ask why a patient like Mr. Anderson would trust Dr. Orasony, not simply to practice competently and not simply to speak the truth as he understands it, but also to offer reliable evidence of the importance of certain human values and virtues. Dr. Orasony isn't looking only for an opportunity to perform treatments or to pass on information. His work in this case includes having a significant impact on Mr. Anderson's conduct. What characteristics of Dr. Orasony are relevant to Anderson's positive response to the dentist in this regard?

It seems doubtful that Mr. Anderson would accept the challenge to place his health ahead of his fear or his ease and to work for a higher degree of self-control if he thought that Dr. Orasony was not himself committed to good health and to the self-discipline necessary to maintain it. Few people are moved to make sacrifices by people who themselves do not make those or similar sacrifices. This is an area of subtle traits of character, but it is an area that is almost certainly crucial to the success of Dr. Orasony's efforts in this case. It concerns Dr. Orasony's integrity and his ability to educate others in the values to which dentistry is committed, not only by his words, but by how he lives and acts.

So there is an eighth category of questions to ask about dentists' professional obligations. What are dentists required to do, and what might they be required to avoid, in order to preserve the integrity of the values that dentistry is committed to and to educate others by living in a manner consonant with those values? Some dentists may well argue that the proper answer to this question is "nothing." That is, there is nothing that a dentist is obligated to do, provided his or her patients have been ethically and competently cared for in other respects. But no matter how the questions in this category are answered, it is clear that there are questions here that must be asked.

EIGHT CATEGORIES OF PROFESSIONAL OBLIGATION

The commentary on the case of Dr. Prentice in Chapter 2 identified two kinds of information that were lacking in that case, with the consequence that a final conclusive judgment could not be made about Dr. Prentice's conformity, or lack of conformity, to his professional obligations as a dentist. First, the case did not give enough information about how Dr. Prentice actually practices, what he actually requires of his employees, and how he enforces these requirements. That is, important factual information about his practice of dentistry was found to be missing.

Second, Chapter 2 spoke of dentists' professional obligations only in very general terms, terms too general to form a conclusive judgment about whether the dentist in the case is practicing in a professional ethical manner or not. This chapter begins to rectify these two problems.

Both of these kinds of information are essential for sound judgments of professionals' practice. But it is the second kind of information that drives the first because it focuses the inquiry and determines which facts about a dentist's actual practice are needed to answer the question about professional conduct. There are innumerable facts available about any dentist's practice. But only certain of those facts are important to judgments about the dentists' conformity or non-conformity to professional obligations. Knowing which facts are relevant depends on having a more detailed account of the contents of dentists' professional obligations.

The account in this book of dentistry's professional obligations will be developed in terms of the eight categories of questions that are the subject of the present chapter. These will be used throughout the book to focus the inquiry and to determine which facts about the case are most relevant to judgments about ethical or unethical conduct.

As has already been mentioned, in order to understand these categories, and to use them most profitably, it is best to think of each category as a set of questions, headed for summary purposes by a "master question" that identifies the focus of the set. Each of these sets of questions, when carefully answered in regard to a particular instance of professional practice or a particular policy or standard regarding practice, will reveal facts about that situation, policy, or standard that are important for a careful judgment about it from the point of view of appropriate professional conduct.

It should already be clear that these eight categories are not completely independent. Some of the questions in each category address matters of importance to other categories. But categorizing questions and data under these headings is a useful way to keep moral reflections and judgments about professional conduct clear and on track. (If other ways of categorizing the contents of professional obligation also prove useful, more power to them, since the goal of this book is clear and careful reasoning about professional obligation, not the preeminence of a particular set of categories.)

This final section of the chapter will examine each of the eight categories a second time, both more generally than in the preceding section and without any effort to connect the discussion with characteristics of Dr. Orasony's conduct in the George Anderson case.

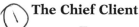 The Chief Client

Every profession has a chief client or clients. This is the person or set of persons whose well-being the profession and its members are chiefly committed to serving.

For some professions, including dentistry, the identification of the chief client seems quite easy. Surely, we might say, the chief client of the dentist is the patient. But who is the chief client of a lawyer? Is it simply the party whose case the lawyer represents or pleads, or to whom the lawyer gives advice? Lawyers are told, however, and announce in their self descriptions and codes of conduct that they have obligations to the whole justice system, and therefore that there are things that they may not ethically do, as professionals, even if doing them would advance the situation of the party they represent or advise. So it appears that the answer to the question about the chief client of the legal profession is complex, involving both the person the lawyer represents or advises and the whole justice system, or perhaps the whole larger community served by that system.

But once this sort of complexity about the chief client is noticed, even what

patients of record, public

appeared to be a simple case proves to be more complex. For the dentist must not only attend to the patient in the chair, but also to those in other operatories and those in the waiting room. The dentist also has some obligations to all of his or her patients of record. In addition, dentists have some obligations to the public as a whole, for example, an obligation to practice with caution so as not to spread infection from patients in their care, and an obligation to make certain that patients who seek dental care in emergency situations do in fact find assistance. So it turns out that the question about who is dentistry's chief client is not as simple as it first appeared. A dentist's obligations to these different clients will be examined at various points in this book.

The Ideal Relationship Between Dentist and Patient

The point of the relationship between a professional and a client is to bring about certain values for the client, values that cannot be achieved for the client without the expertise of the professional. Bringing about these values will require both the professional and the client to make a number of judgments and choices about the professional's interventions. The question addressed in this third category of professional obligation concerns the proper roles of the professional and the client as they make these judgments and choices.

At least four general models of an ideal professional-client relationship can identified. In Chapter 4 these models will be examined in detail in relation to dentistry, and a case will be made that one of them is the ideal dentist-patient relationship. In addition, discussion of the professional-client relationship must include consideration of situations in which the ideal relationship is not possible. The dentist's relationship with patients who cannot fully participate in choices about the dentist's interventions will be the topic of Chapter 7, and in Chapter 8 the dentist's relationship with patients who are uncooperative will be discussed.

The Central Values of the Dental Profession

Every profession is focused only on certain aspects of the well-being of its clients. The rhetoric of many professions often speaks of caring for the whole person. But in fact no professional group is expected by the larger community to be expert in their clients' entire well-being. Expertise is necessarily more narrowly focused. Therefore no profession is committed to securing for its clients everything that is of value for them. Rather there is a certain set of values that are the focus of each profession's expertise and which it is the job and obligation of that profession to work to secure for its clients. These values can be called the *central values* of a particular profession. The central values of the dental profession will be examined in detail in Chapter 5.

Competence

Every professional is obligated both to acquire and to maintain the expertise needed to undertake his or her professional tasks. Every professional is also obligated to undertake only those tasks that are within his or her competence and to assist patients whose needs are beyond their expertise in locating a practitioner who can assist them.

This category of competence is probably the most obvious category of professional obligation. It is also the easiest to describe in a general way. If a professional fails to apply his or her expertise, or fails to obtain the expertise needed for undertaking some task, these failures directly contradict both the point of being an expert and the very foundation of the larger community's award of decision-making power to the professional in the first place.

But the determination of what counts as sufficient or minimally adequate competence on the part of a member of a given profession, both in general and in relation to specific kinds of tasks, is a very complex question. In practice, and almost of necessity, the working out of detailed judgments about requisite expertise is left to the members of the expert group (i.e., the profession itself). But the larger community usually requires that explanations be given regarding the general structure of the reasoning being employed, especially regarding the inevitable trade-offs of values involved in determining what is to count as the standard of minimal professional competence. For such determinations unavoidably include a risk-benefit judgment that balances the greater or lesser availability of expert assistance to those in need against the greater or lesser likelihood that those who pass the standard might not practice in the best possible way.

The Relative Priority of the Patient's Well-Being

Most sociologists who study professions mention "commitment to service" or "commitment to the public" as one of the characteristic features of a profession. Similarly, in the dental profession's published codes of ethics and other self descriptions, the patient's best interest or service to the public has always received prominent mention. But these expressions admit of many different interpretations with significantly different implications for actual practice. It is important to ask just what measure of sacrifice of personal interest and of a dentist's other commitments is professionally obligatory.

The larger community surely does not understand the commitment of the dental professional to be absolute nor to impose, in all circumstances, the utmost of sacrifices for the sake of one's patient. Such an interpretation of the priority issue would be unrealistic in the extreme. In addition, it would be unreasonable of the larger community to risk in this way its having a continued supply of dentists to meet its dental care needs in the future. Therefore while the well-being of the patient is to be given considerable priority, it is not to be given absolute priority. How much priority is it to be given? This question will be examined most closely in Chapter 6 and in Chapter 11.

Ideal Relationships Between Coprofessionals

Each profession also has norms, usually mostly implicit and unexamined, concerning the proper relationship between members of the same profession in various matters and also between members of different professions when they are dealing with the same clients. But there does not seem to be any one account of the ideal relationships between dentists and their coprofessionals simply because so many different categories of such coprofessionals must be considered. There are, for example, other dentists, both specialists and general practitioners, dental hygienists, and also physicians and nurses. Relationships with coprofessionals will be examined most closely in Chapters 9 and 10.

The Relationship Between Dentistry and the Larger Community

In addition to relationships of professionals and their clients and of professionals with one another, the activities of every profession also involve relationships between the profession as a group or its individual members and persons who are neither coprofessionals nor clients. These relationships may involve the larger community as a whole, various signi subgroups of it, or specific individuals. Obviously, a wide range of diverse relationships are included under this umbrella, and which of them are of the greatest importance in a given situation will depend on the particular profession under discussion and the details of the situation. A number of these relationships will be examined in conjunction with the problem areas considered in Part Two.

Integrity and Education

Finally, there is that very subtle component of conduct by which a person communicates to others what he or she stands for, not only in the acts that the person chooses, but also both in how those acts are chosen and in how the person presents himself or herself to others in carrying them out. The two words that seem to communicate the core of this concern are *integrity* and *education*, especially when the two words are paired together because one educates others regarding values far more by how one lives than by what one says.

Dentistry stands for certain values, but a dentist's personal priorities may communicate a different set of values, even though the dentist's choices of treatments and efforts to secure patients' informed consent conform to acceptable standards in these matters. It is this sort of concern, for example, that motivates many dentists to establish in their personal lives patterns of healthy living that are consonant with what they say to their patients. So a final set of questions about dentists' professional obligations asks what they are obligated to do, and what they are obligated to refrain from, in order to remain true to the values that dentistry stands for and to educate others in these values by their own example.

CHAPTER 4

The Relationship Between Patient And Professional

Case: The Dreaded Root Canal

Roger Vianni has been a patient of Dr. Clarke's for 7 years. He is a very talkative man who constantly expresses his anxieties about the condition of his teeth and what Dr. Clarke may have to do about them. Dr. Clarke always responds calmly and sympathetically, but she has learned that gentle words are rarely enough to calm Mr. Vianni's churning anxieties. His fear also heightens his sensitivity to pain and pressure, so local anesthetic has been necessary for even the most superficial procedures, and he invariably has a fresh story for her about an acquaintance who has recently suffered some oral tragedy. How grateful he is, he tells her at each visit, that he has never suffered such things, especially the dreaded root canal.

Luckily, Mr. Vianni has not needed much work up till now. But nearly a year has passed since Mr. Vianni's last visit, and this time he presents with a complaint of significant pain in the upper right quadrant. Dr. Clarke's examination reveals a shallow amalgam in the upper right second premolar that has fractured, breaking the seal and thus needing replacement. But more importantly, and more likely the cause of Mr. Vianni's pain, a sizable carious lesion has developed on the mesiobuccal surface of the adjacent first molar, next to a large silver restoration that was in place before Mr. Vianni became Dr. Clarke's patient. There is, in fact, little sound enamel remaining. Radiographic examination confirms apparent pulpal involvement, with endodontic therapy and then a full coverage restoration as the treatment of choice.

Dr. Clarke is certain, however, that if she describes the root canal procedure and the drilling that would be necessary to prepare the tooth for the crown, Mr. Vianni will simply refuse. It is not that he would prefer to lose the tooth or that he has financial or other reasons for not wanting a root canal and crown. He has often said that he values his teeth greatly and is willing to spend whatever it takes to keep them healthy as long as possible. It is simply that he has such strong reactions to the drill, and especially to the thought of endodontic therapy. The fact that this procedure resolves rather than causes pain and that it can be performed, in the ordinary case, without significant pain or discomfort, will not change Mr. Vianni's reaction. From her previous knowledge of this patient, she is certain that he will either demand that the tooth be extracted or simply leave the office if she explains his situation to him.

Luckily, Dr. Clarke had mentioned the simple problem with the premolar to Mr. Vianni as soon as she had noted it and before she had examined the first molar carefully, and he had mustered up his courage and agreed to its repair, "provided you freeze it up real good." She could very easily anesthetize the first molar at the same time she anesthetized the premolar without Mr. Vianni knowing the difference. She could then perform the pulpectomy on the molar without Mr. Vianni having to suffer from knowing what was going on until all the parts of the procedure that he utterly dreaded were completed. Nor would she have to lie to him since she could truthfully say that she was doing some superficial drilling on the premolar, and she would of course tell Mr. Vianni the whole story of what she had done to save him from anxiety and suffering as soon as the work of preparing the molar was completed. At that point he could choose a porcelain-fused-to-metal restoration preceded by a temporary crown until the permanent crown was fabricated, an amalgam buildup, or even a tooth extraction if that really was his preference. But he would not have to face the anticipation of the root canal that he dreaded so much.

Dr. Clarke is certain that if she could describe the situation to Mr. Vianni without his knowing that it was his own mouth, he would understand and agree that endodontic therapy along with proper restoration of the tooth is the most reasonable and appropriate treatment. The problem is that, in his own case, his judgment would be clouded by his reaction to the idea of receiving root canal therapy and of the drilling that would take place in his own mouth. (While slightly anxious about being sued as a matter of course, Dr. Clarke is actually quite certain that Mr. Vianni would understand her judgment on his behalf and that she is at no risk of a lawsuit if she takes this step.)

Dr. Clarke is certain that Mr. Vianni trusts her to do whatever is best for him. She is also sure that if he could judge the matter objectively, Mr. Vianni would not want to suffer the anxiety of deciding about this treatment for himself. What good reason is there, then, for putting him through the pain of doing so? What should Dr. Clarke do and why?

THE DENTIST-PATIENT RELATIONSHIP

At the center of most issues in dental ethics we find a patient and a dentist and a relationship between them, and we find a decision to be made about treatment, or some other kind of professional action or intervention, for the patient. The previous chapter proposed that for every profession there is an ideal relationship between professional and client that is one of the most important standards of ethical conduct for members of that profession. What is the ideal relationship between dentist and patient? What are the proper roles of the patient and the dentist in the decision-making process that is central to their dealings with one another? This is the topic of the present chapter.

The first thing to note is that not all patients are *capable* of making or participating in decisions about their treatment or other aspects of their health care. Some patients are young children or are severely developmentally disabled. Other patients suffer from other deficits that impair their capacity for decision-making. It will be important to ask, in due course, what a person needs to be capable of participating in a decision-making process and what sorts of deficits justify a doubt about someone's capacity. It will also be necessary to ask how a dentist ought to relate to patients who exhibit such deficits, whether their capacity for decision-making is only partially diminished or they cannot participate at all in decision-making about their dental care. These matters will be addressed in detail in Chapter 7. In the present chapter, however, decision-making and the dentist-patient relationship in situations in which the patient *is* capable of participating will be examined.

There is no single English word that means the same thing as "capable of autonomous choice." But this is a cumbersome phrase to repeat over and over. There is a word in ordinary usage that expresses this idea: *competent*, along with its noun, *competence*. Unfortunately, this term has an important technical meaning in the law that is quite different from its common-sense meaning. In the law, anyone who has reached the age of an adult is *competent;* that is, a person can make decisions and take actions that have legal standing, unless a judge in court rules that this person is no longer capable. Thus a person who is permanently comatose is still legally competent until the person is declared incompetent by a judge after an appropriate hearing and not before then. Similarly, with a few exceptions, a highly intelligent, thoughtful, sensitive 17-year-old is, in the eyes of the law, as incompetent to make health care decisions as an infant. So using this word can lead to some confusion.

It seems best, therefore, to use the terms *competent* and *competence* as well as *incompetent* and *incompetence* only when we need them in their technical legal sense. The word that will be used throughout this book as a shorthand for "capable of autonomous choice" will be *capable*, and the noun *capacity* will be used for "capacity for autonomous choice."

In this chapter decision-making by dentists and capable patients will be examined under three headings. First, four different models of the patient-dentist relationship will be examined, and their accounts of the roles of patient and dentist in decision making will be compared. The focus will then turn to the principle of respecting autonomy, which is a central moral principle in American culture and in many systems of moral philosophy. In the course of examining this principle, we will also ask whether circumstances don't sometimes justify violating someone's autonomy precisely for that person's benefit, a pattern of thinking and acting that is sometimes called *paternalism*. That is, could a dentist ever be morally justified in violating a patient's autonomy for the sake of the patient's oral health? (Admittedly, doing such a thing might put the dentist at legal risk. But even when that is so, legal risk is no guarantee of moral error, and sometimes morality requires a person to take a serious legal risk, so the question about morally justifiable paternalism still needs to be asked.)

The third way of addressing the issue of the proper relationship between dentist and patient will focus on the moral standard of telling the truth and the legal principle of informed consent that is sometimes taken to articulate an ideal moral standard for the dentist-patient relationship.

FOUR MODELS OF THE DENTIST-PATIENT RELATIONSHIP

The dentist-patient relationship can be conceived according to many different models, of which four seem the most important. These will be explained and compared, and the case will be made that one of these, the Interactive Model, is the best description of the ideal relationship between a dentist and a capable patient. The four models are the Guild Model, the Agent Model, the Commercial Model, and the Interactive Model.

The Guild Model

In the Guild Model, the central reality of the relationship between patient and dentist is the dentist's expertise and the patient's lack of it. The dentist has the ability to understand and explain the patient's condition (diagnosis), to predict various future paths that it might take under various circumstances (prognosis), and to intervene with treatments and other forms of care in order to maximize various aspects of the patient's well-being in the outcomes (therapy). The patient, in this model, has none of the expertise needed to do these things, neither the theoretical knowledge on which these actions are based, nor the experience in practice that enables the professional to apply his or her theoretical knowledge effectively in each particular set of clinical circumstances. Indeed, the very reason the patient comes to the dentist is that the patient lacks this expertise and is therefore unable to attend to his or her dental needs unaided.

Consequently, in all important aspects of dental decision making, the proper role for the patient in the Guild Model is literally that of *patience,* as in the word's root sense of undergoing something or being receptive. The patient is one to whom things *are done* because of the patient's inability (due to lack of both theoretical understanding and practical experience in applying that understanding) to make any important contribution to dental decisions about his or her situation.

The source of the dentist's expertise is the profession, the community of dentists who preserve and advance dental knowledge and practice. It is the profession that trains and then certifies that the individual practitioner is qualified to assist patients. It is the profession that determines how individual dentists shall act toward patients, both therapeutically and in other respects. Thus when an individual seeks admission to the dental profession, as has been said, he or she accepts the obligations that the profession sets down as conditions of admittance. Among these obligations is a fundamental commitment to serving the patient's well-being by responding to the patient's dental needs. Just as the technical specifics of appropriate dental care are determined by the profession because of its expertise, so too the specifics of a dentist's obligations to patients are determined (usually by means of a published code of conduct) by the profession. It is by means of a commitment to the profession that the individual dentist undertakes his or her professional obligations.

The patient's need for care has profound moral significance in the Guild Model because it is the patient's need that produces the reason for the profession's existence in the first place, and responding to the patient's dental needs as a representative of the profession is also the fundamental moral commitment of each person admitted to the profession. But it is important to note that because of the patient's utter inability to make the relevant dental judgments in this model, it is the dentist, not the patient, who is to judge what the needs of the patient are in every instance.

There is a serious moral problem with the Guild Model in the eyes of many people, including many dentists. One way to state this problem is to point to the Guild Model's failure to respect the autonomy of patients who are capable of autonomous decision making. A simple statement of this objection is that according to the Guild Model, a dentist is to treat these patients as if they were not capable of autonomous decision-making when they are. Doing so is obviously a violation of the patient's autonomy.

The principle of respecting autonomy and the question regarding whether it may ever be justifiably violated will be examined more fully in the next section. But there is one response to this objection that deserves immediate consideration. Even if these patients are capable of autonomous decision-making in other respects, the defender of the Guild Model would respond, still they do not have the dentist's knowledge and skill, which are precisely what they need if they are to be capable of deciding about their dental care. Therefore the defender of the Guild Model concludes that it is the dentist who should be deciding, especially because the patient is often in pain or considerable distress as well.

What the Guild Model fails to account for is that there are important components of every dental decision that are not included in the expertise of even the most acutely trained and extensively experienced dentist.The reason is that therapeutic alternatives are never value-neutral. All therapeutic choices involve selecting one set of life experiences for the patient over another set, and the knowledge and skills that the dentist brings to the situation are not adequate tools for comparing the value of these possible experiences within the *patient's* life. Instead, the patient's own values must also be brought to bear in the choice of dental interventions. But only with the patient's participation in the dental decision will the patient's values dependably direct that decision.

Therefore the Guild Model's picture of the patient as the passive recipient of expert dental interventions does not fit the ethical reality of patients and dentists in their actual relationships. In fact, this model does not even adequately portray the dentist's proper role in treating patients who are not capable of autonomous choice. As will be explained in Chapter 7, such patients' previous choices or their developing capacity for choices in the future, as well as their relationships to family members and others, have a role to play in dental decision-making that the Guild Model, with its narrow emphasis on dentists' expertise, does not capture.

The Agent Model

A second model of the dentist-patient relationship reverses the dentist's and patient's roles from the Guild Model. In this second model, the whole decision-making activity in dental care is assigned to the patient. Here, the professional simply puts his or her expertise at the service of the patient's aims and values. The dentist's task is only to give effect to the patient's choices, responding as efficiently as possible to fulfill the patient's choices regarding his or her needs or desires. The dentist is to act, in other words, only as an agent for the patient. Hence this is called the Agent Model.

This model is not often discussed in regard to dentistry or the other health professions, probably because it so severely misrepresents our ordinary understanding of a health professional's ethical commitments. The most commonly discussed professional example of it is probably in the image of the lawyer as "hired gun." But the Agent Model is no more defensible as a description of the lawyer's ethical commitments than it is of the health professional's. To construct an example from health care, imagine a dentist, physician, or nurse who would agree to use his or her access to controlled substances to meet the needs of a patient's addiction, simply in order to respond to the patient's choices more completely, without any connection of that action to the aspects of the patient's well-being that the health professional is professionally committed to fostering.

The failure of the Agent Model, then, is that it simply sets aside the idea that each profession has certain central values that it is committed to fostering, by use of its expertise, for its clients. That is, the Agent Model overlooks a central element of the institution of profession as it functions in our society. A patient's particular conception of his or her well-being has an important role to play in decisions concerning the dental care he or she receives, but it is not the sole determinant of how dentists are to act. Therefore the Agent Model is clearly of no use in helping describe the ideal relationship between dentist and patient.

The Commercial Model — dentist has no obligations, commitments

The weaknesses of the Guild Model and Agent Model have prompted a number of people to turn to the Commercial Model in their stead. The consumer movement in health care, as well as proponents of a still wider role for free enterprise in our health care system, have also urged that the Commercial Model is the best guide for health professionals, including dentists, to follow in their relationships with patients.

According to the Commercial Model, the patient is indeed a decision-maker about his or her health care, in contrast with the Guild Model, and the dentist is also a decision-maker, with his or her own values to pursue, and not a mere agent of the patient, as in the Agent Model. In these respects, the Commercial Model may appear preferable to each of the others. But other features of the Commercial Model make its claim to be the ideal relationship more problematic.

According to the Commercial Model, a member of a profession is simply another producer selling his or her wares in the marketplace. Thus a dentist has a product to sell, and patients may want to buy it. The two parties may make whatever agreements with interested purchasers that they are willing to make. By the same token, both the dentist and the patient may refuse any arrangements that either one chooses to refuse. In other words, according to the Commercial Model, the only moral standards that apply to dentistry are those that apply to every other bargainer in the market place as well. These standards seem to be not to coerce, not to cheat or defraud, and to keep the contractual commitments one makes with others. Other than these obligations, according to this model, the dentist has no other obligations to any patient except such obligations as the dentist and the patient voluntarily undertake. According to the Commercial Model, in other words, there are no specifically professional values or obligations on the part of the dentist; there is nothing to which a dentist is obligated *because* he or she is a dentist.

In addition, as in all market relationships, the dentist and the patient are competitors first and foremost. That is, each is trying to obtain from the other the greatest amount of what he or she wants (money, satisfaction, effort, time, and other aspects of well-being) while giving up in the exchange as little as possible. The dentist is concerned about the patient's well-being only as a means of improving his or her own. Thus the dentist has no obligation to any patient to preserve or foster the patient's oral health or any other aspect of the patient's well-being until the dentist specifically contracts to have such an obligation. No patient should presume such an obligation or commitment in advance of a specific contract to this effect between the dentist and that patient.

In the Commercial Model, further, the patient's need for care is not a direct determinant of a dentist's action. The patient's need has no special ethical import for the dentist, and there is certainly no antecedent obligation to meet a patient's needs; there is only whatever obligations the dentist and patient themselves subsequently negotiate regarding their relationship. Need does function, of course, as a potent motivater for patients to seek and contract for dental care. As such, need can be used effectively by the dentist to market his or her wares to the patient. But in the Commercial Model, when a dentist says to a patient, "this procedure will answer your need for. . .," these words should not be received by the patient with any special degree of trust, no more so than would the comments of a person selling anything else.

Obviously, in this model the client is not a passive recipient of expert professional services, as in the Guild Model. The patient first judges the value of the information that the dentist can supply and then chooses whether or not to purchase it. Then, after judging alternative courses of action on the basis of this information, the patient judges the value of various therapeutic interventions by the dentist or others and chooses either to purchase them or not. The patient in the Commercial Model is regarded as an example of *homo economicus*, the rational consumer, who weighs all the elements of cost and benefit relevant to a given exchange and chooses the available product or service that yields the best combination of these.

The Commercial Picture of dentistry as a profession was rejected in Chapter 2. But it might be possible, or at least not simply contradictory, for a normative profession to have a commercial relationship as its ideal of the relationship between patient and health care professional. Because a number of authors, including a number of dentists, propose this as the ideal relationship, it deserves careful examination. First, is the Commercial Model a realistic possibility for the relationship between patient and dentist? Second, if dentists and patients could function in this way, does this model describe an ethically ideal relationship between them?

There are evident limits on the extent to which patients not extensively trained in dental science can understand the subtle differences between alternative oral conditions and alternative interventions to address them, even if they do receive a great deal of dental information first. Nor have patients had the benefit of the experience of dental practice, which is every bit as important in dental judgments at chairside as scientific theory and familiarity with the current literature. It is therefore a legitimate question to ask whether the average patient can fully play the rational consumer's role in comparing alternative therapies.

Another consideration is that many patients in our health care system do not contact a dentist until they believe they no longer have the option not to seek dental care. But it seems clear that one cannot function as a rational consumer, comparing all alternatives in terms of cost and benefit, if one has already set aside the option not to buy at all. The rational consumer must be able to leave the relationship if none of the products offered is on his or her optimal cost-quality curve.

One response to these arguments is that dentists need to be more effective at communicating with patients and that more concern is needed for patient education. But this response has, in fact, already begun to view the patient-dentist relationship in a manner different from the Commercial Model. No doubt the dentist who communicates and educates better has a better product to sell and will ordinarily sell more of it for a better price. But that is very different from saying that the dentist has an obligation to communicate and educate effectively because of the (moral) importance of effective patient decision-making. This response suggests a different picture of the patient-dentist relationship, one in which the dentist and the patient work out their judgments and choices together, at least to some extent, rather than competing, each trying to maximize his or her gain. That alternative picture will be examined more fully in a moment.

Another response is that the patient ordinarily views life and health as values much too important to put into the hands of someone who is simply a competitor. The reality of the patient-dentist relationship is therefore unavoidably more than one of competition. Even if the dentist tried to be simply a competitor and the patient was intensely competitive, it is doubtful that the two could maintain a relationship on these terms for long, and it is probably beyond the ability of most individuals to even try to do so. It cannot be the case that it is simply a matter of good business and important only for that reason that dentists act for the sake of their patients' well-being and that patient's trust them to do so.

At the same time, this should not drive us back to the Guild Model because what counts as the patient's well-being is not something fully known by the dentist, either by training or by experience. The dentist's commitment to the goal of fostering (important aspects of) the patient's well-being cannot be carried out independently of empathetic communication and shared judgment with the patient. The point here is not only the negative one that the Commercial Model and the Guild Model each falls short. It is also a positive one: that some sort of shared judgment and choice between dentist and patient is unavoidable in a patient-dentist relationship that takes account of the full reality of the patient.

Another point to bear in mind is that persons who are sick almost always experience their illness as a lessening of their ability to direct and control their bodies and their lives. The reason is not just that illness involves symptomatic deficits of function, although this is certainly true in most cases to varying degrees. Even more important is the fact that illness, the experience of being sick, is itself an experience of not being in control of one's body. One's goals, one's plans, and one's capacity to achieve at all are compromised. Even patients who are not presently ill still come to dentists in large part to prevent such loss of control from occurring.

In other words, one important reason why patients come to dentists is to recover their lost autonomy (or secure it from being lost), even as they also are trying to exercise their autonomy in choosing particular dental treatments while in a dentist's care. They come to dentists hoping that the dentist's expertise will restore their lost control and their full ability to direct their lives. In this respect, they do not come simply as bargainers, co-equal with dentists in the marketplace. Instead, their sense of themselves is, in part, that they have lost or are at risk of losing the ability to fully control (an important aspect of) their lives without assistance. But at the same time, they do not necessarily come incapable of autonomous choice either, that is, they are not incapable of playing a role in the choices and actions necessary to restore control over their bodies and lives.

The Interactive Model

In the model of the patient-dentist relationship that is gradually being formulated here, dentist and patient are equal partners in their relationship in three important respects. They are equal, first, in that each has standing in the relationship as a distinct chooser who deserves the other party's respect as such. Second, each is someone who has, by life-choices and commitments of many sorts, a set of values that he or she is trying to live by. So each is obliged to respect the other in this regard as well. Third, each comes to decision-making about the patient's oral health possessed of understanding about the decision that the other lacks and that can only be made up for by communication and mutual cooperation. The dentist has the expertise on which the patient's oral health and the patient's retention or recovery of lost autonomy in regard to oral health depend. The patient has the understanding of his or her own values, goals, and priorities, without which the decision to accept the professional's interventions cannot be coherently justified.

Unlike the Guild Model, the Interactive Model stresses the value of the patient's autonomy to the maximum degree that the patient is able to exercise it. It views the preservation and maximization of the patient's autonomy as one of the principal goals of dentists. But unlike the Commercial Model, the Interactive Model does not simply assume that patients are effective market decision-makers. Most patients not only lack the dentist's expertise but are also sick and so are not as fully in control of their circumstances as the dentist is of his or hers. Rather than granting the dentist a competitive edge in these respects, as the Competitive Model would if it were taken seriously as the ideal dentist-patient relationship, the Interactive Model sets aside competition in favor of collaboration. The dentist, to the extent that he or she is able, is committed to working to enhance the patient's autonomous decision-making capacities.

We can summarize this by saying that in the Interactive Model, the dentist and patient have equal moral standing within their relationship. But their equality, their equal claim to voice and vote within their relationship, derives from different grounds on the two sides. It derives from the value of autonomy and the fact that it is the patient's body and life that are being affected, on the patient's side, and from the fact of expertise regarding the patient's needs and enabling the patient to regain or maximize control over his or her body and life, which is precisely expertise concerning the central values of dental practice, on the dentist's side. In the Interactive Model both parties have unique and irreplaceable contributions to make in their judgments and choices together, and both the patient's and the dentist's values serve as determinants of what they do together.

It is a characteristic of American culture, and of most philosophical writing within our culture, to look upon all choices as the work of individuals alone. A little reflection suggests that spouses, families, friendships of two or three persons or more, and other groups in fact make choices together, as a unit. The Interactive Model of the patient-dentist relationship proposes that the choices that issue from their transactions are, in the ideal situation, made by both together in this way. To be sure, this ideal situation is often not realized in practice, either because of extensive limits on the patient's ability to participate (see Chapter 7) or because one or both parties do not have the achievement of an interactive relationship as a goal to work toward. But as a first step in understanding the fundamental elements of the patient-dentist relationship, it is important to note that such a relationship is possible and that, when it occurs, it overcomes the clear limits of the Guild, Agent, and Commercial Models of this relationship. The authors propose that the Interactive Model is the best articulation of the ideal relationship between dentist and patient.

AUTONOMY AND THE QUESTION OF JUSTIFIABLE PATERNALISM

Both in contemporary Western culture and in most theories of moral reflection developed in the West, respecting a person's autonomy when the person is capable of autonomous decision-making is a very important moral principle. The several capacities that, taken together, make a person fully capable of autonomous choice and action will be examined in Chapter 7. For the present, a shorter description of autonomy will suffice. *Autonomy* will be taken here to refer to a person's choosing and acting on the basis of his or her *own* values, principles, or ideals of conduct, goals, and purposes. The wording of this description is deliberately open-ended to include a wide variety of bases of action that a person might choose from. The central point is that the person chooses and acts from his or her *own* bases of action. In fact, this is exactly what the etymology of the word *autonomy* conveys. In ancient Greek, *auto* stands for "one's own," and *nomos* stands for "rule, principle, law." Thus *autonomy* would be "living or acting according to one's own rule, principle, or law."

A number of philosophical arguments aim at showing why the principle of respect for autonomy is such an important principle for moral reflection and action. One set of these employs a consequentialist, or utilitarian, mode of moral reasoning. That is, these arguments defend the importance of this principle by trying to show that actions that are respectful of autonomy are ordinarily more beneficial for the parties involved than alternative courses of action would be.

There are three utilitarian arguments that support a principle to respect people's autonomy. The first of these can be called the "short-term efficiency argument" for respecting autonomy. It points out that, in most circumstances, capable adults are the best judges of what will maximize their own well-being. Of course, people sometimes misjudge what is best for themselves, but in the vast majority of such cases, when this happens, it is because they are not capable of autonomous choice on the matter at the time. When people are capable, however, then it is almost always going to be a more efficient producer of their maximal well-being if we have them choose about matters that affect them than if someone else chooses in their stead.

Consequentialist, or utilitarian, arguments focus on identifying the course of action that will maximize values or well-being for everyone affected by what is done. In this case, we are comparing two principles of conduct that could be adopted by people generally in all the actions they undertake. The argument is that far more well-being will be realized by those persons affected if people are not interfered with by others and are allowed make their own choices about the things affecting them, when they are capable, than will be realized if others make these choices instead. In sum, to maximize well-being, don't interfere with capable people's choices.

The second consequentialist argument for respecting autonomy calls our attention to how painful we find it when someone interferes with our chosen actions, and to the fact that the more we consider our actions to be based on our *own* values, goals, priniples, and ideals, the more painful it is. By contrast, when we choose a course of action and carry it out without interference, we often experience a very special kind of satisfaction from being the one who chose the action and carried it out in accord with our *own* values, goals, principles, and ideals. The positive value associated with choosing and acting autonomously, and the negative value associated with being interfered with, are considered by some people to be among the strongest positive and negative experiences of value in human life, and in any case, these are important matters for almost everyone capable of autonomous choice.

Consequently, respecting someone's autonomy yields satisfaction for that person directly, and interfering yields a form of pain or suffering. So to maximize values and well-being, the best principle is: don't interfere with capable people's choices.

The third consequentialist argument is a "long-term efficiency" argument. Consider those persons, perhaps young men and women, who have been brought up in households or other circumstances in which they have had little or no opportunity to make choices for themselves on the basis of their own values, goals, principles, and ideals because someone else made all of their choices for them. Almost always, when they first encounter the need to make choices for themselves, they find it very difficult, even painful. In addition, they are not very good at it at first and are prone to make errors of judgment that do not in fact maximize well-being for themselves or for others. Therefore those who have had greater opportunity for actions that were based on autonomous choices and were not interfered with will grow increasingly efficient in their choosing, and those with less opportunity for such choices and who have been interfered with more will not.

The same is true of whole communities of people. Where opportunities for the exercise of choice are newly won, for example, there it takes time and experience to make the choice making process reasonably efficient. So both for individuals and for groups and even whole nations, respecting people's autonomy is far more likely to produce far greater benefits for people's well-being than interfering with their autonomy would. Again, the lesson for one aiming to maximize values is to respect people's autonomy.

Do these three arguments mean that it is always simply wrong to interfere with a capable person's autonomy? Consequentialists are rarely willing to claim that they can imagine every possible set of circumstances in which even a quite general principle like "respect people's autonomy" might be challenged. Thus they are not in the habit of saying "always" when such principles are being discussed. There are ethical theorists from other traditions of moral philosophy, however, who would say that the principle of respecting autonomy is so fundamental to morality that it may never be morally violated. They will be considered shortly.

But more specifically, there is at least one kind of situation in which, in most utilitarians' judgment, interfering with an autonomously chosen action will lead to better outcome for the people affected than not interfering will. This is the circumstance in which one party, *A*, is autonomously acting to harm or to threaten harm to another party, *B*, who does not choose to be so harmed. In such a case, interfering with *A's* autonomy preserves *B's* autonomy from interference and also preserves *B* from harm; that is, it is very possible that the negative outcomes are less if *A* is interfered with than if not.

In actual life, it will always be necessary to carefully weigh the form of interference with *A's* action that is contemplated in the case and also the precise nature of the interference with *B's* autonomy and of the harm that *B* is at risk of suffering from *A*. For utilitarian or consequentialist moral reasoning is always of the form, "such-and-such action is justifiable if, among the actions available, it produces the greatest benefits (or, in this case, the least harms) possible under the circumstances." But it is clear even from this brief argument that, from a utilitarian perspective, the general principle of respecting capable people's autonomy must be supplemented with another principle, often called the *Harm Principle*. It holds that it is often justifiable to interfere in the actions of someone who is interfering with and harming or threatening harm to someone else.

As was mentioned, some moral theorists consider the principle to respect autonomy to be exceptionless. For example, the late eighteenth century German philosopher, Immanuel Kant, claimed that violation of another person's autonomy is, in effect, contradictory. The other person's autonomy, he argued, is no different in kind or worth from my own. So how could I consistently refuse to permit anyone else to choose my actions for me, while simultaneously preventing someone from choosing his or her own action by my interference? The contradiction here demonstrates, Kant held, that violating autonomy is always not only irrational, but profoundly immoral. Other moral theorists defend the same conclusion by arguing that every capable human being has a fundamental right to respect for his or her autonomous decisions. Because no violation of this right can ever be justified, they argue, there are no exceptions to the principle that autonomous decisions of a capable person must always be respected.

Both kinds of defenders of an exceptionless principle of respecting autonomy recognize that situations can arise in which a person who is violating or threatening to violate another's autonomy must be confronted. They acknowledge that it would certainly be strange if the rest of us would be acting immorally if we interfered with such a person in order to protect the autonomy of his or her victim. This situation is usually explained in their accounts of moral reflection by saying that acts that violate the autonomy principle have already been proven irrational (because they isolate that principle); therefore such acts are not themselves truly autonomous (since thinking rationally is one of the components of autonomous decision-making). Consequently, they argue, people who interfere with such acts are not actually violating the perpetrators' autonomy.

A harder question for both consequentialist thinkers and those who defend an exceptionless principle of respecting autonomy is whether it is ever justifiable to interfere with a person's autonomously chosen action when that action is harming or is very likely to harm only *the chooser*. Such interference is often called *paternalistic* in the literature of moral philosophy, and the view that it is sometimes morally justifiable to interfere to benefit or to prevent harm to the one interfered with is often called *paternalism*.

The term *paternalism* and its less sexist equivalent, *parentalism* are not *literally* appropriate to the issue here. They speak literally of interference with a small child, and small children are not capable of autonomous choice. In addition, the word *paternalistic* is sometimes applied to interventions with a person who does not know, or is assumed to not know, that his or her action will be harmful. This makes for considerable confusion in the use of the term *paternalistic*. For the sake of clarity, interventions with someone who is known to be or is presumed to be unaware of some likely harm will not be called *paternalistic* here. Instead, an act will be called *paternalistic* in this book only when it prevents a choice or action of a person presumed to be acting autonomously, and therefore knowingly, in a manner that is harmful to or prevents a benefit to that person.

Terminology aside, however, the question remains whether it is ever justifiable to interfere with someone's autonomously chosen action in order to prevent him or her from self-harm or to provide a benefit. At the heart of this question is a question about the relative importance of the value of autonomy, or of the moral principle of respecting autonomy, or of the moral right that autonomy be respected. Is autonomy the most important standard of morality so that if both autonomy and some other moral value were at stake in some action, choice of the other value over autonomy would always be wrong? Or are there other values that are equal to autonomy or of even greater importance than autonomy such that these other values could be morally chosen over autonomy when both could not be maximized or respected at the same time? In that case, some paternalistic actions would be morally justifiable.

Even if autonomy does rank higher than any other moral consideration, is it also supreme, so that even a potent combination of all the other lower-ranking values could still not justify an act that fails to respect someone's autonomy to prevent that person's own harm? If this were the case, then no paternalistic act could ever be morally justified.

Philosophers and other moral theorists have wrestled with these difficult questions for centuries and, as yet, no final answers about the relative importance of autonomy and other moral standards in human morality exist. On the other hand, the specific commitments that dentists make when they become members of this profession, it has been argued, do require them to respect and support their patients' autonomy by striving for the ideal of a full interactive relationship with each of them. But this much clarity about dentists' professional commitments still does not resolve the question about the *relative* importance of patients' autonomy for a dentist, that is, in comparison with the other central values of dental practice when circumstances arise in which they cannot all be maximized or respected at once. The relative importance of the various central values of the profession will be discussed in the next chapter.

TRUTH-TELLING AND INFORMED CONSENT

A series of important court cases—for example, *Schloendorff* (1914), *Salgo* (1957), and *Canterbury* (1972)—and legislative acts in many jurisdictions have made *informed consent* the legal standard for judging the relationship between a patient and a health care provider. Very briefly, the law requires that this relationship include a choice by the patient, if he or she is legally capable of choice *(competent)*, and that this choice be *informed* by the provider, who must explain to the patient each of the courses of action that are available to the patient in the professional's expert judgment (including taking no action), as well as the likely outcomes of each.

The phrase *informed consent* is also often used to name the *ethical* standard for judging the relationship between a patient and a health care provider. Certainly in dentistry informed consent is the most common description of a professionally correct relationship with a patient. But it is worth asking whether this notion really is adequate for the job.

One component of the dentist-patient relationship that has not been stressed so far in this chapter is telling the patient the truth. Truthfulness is an important component of an ethical life, and it has a special importance in the relationship between health professional and patient because they depend on each other for information they need to play their respective roles in the relationship. The dentist depends on the patient for important information about the patient's general health, medical condition, medications being taken, and patterns of hygiene and self care. The patient depends on the dentist for an understanding of the condition of his or her mouth, of the need for intervention by the dentist, and of the likely outcome of alternative treatments. Neither party could function effectively, and dental care would be of far lower quality, if patient and dentist alike could not count on truthfulness in their relationship.

For many dentists, the word *informed* in the phrase informed consent is a reminder of this obligation to truthfulness on the part of a dentist. But in the phrase informed consent, only the *patient's being informed* is implied, and only the *dentist's obligation to communicate* truthfully and effectively implied. This is also what is emphasized in the legal cases that have given us this phrase. But in actual practice, *both* parties must be informed and *both* parties must communicate truthfully and effectively. The ideal relationship requires two-way communication and understanding. It requires an interactive relationship, and our ordinary understanding of informed consent does not point us clearly enough in this direction.

In a similar way, the word *consent* is often taken to emphasize the importance of the patient's autonomy in the dentist-patient relationship. But it is not only the patient who must choose, and not only the dentist who must respect another's appropriate control of the situation. The ideal relationship requires choosing on both sides and mutual respect for autonomy on both sides as well.

It might seem that the only point being stressed here is that patients have obligations. But the point of arguing that informed consent is much too narrow a description of the ideal dentist-patient relationship is not principally to stress the obligations of patients. It is to enrich our understanding of what dentists must do to bring about the mutuality of effective communication and mutual choice that is the ideal interactive relationship. A point made earlier needs to be stressed again to make this clear.

Whether they are currently experiencing pain or dysfunction or they are only aware of its possibility and hope to forestall it by preventive care, dental patients seek the dentist's help because they cannot fully control this important part of their bodies without it. They come to the dentist aware that they are not in complete control of their bodies and aware that the dentist's expertise can significantly restore or prevent their loss of control. This fact, plus the more variable factors of actual pain, fear, and inequalities of education and social position, mean that even within the most interactive relationship, initiative in controlling the situation rests with the dentist.

Consequently, it is not enough—it falls far short of the ideal—if the dentist merely initiates the provision of information, however truthful, and asks the patient to consent or not to a recommended course of action. The achievement of mutually effective communication and mutual choice will depend on the dentist taking the initiative not only in doing his or her part in this interaction but also in prompting and assisting the patient to do his or her part as well.

In the Guild Model of this relationship, the patient's tendency to passiveness in the relationship is viewed as appropriate. In the Interactive Model, the patient's tendency to passiveness—to merely being informed and consenting to the actions recommended, or to even less of a role than this—is viewed a something to be overcome if possible. It is to be overcome gently, with prompts, support, and assistance, rather than with pressure or negative judgments, because only in this way is the dentist genuinely respectful of the patient's actual choices—about the relationship as well as about treatment—as they are being made. But every response by the patient in the direction of sharing in the process of communication and mutual decision-making is valued as progress toward the dentist's professional ideal, rather than as a mistaken intrusion into the dentist's area of control.

A dentist must certainly attend to the standard of informed consent because it defines the minimum of legally acceptable relationships between the dentist and his or her legally competent patients. Moreover, insofar as the phrase informed consent expresses for many dentists their professional commitment to ethical norms of truthfulness and respect for patients' autonomy, it expresses a worthy ethical standard as well. But dentists must also ask themselves if informed consent is a full statement of the ideal relationship between dentist and patient. The proposal defended here is that it falls far short because, in its ideal form, this relationship is one of *mutual* communication and *shared* choice, even though the initiative for bringing the relationship with a particular patient as close as possible to this ideal most often rests principally with the dentist.

THINKING ABOUT THE CASE

Determining what ought to be done in the case of The Dreaded Root Canal would first require determining whether Mr. Vianni is capable of autonomous decision-making regarding the decision at hand. A fuller description of what is involved in autonomous decision-making will be given in Chapter 7. But two of its elements have been described here. First, the autonomous decision-maker can understand the alternative treatments that the dentist explains and their likely outcomes, as well as the likely outcome of no treatment at all. Second, the autonomous decision-maker can act on the basis of his or her own values, goals, purposes, and principles of conduct.

The case gives no reason to doubt that Mr. Vianni can understand simple concepts such as the structure of a tooth and the various steps involved in a root canal procedure. Nor does he exhibit any deficit in general intelligence. So the question regarding his ability to make an autonomous decisions about his dental treatment rests more on the question of whether his likely refusal of endodontic therapy, if he is presented with this treatment option in the usual way and asked whether he will choose it, would be in accord with his own values, goals, or purposes. Mr. Vianni is highly fearful of endodontic therapy and is so anxious about use of the drill that it sharply heightens his sensitivity to pain and discomfort. That is why Dr. Clarke expects that he would refuse the root canal.

Although Dr. Clarke might judge a refusal of endodontic therapy by Mr. Vianni to be a serious error on his part, the case could be made that this move would be consistent with his genuine and frequently expressed desire to avoid this procedure and other procedures involving extensive drilling. The case might be made, then, that Mr. Vianni is a capable decision-maker in this matter and that any move by Dr. Clarke to withhold information about his treatment alternatives until one set of them has been completed would be a violation of the principle of respecting autonomy.

On the other hand, if autonomy is choosing and acting on the basis of one's own values, Dr. Clarke is certain that the treatment most in accord with Mr. Vianni's repeatedly expressed valuing of his oral health is endodontic therapy and a proper crown. In fact, she could argue that it is failure to perform this procedure that would violate the principle of respecting Mr. Vianni's own values. In temporarily screening him from certain facts, she might argue, she would only be assuring that he would evaluate those facts according to his own values, rather than on the basis of fears and anxieties that are not only unreasonable from an observer's point of view, but are in fact inconsistent with Mr. Vianni's own values.

But if Dr. Clarke genuinely believes that Mr. Vianni is psychologically incapable of choosing in accord with his autonomy in this matter, then Dr. Clarke must act on the basis of some other principle than respect for autonomy. On this interpretation of Mr. Vianni's situation there is no autonomous decision on the part of Mr. Vianni for her to respect. That is, on the reading of the situation, Mr. Vianni is in fact *not* capable of autonomous decision-making regarding this form of treatment.

Determination of a patient's capacity for autonomous decision-making ultimately requires a more detailed understanding of autonomy than this chapter has offered. In addition, the principles that should guide a dentist in determining treatment and other interventions for patients who are incapable of autonomous decisions must be carefully examined. These tasks will be undertaken in Chapter 7. Therefore for present purposes let us presume that Mr. Vianni is in fact *capable* of autonomous decision-making in the matter of his first molar, although he is moved by powerful fears and anxieties regarding the best treatment available able to him, endodontic therapy. Let us ask whether, in such a case, Dr. Clarke could be ethically justified in violating the principle of respecting autonomy in order to provide Mr. Vianni with the best possible treatment for his situation. Are there are any features of the case that would justify such a violation, anything about the case that is of greater moral significance than respecting Mr. Vianni's autonomy?

Before proceeding, it is important to note that if Dr. Clarke were to do this, she would be engaging in legally risky action because Mr. Vianni is certainly legally competent and so has a legal right to either consent to or refuse endodontic therapy. But the present point is not to ask if such an action would be legally correct or legally risky but to ask whether it would be professionally unethical. Is the dentist's commitment to the patient's autonomy such that for a patient capable of autonomous decision-making, the dentist may never choose any value for the patient ahead of the patient's autonomy?

It is also important to avoid the kind of spurious position that holds that a patient is automatically and certainly incapable of autonomous decision-making simply and solely because he or she disagrees with the dentist about the treatment to be chosen. The determination of a patient's incapacity must depend on evidence in addition to disagreeing with the dentist. In the present case, the patient is fearful and anxious, but fear and anxiety are often reasonable responses to a situation, not signs of incapacity. For the time being, we are assuming that this is the case with Mr. Vianni in order to ask whether, even though we assume Mr. Vianni is capable of autonomous decision making, there are still values at stake in this case that are important enough that a dentist may ethically choose them for the patient rather than respecting his autonomy.

With the issue thus focused, it is important to notice one additional feature of the case that has not yet been stressed in this commentary. Mr. Vianni's fear and anxiety are not news to Dr. Clarke. Nor is it news that there is little sound enamel left on the first molar, or that it contains a large restoration that is getting very old. It would have been prudent of Dr. Clarke to warn Mr. Vianni, gently but regularly as she got to know him, that this tooth would probably not hold up forever and that endodontic therapy, performed in a pain-free manner, would be the best therapy for it.

More importantly, Dr. Clarke should not have waited until now to wonder what to do about Mr. Vianni's fears and anxieties. She should have established a plan with him some time before to begin addressing these concerns of his, so that he could be better prepared for the major restorative or endodontic or periodontic work that he would likely need as he grows older. Dr. Clarke has been willing to leave the relationship very one-sided, very much according to the Guild Model, instead of working to address the factors in Mr. Vianni that were making it so. She does not seem to have worked as hard at producing an interactive relationship as Mr. Vianni's limitations required.

Of course, Dr. Clarke might well be able to say that she did try to bring their relationship around to being more interactive and that Mr. Vianni was unwilling or unable to let that happen. She might also be able to say that there is only so much time and effort that she owes this particular patient. It might be that she has already met or even gone beyond the basic commitments of time and effort that every patient has a right to, within the ordinary dentist-patient relationship, so that devoting further time and effort to a more interactive relationship for Mr. Vianni would have either taken time owed to other patients in need or taken time from other commitments and other aspects of Dr. Clarke's life that legitimately compete with this patient's needs.

These two issues, how much time and effort a dentist owes to each patient, in comparison with other patients also in need, and how much sacrifice of other commitments and concerns a dentist owes to his or her patients, are very important questions that do not admit of easy answers. They clearly play an inportant roel in this case, and they will be discussed more fully in Chapter 6 and in later chapters in this book.

But the importance of these issues does not eliminate or provide an answer to the question that is the central focus of this chapter: what is the ideal relationship between dentist and patient? If the interactive relationship is the ideal, as has been proposed here, then it is the relationship that a dentist ought to try to achieve with whatever resources of expertise, time, effort, hard work, and common sense he or she has available. It will often be impossible to achieve this ideal fully, given the patient's situation and the resources available to the dentist. But that does not lessen its claim to being the ideal that dentists are to strive to achieve. For with whatever resources the dentist has available, and to the extent possible, given the patient's actual situation, it is an interactive relationship that the dentist should be working to bring about.

So what should Dr. Clarke do, on the assumption that Mr. Vianni is capable of autonomous decision-making about endodontic therapy? One option might be to work for additional time in order to persuade Mr. Vianni to choose the best treatment. She might, for example, provide temporary pain relief and antibiotic therapy (to prevent further infection) in order to have several days' time to actively address Mr. Vianni's unreasonable fears of endodontic therapy. The risk of this option is that the task of refocusing Mr. Vianni's attention on his commitment to dental health and the benefits of endodontic therapy in the present situation may well take more time than Dr. Clarke's temporizing efforts can provide. She will have lost the option of beginning endodontic therapy here and now, and she may not be able to persuade him to choose endodontic therapy anyway.

It is also worth asking if Dr. Clarke would really be working effectively for a more interactive relationship if she opted for this path. Much would depend on how she used the time that temporizing would provide. If it were devoted to an extensive effort to persuade him to choose endodontic therapy, it is doubtful that the fundamental equality of the two parties and the mutual respect of each other's values, on which an interactive relationship rests, would be effectively honored. On the other hand, it might be possible, if time for thoughtful conversation were available (although it might be the case that neither party would have time for this anyway), that the value of Mr. Vianni's oral health, which both parties wish to honor, could bring them to a shared decision about his treatment. An interesting question is whether, if a shared decision were reached, it would have to be a decision for endodontic therapy.

Still assuming that Mr. Vianni's refusal of endodontic therapy would be an autonomous one, Dr. Clarke might simply hold that the moral and professional importance of respecting Mr. Vianni's autonomy require that she seek his consent without any deception and, if consent is refused, abide by that choice. How she should proceed after that would depend on her judgment about the suitability of alternative therapies, for example, simple extraction or extraction with a restoration to fill the space and to maintain the occlusion and integrity of the dentition.

If she chooses this option, it is worth noting, Dr. Clarke might be able to view the choice as one that she and Mr. Vianni have made together. But without conversation of the sort mentioned in the previous paragraph, it seems more likely that she will view herself as unwillingly supporting a mistaken choice by Mr. Vianni. The mere fact that a patient's autonomous choice has been respected by the dentist does not automatically mean that the ideal of an interactive relationship has been approached. As was indicated earlier, the proposal that the ideal relationship between dentist and patient is an interactive one often asks far more of both parties than is necessary to achieve informed consent.

Finally, even on the assumption that Mr. Vianni's refusal would be an autonomous one, Dr. Clarke might still hold that she ought to initiate endodontic therapy here and now, without fully informing Mr. Vianni until the worst is past, because there are values that she is committed to as a dentist and that are an accepted part of the dentist-patient relationship that Mr. Vianni has chosen that are more important than respecting his autonomous choice in this matter. The justification of this view would require some careful analysis of the central values of professional dental practice to support the claim that Dr. Clarke's professional obligations would require her to rank some other value ahead of a patient's autonomy. A discussion of the central values of dental practice, and of their proper ranking, follows in the next chapter.

CHAPTER 5

The Central Values of Dental Practice

Case: The Cheapest Will Have To Do

Ina Kirchland came to Dr. Luban's office in considerable pain and was squeezed in between the 9:40 and the 10:00 appointments. Although Mrs. Kirchland's teeth are generally in good shape, her upper left first premolar has been a problem for some time, and Dr. Luban had foreseen that the day would come when it would be a matter of either doing a root canal or removing and replacing the tooth. A quick examination makes it clear that because the coronal portion of the tooth has fractured that time has now come.

Mrs. Kirchland is a 68-year-old widow in good general health. She does not have much money, and she does not have dental insurance. She lives on her deceased husband's social security benefits, which she supplements to some extent by doing day care in her home several afternoons a week. Her resources for dental care, as for everything, are very limited, and her constant anxiety about how to make ends meet has been articulated at the outset of every dental appointment in recent years.

Dr. Luban would certainly prefer to see Mrs. Kirchland get a root canal with post and crown, but it is obviously much more expensive than a simple extraction would be. Of course, it would be important for her to fill that space. She could elect an extraction with a fixed bridge to fill the space, but that would be more expensive still, and Dr. Luban judges that this is not a useful alternative for her. Another possibility would be an extraction with a removable partial prosthesis to fill the space. An extraction and fabricating a removable prosthesis would cost Mrs. Kirchland less than endodontic therapy and a crown. But the prosthesis would require constant care for the rest of her life, and it may need replacement later on if her mouth changes significantly with age.

If Dr. Luban simply presents Mrs. Kirchland with just the facts about these three options—root canal with post and crown, extraction with a prosthesis, and simple extraction—he is quite certain that she will simply choose the cheapest therapy, even with the serious risk of moving teeth and malocclusion. "I am getting old," she has said many times, "the cheapest and simplest will have to last me."

It is also the case that endodontic therapy can be tricky; a strange twist to the canal might later mean removal of the tooth anyway. Dr. Luban certainly has to mention this possibility in some way as well, but too much of this may cause the simple extraction to look even better to Mrs. Kirchland.

On the other hand, he can definitely control how much to stress this aspect of root canal therapy in his explanation. In fact, he can probably make his explanation of the alternatives persuasive in any direction he chooses. By pressuring Mrs. Kirchland strongly about the benefits of endodontic therapy with post and crown, the risks of extraction alone, and the inconvenience of caring for a prosthesis and the possibility of its needing to be replaced later on, Dr. Luban could probably lead Mrs. Kirchland to choose the root canal. But he has serious reservations about doing this because a choice by Mrs. Kirchland under such circumstances might not be a very free one.

Another possibility is to not even mention the possibility of a simple extraction. But wouldn't that leave Mrs. Kirchland even less free to choose? Doing so would mean that she would not know about a possible treatment that is still within the range of clinically acceptable therapy, even though it is not the preferred treatment for her clinical situation.

Yet Dr. Luban is certain that the root canal with post and crown is really worth her money, and he has doubts that even a choice of either cheaper therapy would be a very free choice on her part, given her view of her financial situation and her evident anxiety about it.

What should Dr. Luban do and why?

STUDYING A PROFESSION'S CENTRAL VALUES

The practice of each profession, that is, the application of its expertise for the benefit of its clients, is necessarily focused only on certain aspects of the well-being of those clients. No professional group is expected by the larger community to be expert in their clients' *entire* well-being. Consequently, no profession is committed to securing for its clients everything that is of value for them. Of course the achievement of any values for a profession's clients will depend on an understanding of the relation of these values to each client's whole person. It is precisely in this way that the expressed concern of many professions about being attentive to the "whole" client can contain an important element of truth. But there is always necessarily a certain limited set of values that are the specific focus of each profession's expertise, and it is therefore the principal job and obligation of that profession to secure these for its clients. These values can be called the *central values* of that profession's practice.

The aim of this chapter is to propose an answer to the obvious question: What are the central values of dental practice and of the dental profession? What specific aspects of human well-being is it the task of each member of the dental profession to secure for its clients? In addition, if there are a number of central values, are these of equal importance, or do some of them take precedence over others when all of them cannot be achieved simultaneously? That is, do they form some sort of hierarchy?

Before considering these questions, however, two other questions must be addressed. First, who determines a profession's central values? Second, how then can we identify the values that are currently accepted as the *central values* for a particular profession's practice in a particular society? Clearly, it is not the individual practitioner who determines what values are central values for the dental profession and dental practice in a given society. Of course, each individual dentist does make a personal choice to accept the obligations of professional practice as a dentist, and in this respect each dentist's commitment to the central values of dental practice is his or her own doing. But the contents of this commitment, as Chapter 2 explained, are rather the product of an on-going dialogue between the dental community and the community at large. So when a person chooses to become a dentist, it is the values identified as central values in that on-going dialogue that he or she accepts and commits to, not some set of values of the individual practitioner's own devising.

The person who becomes a dentist may even consider the values currently accepted as central values for dental practice in that society to be in need of revision or significant adjustment. Such a person may therefore choose to work, as a member of the dental community, to change or adjust the values that both the dental community and the community at large accept as central for dental practice. Some subtle ethical questions can arise for such a dentist about the extent to which a member of a profession may, and sometimes even ought to, engage in conscientious refusal to serve values that he or she judges incorrect for that profession's practice. But the starting point of all such reflections and choices must be the fact that the content of professional norms for a given profession in a given society is the product of an on-going dialogue between that professional group and the larger community. It is not the product of unilateral choices on the part of an individual practitioner or even on the part of the professional group alone.

How then can we identify the values that are currently accepted as central for the dental profession and dental practice in our society? The short answer to this question is that we must carefully examine the *conduct* and the *discourse* of the members of the society as these pertain to dental practice. That is, we can begin to identify the central values by carefully examining the conduct of members of the dental profession and their patients as these parties discuss and then make decisions about dental treatment. Regarding discourse, some of these values can be identified by examining the kinds of reasons that these parties give and accept, as well as the kinds of reasons that are given and accepted in the society at large, as justifying dentists' and patients' decisions in practice and their relationships with each other.

In spite of its length, this is the "short" answer because the long answer involves the actual work of sifting and sorting all the data about conduct and discourse that were identified as relevant in the previous paragraph. In fact, without noticing it, all of us who deal with the dental profession in our society, and certainly both the established and the aspiring members of the dental profession itself, constantly absorb and contemplate these data to form an understanding of what is taken for granted about the central values of dental practice in our society.

Ideally, those who are most concerned about the dental profession and dental practice perform this work of sifting and sorting much more explicitly and self-consciously. They then try to articulate what they observe in accepted patterns of conduct and discourse so that other concerned parties can evaluate their proposals and offer the evidence of their own observation and experience until a genuine consensus about the contents of accepted professional norms can be formed. The accounts of the accepted norms of dental practice that appear in the codes of ethics of professional organizations, and the sets of advisory opinions about such codes, are examples of such efforts.

The account of the accepted norms of dental practice offered in this book, and the discussions in articles and books by other scholars of dental professional ethics, are also intended to be part of this process.

The codes of ethics proposed by organized dentistry have a special importance in this effort because they are commissioned and supported by large groups of dentists. Thus their authors have far more claim to be representative of the dental community than the two authors of this book have or the authors of other scholarly articles and books have. At the same time, it is extremely rare that members of the nondental community are represented at all in the processes that lead to such codes. Consequently, the codes are often representative of only one side of the dialogue. On the other hand, a book like this or a scholarly article on a particular topic in dental professional ethics can examine the accepted norms of dental practice and raise questions about the reasons supporting them and possible alternatives to them in far more detail than any published code or set of advisory opinions can do. Thus both kinds of efforts are needed to help make the contents of the on-going dialogue more articulate. The role of organized dentistry's codes of ethics will be discussed more fully in Chapter 15.

From what has been said, it follows that the many statements about professional norms and obligations made in this book should be read as hypotheses about the contents of the current dialogue between the dental community and the community at large regarding the norms and values that the two groups accept as shaping the dental profession and dental practice in our society. Yet while these are "only" hypotheses, the accounts of professional norms and obligations offered here are not mere constructions of the authors' imaginations. They are based on extensive and careful analysis of our society and its dental community using the most sophisticated concepts about the nature, basis, and implications of professional obligation available, many of which are also summarized in this book so they too can be thoughtfully evaluated by the reader.

If the data needed for determining a profession's central values and other norms are to be found in broad patterns of conduct and discourse within a society, it might seem that only a trained sociologist could correctly identify dentistry's central values. But the answers to many questions about the nature of important social roles are so evident in the practice, expectations, and concrete relationships of persons in a society that ordinary people carefully performing ordinary judgments about such matters can handle them very well. In such cases, formal sociological demonstrations perform only a confirmatory role.

Consider this example from a different part of the health care system. A hospital, through its administrators, employs and pays house staff physicians, nurses, nurses' assistants, laboratory personnel, and many other health workers. These are all answerable to their own supervisors and to a number of other officers in the hospital's chain of command. In addition, many of their tasks are determined by "orders" from attending physicians. Nevertheless, there is no doubt in anyone's mind that their proper clients, the persons to whose well-being these workers are chiefly to attend, are none of these parties, but rather the hospital's *patients*. Sociologists can offer formally constructed confirmations of this, but we do not need their expertise to reach a dependable judgment about this aspect of health professionals' obligations.

The questions being addressed in this book may not all have answers that are this evident in practice, for some of these questions are very complex and involve factors of many different kinds. But it is important to distinguish between a question's complexity—the need for careful analysis and reflection before a person can answer it—and the features that necessitate formal sociological examination. The reader may conclude, at various points in this book, that a question we try to answer cannot be adequately answered without the assistance of formal sociological research. In such instances, if there are any, the answers we propose here will be no more than hypotheses for further sociological investigation. But the authors believe that the claims made in these pages about the contents of dentistry's professional norms are in fact well supported by the data; that is, they are supported in the conduct and discourse, the actions undertaken and the reasons given, of dental professionals, their patients, and other members of the larger community.

THE CENTRAL VALUES OF DENTAL PRACTICE

As dentists care for patients, they make numerous decisions that are inherently value-laden. Most of these do not involve conscious examination of competing values by the dentist because they are the fruit of well-established habits of professional practice. But whether the value content of a particular judgment is explicit or implicit, a dentist cannot practice without numerous decisions in which values play an important role. The practice of dentistry, in other words, is not only a matter of technical judgment and skill; it is also an activity in which the <u>dentist strives to bring about certain values either directly for the patient or as part of his or her relationship with the patient</u>.

To make the same point in another way, consider a dentist who focused his or her efforts principally on entertaining the patient and receiving the patient's plaudits as a result, even if this meant foregoing procedures needed for the patient's oral health. Or consider a dentist who worked chiefly to give patients the excitement and exhilaration that some people experience when they face a serious risk to life or health head-on and who therefore made little or no effort to control or <u>minimize the risk to the patient in advance</u>. Such dentists would have a limited clientele, of course. The risk-adverse would not be interested in the latter dentist, and patients who go to dentists for more familiar reasons would probably avoid both of them. But many people enjoy being entertained, and there seem to be people who enjoy risk-taking enough that each kind of dentist might still have regular patients. Would either of these practitioners be practicing in a professionally acceptable way, even if they had patients?

The answer to this question is clear. Neither of these ways of employing dental expertise is professionally acceptable under the accepted standards of dental practice in our society. Regardless of whether a person could actually earn a living doing such things, these ways of acting are not proper ways for a person who claims to be a dentist to act. They are misdirected; in fact, precisely what is wrong with them is that they are directed at the wrong values.

As in every profession, there are certain values that are central to the proper practice of dentistry, and every dentist is committed, as a professional, to working to achieve these values above all in his or her practice. What are these central values of dental practice? There are six values that appear to be accepted as the central values for dental practice in our society:

1. The Patient's Life and General Health
2. The Patient's Oral Health
3. The Patient's Autonomy
4. The Dentist's Preferred Patterns of Practice
5. Esthetic Values
6. Efficiency in the Use of Resources.

The question whether these six are hierarchically ranked will be discussed later in this chapter. But before that, each of the six must be explained in its own right.

The Patient's Life and General Health

One value that certainly plays an important role in dentists' judgment in practice is the value of the patient's life and general health. Although this value is not discussed as much as patients' oral health, nevertheless every patient that a dentist examines and every treatment that a dentist recommends or performs must be evaluated on the basis of this value. A dentist who recommended a treatment that placed a patient's life at risk without any consideration for this fact would certainly be acting unprofessionally. Moreover, a dentist who paid no attention to the connections between a patient's oral condition and other aspects of the patient's health would similarly be guilty of a serious professional failure.

It will be important to reflect on the relative importance of this value—the patient's life and general health—in comparison with other values in dental practice. Is it correct to say that the patient's life and general health should take priority over all other values that a dentist strives to achieve, or are other values more important than this in the practice of dentistry? This question will be examined in detail in the next section. But first a description is needed of the other five central values for dental practice.

The Patient's Oral Health

Here is the most obvious value that dentists aim to achieve for their patients. Although it may appear to be a fairly simple idea, *oral health* is actually quite a complex notion. There are general standards of appropriate oral function, of course, but the specific character of appropriate functioning for a particular patient will depend on many variables, including the patient's age, the pattern of development of the patient's dentition, other health conditions, the patient's functional needs, the patient's underlying anatomy, and so on. Oral health also includes the notion that oral functioning is pain-free. But pain and discomfort are also relative terms, and the specific standard that a dentist should apply to a given patient will also depend, at least in part, on variables like those already mentioned. Nevertheless, in spite of the complexity of its content, oral health plays a very important role in the judgments dentists make every day in practice. For present purposes, "oral health" will be defined as "appropriate and pain-free oral functioning."

The complexity of the notion of *oral health* is in fact just an extension of the complexity of the idea of *health* itself. *Health* is not merely a factual concept. It is an evaluative concept as well, which is used to identify certain characteristics and conditions of humans as the ones humans are better off having. It is beyond the scope of this book to study the larger concept of *health* in any detail, but all who are health care providers, including members of the dental profession, would do well to think carefully about the meaning of this concept and its implications for their professional practice.

The Patient's Autonomy

Autonomy was discussed at some length in the preceding chapter. The brief definition adopted there, "choosing and acting on the basis of one's own values, goals, purposes, and principles of conduct" will continue to be operative here.

The prominence of the professional-legal principle of *informed consent* and the reasons given in Chapter 4 for considering the Interactive Model as the ideal model for the dentist-patient relationship should be reasons enough for including autonomy on this list of central values for dental practice. However, once the relative importance of these central values becomes the focus of discussion in the following section on ranking dentistry's central values, the question of the relative priority of the patient's autonomy will be seen to be more complex than this.

The Dentist's Preferred Patterns of Practice

The dentist who practices in a technically competent manner still has many choices to make. Among these choices are some that might be noticed by a thoughtful lay person; for example, the dentist must choose among various kinds of dental chairs and various ways of laying out an operatory. But there are many more and many that are much more important. There are choices among various styles and brands of hand instruments, among various kinds and brands of medicaments, of dental materials, and so on. There are a wide range of choices to be made regarding major dental equipment because the available technology changes and advances so rapidly. Still more complex than these are the dentist's choices among various acceptable approaches to most of the diagnostic, operative, and other procedures in dental practice. A dentist must make choices in all these areas, weighing the options in terms of patient outcome and patient comfort, of course, but also in terms of the dentist's own output of time, effort, and dollars, as well as the dentist's degree of comfort with and trust in each particular alternative.

It might seem that no special values are involved in these choices other than those mentioned under the other five headings in this section. That is, once the other five values have been fulfilled, it might seem that nothing else is at stake but the dentist's own preference, which has no special ethical standing beyond the legitimacy of a professional choosing as he or she wishes when matters are otherwise undirected. But in fact, there is a subtle professional value at stake in these choices that needs careful articulation because it is so easily overlooked.

No one can effectively apply complex expertise to concrete situations, such as the specific clinical needs of a particular patient, if every detail of that application must be self-consciously judged and chosen each time it arises. For this reason, becoming a competent and effective professional is, in significant measure, becoming capable of applying many aspects of one's expertise *habitually*, without self-conscious attention. The initial development of such habits—habits of perception, valuation, judgment, and action—is the principal goal of the future dentist's training in dental school, and the development into habits of more and more details of competent practice is the chief effect of a young dentist's early years of practice. It is only when most of the ordinary details of a particular procedure—whether diagnostic or operative or something else—can be addressed without self-conscious reflection and judgment that a dentist is able to then attend effectively to the unusual, the unique, and the problematic in this particular patient or respond effectively when an apparently ordinary situation for some reason goes awry.

Consequently, a dentist's comfort with, trust in, and preference for a particular pattern of practice—in any area in which, within the range of technically competent practice, important choices remain—is not something merely subjective and professionally value-neutral. Instead the dentist must judge whether a particular pattern of practice is one that he or she is able to effectively habituate and whether it is one that the dentist wants to have as part of his or her habitual way of practicing. Such judgments are objectively significant for professionally adequate dental practice, and respect for such judgments is therefore a central value of dental practice.

The same is also true, at a different level of generality, of what is sometimes called a dentist's "philosophy of practice." Dentists who practice in a technically competent manner differ not only in their choices regarding particular elements of dental practice, such as choice of hand instruments or disinfectants or how to approach a three-unit bridge. Within the range of technically competent practice, dentists can also choose different "philosophies" of dental treatment.

For example, one dentist may do everything possible to save and work with natural teeth, refusing to extract natural teeth unless there is no other clinically acceptable option and, in all other cases, referring to other dentists any patient who is unhappy with so narrow a range of clinical options. Another dentist may be less restrictive in this regard, urging the patient to preserve natural teeth, but willing to provide any technically acceptable form of treatment that the patient might choose. Yet another may routinely present the several technically acceptable treatments for a given oral condition as simply being equally commendable. So long as all three of these dentists are functioning within the range of technically acceptable practice, none of them are in violation of the central values of life and general health or oral health. (It is also true, however, that different dentists may have different opinions about what constitutes "technically acceptable practice." In general, if it is determinable, the proper criterion here will be the judgment of the dental community as a whole.)

A dentist's philosophy of practice is a drawing together of many narrower choices within the range of what is technically competent, and it focuses and determines choices in a number of aspects of practice. Like the choices already discussed, it affects dental practice through becoming habituated, so that fundamental questions about the proper goals of dentistry—within the range of what is technically competent—do not have to be debated by the dentist in regard to every patient. For the same reasons already given, then, respect for a dentist's choice of philosophy of practice is also part of the central value under discussion here.

These choices of habitual patterns of practice within the range of what is technically competent will here be called "preferred patterns of practice." The relative importance of the value of respect for a dentist's *preferred patterns of practice*, in comparison with other central values in dentistry, will be discussed below.

Esthetic Values

A dentist who paid no attention to the oral and facial appearance of patients or to their judgments about their oral and facial appearance would surely be failing professionally. There are also accepted standards of form (regarding the size of teeth, their shape, color, placement, and so on), over and above considerations that are directly related to oral health, that the dental profession subscribes to and that a dentist learns initially in dental school and more fully through practice and contact with other dentists. A dentist would be failing professionally who paid no attention to these standards in his or her practice. Clearly, then, the central values of dental practice include esthetic values.

It is important to note, however, the differences between the two kinds of esthetic values involved here. Regarding patients' judgments of oral and facial appearance, there is no single standard of appropriate appearance that all patients or even the generality of patients apply. Therefore to a significant degree, the dentist honors this aspect of esthetic values in dental practice principally by guiding each patient to judge oral and facial appearance according to his or her own standards.

Of course, the dentist's own standards of appearance will probably play some role in the dentist's advice and guidance of the patient. Certainly the dentist's interpretation of the community's standards of appearance should play a role, since serious violation of these standards might have an impact on the patient's psychological well-being, which the dentist must consider as one element of the patient's general health. Even more importantly, acting on the patient's judgments of good appearance never justifies doing serious damage to healthy teeth. This will create difficult judgment calls for many dentists, for example, determining whether the removal of part of a tooth to apply gold to it, solely because of the patient's positive esthetic judgment about the gold, is professionally justifiable. In any case, there is no standard set by the profession that is operative in such matters except to honor the patient's judgment unless it appears to be truly harmful to the patient's own well-being.

On the other hand, there is an accepted standard, or set of standards, within the dental profession regarding the proper shaping of a restoration and numerous other matters of form in restorative work, prosthetic work, and many other aspects of dentistry. These standards pertain to form rather than function, and so concern esthetic matters rather than oral or general health. Nevertheless they constitute an objective criterion for judging practice, *objective* because these are the actually accepted standards for practice within the dental community in our society.

Efficiency in the Use of Resources

There are two points to be made about efficiency as a central value of dental practice.

First, efficiency is a common value, and it might not seem to have any more importance for the professional practice of dentistry than it has for any other occupation. But in fact it does have a special place in dental practice. The expertise of the dentist and the specialized physical resources used by dentists have been developed at considerable effort specifically to respond to a certain set of important human needs. The special importance of these needs to dentistry's patients, along with the fact that dental expertise and other dental resources are not in unlimited supply and the fact that special effort has been necessary to make them available at all, all indicate that a dentist who used these resources to no particular good or who squandered them thoughtlessly even when pursuing an appropriate benefit for a patient, would be acting unprofessionally.

Of course, few dentists would seriously considering doing such things. Thus the more important point about efficiency as a central value for dental practice is that, for the reasons just mentioned, dentists are fully justified in appealing to the value of efficient use of resources in their judgments in practice. There is nothing unprofessional in a dentist's working to control costs—in time, effort, or materials—provided the other central values are also given their due. Anyone who would criticize a dentist for being concerned with efficiency in the use of professional expertise or of the specialized physical resources of dental practice, when the dentist was also according the other central values of dental practice their proper place, would be making a mistake.

RANKING DENTISTRY'S CENTRAL VALUES

What is the proper ranking of these six central values? Does one or another of them consistently take precedence over some or all of the others?

In many dental practice judgments, the ranking of these values will not be very important because only one of them will be significantly at stake. But when two or more of these values are simultaneously at stake, and when the alternative interventions available to the dentist are such that these several values cannot all be maximized at once—that is, when the central values of dental practice conflict with one another by pointing to mutually exclusive courses of action—then the question whether they are ranked in priority and so form a hierarchy of importance becomes crucial.

To stimulate careful discussion of these issues, the following ranking of the six central values is proposed, beginning with the most important:
1. The patient's life and general health
2. The patient's oral health
3. The patient's autonomy
4. The dentist's preferred patterns of practice
5. Esthetic values
6. Efficiency in the use of resources
The following discussion identifies our reasons for proposing this particular ranking of these values as normative for dental practice.

To begin with the first, a dentist who recommended a treatment that involved significant risk to a patient's life or severely compromised a patient's general health for the sake of any of the other values on the list would be acting unprofessionally. In fact, the only circumstances in which a dentist might ethically recommend a treatment posing serious risk to life or health are those in which the oral condition to be treated itself poses significant risks to life or health and the proposed dental treatment might diminish those risks in the foreseeable future. That is, risk to life or general health via dental interventions is justifiable only for the sake of life or general health itself. Consequently, it seems clear that the patient's life and general health are the highest ranking of the central values of dental practice.

Appropriate and pain-free oral functioning is the dental value appealed to most frequently in dental practice and is the next most important value in dental practice. Relatively minor trade-offs of oral function may be acceptable for the sake of the patient's autonomy, esthetic values (the patient's), and possibly efficiency in the use of resources. But a dentist who accepted a trade-off that would leave a patient with significantly impaired or painful oral function, even for the sake of values lower on the list, would be practicing unethically. Therefore the patient's oral health ranks second on the hierarchy of central values.

The relative importance of the patient's autonomy in the hierarchy of central values for dental practice is, in one respect, easy to state, but in several other respects it is a complex matter. If a patient asked a dentist to perform a procedure that, in the dentist's professional judgment, would significantly harm the patient's oral health or harm the patient's life or general health, and if the dentist acted on the patient's request out of respect for the patient's autonomy and did the procedure, the dentist would be acting unprofessionally. Instead, the dentist must refuse to respect the patient's autonomous choice if the action chosen is contrary to the patient's oral or general health. It seems obvious, then, that the patient's autonomy ranks lower in the hierarchy of central values than both the oral health of the patient and the patient's life and general health.

In addition, if there are alternative treatments for a patient that all support the patient's oral and general health, and if the dentist fails to respect the patient's autonomous choice among these alternatives in order to maximize esthetic values or efficiency in the use of resources, it seems clear that the dentist would be acting unprofessionally. These values, though central to dental practice, are nevertheless below the patient's autonomy in the hierarchy.

The issue grows more complex, however, when the value of the patient's autonomy is compared with value of dentists' preferred patterns of practice. In fact, some dentists simply hold that dentists' preferred patterns of practice have a higher position in the hierarchy of central values than patients' autonomy, in spite of all the arguments (summarized in the previous chapter) about the great moral importance of respect for patients' autonomy.

In examining this issue, however, it is important to remember that the content of a profession's norms is not the work only of the members of the profession; it is the fruit of an ongoing dialogue between the profession and the larger community. So the value of preferred patterns of practice is not to be measured by how attached a dentist might be to his or her patterns of practice, but rather by the benefits it secures to dentists and patients together. Significant reasons for considering habituated patterns of practice that are very important to effective dental treatment were summarized in the previous section. Nevertheless, it seems unlikely that the larger community, which is mostly the community of patients, would routinely hold that patients' choices between alternative treatments (when these are all supportive of their oral and general health) may be justifiably set aside if the sole reason for setting them aside was simply that the dentist has a habit of practicing a certain way and habits are important. The mere fact that a dentist has a preferred pattern of practice does not seem a strong enough reason for failing to act on a patient's autonomous choice, providing oral and general health are not put at risk by doing so. So the patient's autonomy seems to rank higher on the hierarchy than the dentist's preferred patterns of practice.

Of course, there are other situations in which the patient's oral or general health depends on the dentist's following a preferred pattern of practice. That is, there are situations in which the value of a preferred pattern of practice in a particular situation is not in its being a preferred pattern of practice as such, but in that pattern's being necessary for the oral or general health of the patient.

Suppose, for example, that it is part of Dr. Jones' philosophy of dental practice that she does not believe in amalgam buildups, even in situations in which this sort of restoration would be within the range of minimally acceptable treatments. In such cases, Dr. Jones prefers to place a gold or porcelain-fused-to-gold crown. Consequently, when clinical circumstances arise in which she needs to mention an amalgam buildup as a treatment option, she invariably mentions that she does not recommend or perform them and would therefore need to refer the patient to another dentist if the patient were to choose that option.

But now, Mr. Smith, whose regular dentist of many years has recently died, is in Dr. Jones' chair and is asking for an amalgam buildup rather than a more expensive crown because his previous dentist was willing to provide them. In this particular case, however, Dr. Jones is certain that the amalgam buildup would be unstable and would fracture in a short time. She therefore declines to provide it, not because she prefers alternative therapies, but because, in this instance, it is the wrong therapy. That is, it would be a violation of Mr. Smith's oral health to provide this treatment under these clinical circumstances, regardless of Mr. Smith's wishing otherwise. In such a case, the pattern of practice *is* more important than the patient's autonomy, but not because it is a preferred pattern of practice. Consequently, such situations are not evidence against the proposed hierarchy in which the patient's autonomy ranks above preferred patterns of practice and below the patient's oral and general health.

A more complex question about the value of the patient's autonomy in dental practice arises from the intersection of three ethical characteristics of dental practice. (1) The dentist may not ethically treat a patient capable of autonomous choice without the patient's participation because of the primacy of relating to the patient interactively as has already been discussed; (2) the patient, in choosing treatment, is not bound by the ethical standards of the dental profession, including the hierarchy of central values, as the dentist is; (3) but the patient is still dependent on the dental professional to provide such dental treatments as the patient might want, and so has access through the dentist only to those treatments that the dental profession deems appropriate in terms of the patient's oral and general health because these are the dentist's professional norms.

It is common to begin explaining this complex feature of ethical dental practice by focusing on the fact that the dentist cannot ethically treat the patient who is capable of autonomous choice without the patient's participation. This seems to entail that the patient's autonomy is the most important value for dental practice. Thus when the point is then made that the dentist may not ethically offer or perform treatments that violate the patient's oral or general health, the dentist appears to be required to violate what seemed to be the highest ranking value of dental practice. But a different approach to this matter, the one being taken here, represents the actual ethical situation far more accurately.

The first point to be made about the hierarchy of central values is that the patient's general and oral health are be placed ahead of every other value, so that patients' requests for interventions that violate these values may not be ethically honored. With this as the starting point, the additional fact that no intervention supportive of the patient's general and oral health may be undertaken without the patient's participation simply supports the proposal that the patient's autonomy is the next ranking value in the hierarchy. Autonomy may not be chosen ahead of the patient's general or oral health, but whenever there are alternative treatments that equally support general and oral health, respect for the patient's autonomous choice is the next ranking ethical requirement. This is also the reason why the dentist must inform the patient of all available treatments that are consistent with the patient's oral and general health, since an understanding of the whole range of one's alternatives is obviously important for autonomous choice. But the dentist does not have the obligation to inform the patient of other conceivable interventions that would compromise the patient's oral or general health because the dentist may not undertake such actions anyway. Thus autonomy again ranks below oral and general health and above the dentist's preferred patterns of practice.

For many people, it may be a close call whether esthetic values outweigh or are equal to the value of preferred patterns of practice. But it does not seem unreasonable to propose that the intrinsic value of the *patient's* judgments of oral and facial appearance, for which there is no objective standard, makes them less significant than the continued capacity of the dental professional to apply his or her expertise for the patient's benefit through preferred patterns of practice. Since these are something of objective value, they seem more important than this more subjective component of esthetic value.

But what about the dental profession's esthetic standards, which, as has been explained, have an important objective status? There will certainly be situations in which, for example, the proper shaping of a restoration will be of sufficient importance that the dentist would be required to make an exception to his or her preferred patterns of practice if these two values somehow were in conflict. It seems unlikely, however, that such a conflict would occur and thus unlikely that the profession's esthetic standards would be more important in a given case than respecting the dentist's preferred patterns of practice, unless some important component of the patient's oral health were also at stake. In that case, of course, whatever is necessary to avoid violating the patient's oral and general health is the required course of action, but this is because of the higher rank of the patient's oral and general health, not because of the esthetic values themselves.

In any case, then, where only the patient's judgments about appearance or the profession's accepted standards of form for rebuilt oral structures are at stake, rather than genuine considerations of the patient's oral or general health, these esthetic standards seem less important than the continued capacity of the dental professional to apply his or her expertise for the patient's benefit. That is, esthetic values rank below respect for the dentist's preferred patterns of practice in the hierarchy of central values for dental practice.

The last remaining question about the hierarchy of central values concerns the relative ranking of esthetic values and the value of efficiency in the use of resources. Here at the bottom end of the hierarchy it may be that the ranking of these last two values is too close to call. But the conduct of a dentist who would pay no attention to the profession's accepted standards of form, or who would not attend to a patient's valuation of a particular aspect of facial appearance solely to avoid expending the personal, financial, and other resources that would be involved, nevertheless seems inappropriate.

That is, esthetic values should be considered to take priority over a general commitment not to waste resources. The reason is that if esthetic values are indeed central values for dental practice, then employing resources to accomplish them is *not a waste*. The only way in which resources devoted to esthetic improvement of a patient could be considered a waste, and hence unjustifiable in terms of efficiency, would be if esthetic values were in fact not among the central values of dental practice.

Of course, it is quite possible to imagine a situation in which immense resources will be necessary to accomplish a patient's goals regarding facial appearance, and for the moment let us assume that accomplishing the patient's goal would not involve significant damage to the patient's healthy teeth. The question arising about such a case is whether a professional commitment to esthetic values means that the dentist is professionally required, if competent in the matter, to undertake whatever the patient asks for in this regard. Even if the dentist would be fully paid for time, effort, and materials, does the priority of *esthetic values* over *efficient use of resources* mean that the dentist is required to undertake whatever esthetic tasks the patient can imagine?

The answer to this question is *No*. But the reasoning behind this answer does not relate to the ranking of the central values of dental practice. It relates to a different aspect of the ethics of dental practice, the question of the extent to which the central values and other norms of dental practice can outweigh other moral considerations that may be relevant to a given situation. Included in this will be the question of how much sacrifice of personal effort, resources, and so on a dentist is required to commit to the well-being of his or her patients and whether the degree of sacrifice required will be less in regard to lower-ranking values in the hierarchy.

Every profession presents itself to the larger community, in its rhetoric and self-descriptions, as being a group of experts who are committed to serving the interests of their clients above all else. But this commitment cannot possibly be unlimited for a number of reasons. Thus how extensive is this commitment and, if it has limits, what are they? Moreover, if it entails some genuine sacrifice of his or her own interests on the part of the dental professional, as it almost certainly does, then what sacrifices does it require? These questions will be discussed in the next chapter. But correct answers to them do not challenge the claim being made here, that the value of efficiency in the use of resources is the sixth ranking value in the hierarchy of central values of dental practice.

The drafters of the 1990 revision of the Code of Ethics of the Canadian Dental Association incorporated these same six central values into their description of ethical dental practice and ranked them in the order in which they have been ranked here. At the conclusion of the list, however, the drafters offered two comments. First, "under certain circumstances, a lower ranked value may justifiably be chosen over the next higher. These circumstances will depend upon the clinical situation that may arise." Unfortunately, the drafters did not provide any examples of such circumstances. Second, "other external factors may be present, but will rarely be of such ethical significance as to outweigh the prioritized values, particularly the higher values." That is, the drafters did not see any other central values of dental practice that needed to be added to the list.

Anyone who is concerned about professional ethics in dental practice should carefully consider the theme of the central values of dental practice. They should examine proposed accounts of these values, like the hierarchy of central values offered here, and should ask, first, whether any important values have been omitted from the list, and second, whether the proposed ranking of values is incorrect or admits of important exceptions.

THINKING ABOUT THE CASE

Now we can apply this proposal about the hierarchy of central values of dental practice to the case presented at the beginning of the chapter.

First of all, Dr. Luban's question about Mrs. Kirchland's capacity for autonomous choice, given her anxieties about money, is an appropriate question to ask, provided Dr. Luban does not simply assume one particular answer to it. The dental professional's proper relationship to a capable person differs significantly from his or her proper relationship to a patient with diminished capacity to participate, as Chapter 7 will explain. Moreover, profound fear is able to diminish a person's capacity for autonomous choice. So Dr. Luban's question about Mrs. Kirchland's capacity is reasonable.

But Dr. Luban has known Mrs. Kirchland for many years and has not observed any other signs of diminished capacity then or now. Nor has he previously considered her continuing concerns about finances and her need, in her judgment, to be satisfied with "the cheapest and simplest," to be signs of diminished capacity. Therefore these patterns cannot be consistently viewed as marks of diminished capacity in the present situation without strong additional evidence to support such a shift in judgment. Nor, obviously, can the mere fact that a patient chooses less-than-optimal therapy or therapy different from the health professional's recommendation be taken as conclusive evidence of the patient's incapacity for autonomous choice.

In the absence of additional evidence of lack of capacity, which the case does not provide, Dr. Luban must judge Mrs. Kirchland to be as capable of autonomous choice as she has ever been.

Dr. Luban should not overlook, however, that Mrs. Kirchland is presently in "considerable pain," pain serious enough that she has asked for an emergency appointment (and done so in spite of her limited financial resources). Pain, especially severe emergent pain, is a significant inhibitor of the exercise of autonomous choice. In fact, Mrs. Kirchland is likely to be far more interested at this moment in relief of her pain than in any other benefit that Dr. Luban could offer, including the long-term treatment of this tooth.

Thus the value of the patient's life and general health and the value of the patient's oral health and the third ranking value of the patient's autonomy all require Dr. Luban to address Mrs. Kirchland's emergent pain first of all. Only when she is out of serious pain will she be able to make a thoughtful choice among the available long-term therapies.

Dr. Luban may have a strong preference that Mrs. Kirchland settle on a treatment plan during this visit rather than rescheduling an appointment for a visit that might well be only a consultation to settle that. However, even if Dr. Luban is able to provide quick relief of her pain, Mrs. Kirchland's state of mind may not be well suited to moving directly into conversation about expensive long-term treatments. Thus Dr. Luban's preferred patterns of practice will have to give way to his efforts to help Mrs. Kirchland make as autonomous a choice in this matter as she can, and that may require rescheduling an appointment on another day.

On the other hand, since Mrs. Kirchland has been squeezed into a full day of patients, Dr. Luban may prefer to reschedule her to determine the long-term treatment for this tooth. What if, in that case, she wanted to hear about the pros and cons of the different therapies and discuss it all right away? In such a scenario, it is not only Mrs. Kirchland's autonomy that is at stake, but the oral and general health and the autonomy of a number of other patients. Dr. Luban has obligations to the patients in the other operatories and those in the waiting room, not only to the patient before him in the chair. Nor is there a clear guideline for dentists to use in ranking the competing needs of different patients. The priority of general and oral health require that emergencies be addressed. However, among nonemergency patients, including Mrs. Kirchland, after pain relief has been administered, rules of thumb like "patients with appointments get priority" and "first come first served" are reasonable, but do not completely resolve the question of how the dentist should distribute his or her time and energy among them. Arguably, as long as each patient's general and oral health and autonomy are being adequately served, a dentist may distribute it as he or she chooses. But it is worth asking if this is the proper way to understand this matter.

Suppose that Dr. Luban is able to provide Mrs. Kirchland with quick relief of her pain by perhaps a pulpectomy and medication, and she is able to return later the same day during the time of a canceled appointment. Unburdened by pain, she is ready to work out a long-term treatment plan. But her financial situation has not improved (and in fact is now worse, since she owes something for the emergency appointment and pain relief). What guidance could Dr. Luban receive from the proposed hierarchy of central values for his conversation with Mrs. Kirchland?

First, Dr. Luban may not recommend or do anything that he believes would violate Mrs. Kirchland's general or oral health. (The norm of competence requires, of course, that his judgment be well informed and that he not undertake anything that is beyond his competence.) Second, the value of the patient's autonomy requires that Dr. Luban must explain to Mrs. Kirchland all of the treatments, including the option of no treatment if appropriate, that are at least minimally adequate responses to Mrs. Kirchland's needs, where adequacy is judged by the standards of dental professionals in our society generally. He must explain them in language she can understand, both treatment and likely outcome and the likelihood of the various possible outcomes and complications, accompanying pain or discomfort, and costs. All of this is well known.

But the value of the patient's autonomy, like the ideal of an interactive relationship, requires more than just informing the patient of these matters. It requires further that to the extent possible given the time and human and other resources available, Dr. Luban not only must not violate Mrs. Kirchland's autonomy but must work to *enhance* it. In the case at hand, one of the chief hindrances to maximally autonomous choosing is Mrs. Kirchland's financial situation. Is there anything that Dr. Luban can do to address this difficulty so she can choose more autonomously?

One possibility is that Dr. Luban could offer Mrs. Kirchland a payment plan to reduce the financial impact of her choice. Perhaps he could make adjustments in the cost of the more expensive options, especially for the treatment of choice. Perhaps he could make even greater sacrifices, providing treatment at cost or less than that, accepting day-care services in partial or complete payment for the needed dental care, or other options. The hierarchy of central values does not provide definitive guidance to Dr. Luban about which of these alternatives he ought to undertake, partly because the questions at issue include the question of how much sacrifice of other considerations a dentist is professionally committed to undertake for the sake of his or her patients to receive the best possible treatment. This question will be addressed in the next chapter. But in any case, simply offering her the needed information and waiting for her to consent is unlikely to be enough. The value of Mrs. Kirchland's autonomy within the hierarchy of central values most assuredly requires Dr. Luban to at least *ask* himself these questions to see what options are available to him to *enhance*, not merely refrain from violating, her capacity for autonomous choice.

Third, a patient's oral health depends significantly on correctly understanding relevant facts. Mrs. Kirchland apparently views herself as quite elderly, and her comment that the cheapest and simplest will have to do suggests that she does not recognize that, at 68, she could easily need her teeth to be functional for another 15 to 20 years. Consequently, the value of Mrs. Kirchland's oral health requires Dr. Luban to try to educate her—probably gently, but the manner depends on the particular patient, dentist, and their relationship— about these facts. In addition, he should try to do this independently of the particular treatment decision at hand. She should rethink her whole view of herself as being at the end of her life, and he should try to guide her to challenge the view that care of her teeth, and perhaps other aspects of her health, is not as important as it used to be.

Finally, to take up the hardest aspect of this case, suppose that Dr. Luban and Mrs. Kirchland have a long and careful conversation about all these matters, and suppose that at its conclusion, Mrs. Kirchland chooses a treatment that is inconsistent with Dr. Luban's philosophy of dental practice. Suppose, for example, that she chooses the extraction and partial denture rather than endodontic therapy, and suppose that Dr. Luban, in a way that the original case did not indicate, is strongly committed to preserving natural teeth. Suppose, for example, that he strongly prefers that patients who are candidates for endodontic therapy, but who do not choose it, be referred to other dentists who provide a form a treatment contrary to his philosophy of practice. Does the hierarchy of central values provide any guidance to Dr. Luban in this sort of situation?

If respect for Dr. Luban's preferred patterns of practice, including his philosophy of practice, ranks below Mrs. Kirchland's autonomy on the hierarchy of central values, as the account of central values given in this chapter proposes, this might seem to require that Dr. Luban provide a treatment that violates his philosophy of practice. But it is important to remember the setting in which Mrs. Kirchland seeks treatment for her tooth. In most urban areas of the North America most people have fairly ready access to a large number of general dentists. In such a setting, Mrs. Kirchland could easily receive treatment consistent with her own choice from a dentist who does not share the philosophy of practice now attributed to Dr. Luban. In fact, there are probably specific dentists whom Dr. Luban trusts and to whom he refers patients under just these circumstances.

In this way, because of the ready availability of dentists with different philosophies of practice, neither the value of Mrs. Kirchland's autonomy nor the value of Dr. Luban's preferred practice values would need to be compromised. But suppose other dentists were not conveniently available, or suppose the treatment at issue was an emergency treatment so that there was not time to refer the patient to a dentist with a different philosophy of practice. In such a case, the setting would not eliminate the conflict of central values, as it was seen to in the previous paragraph. What ought Dr. Luban do then?

If the account of the hierarchy of central values offered above correctly represents the content of the dental profession's norms in our society at this time, then in a situation of this last sort, Dr. Luban would be professionally required to act according to it. First, if the situation were an emergency, or other practitioners were not available, then the values of the patient's life and general health and the patient's oral health would require Dr. Luban to personally address Mrs. Kirchland's needs, rather than referring her to another dentist. Second, if several treatments were within the range of technically acceptable treatments for Mrs. Kirchland's condition, then the value of her autonomy requires that all of them be presented to her for choice. Dr. Luban may appropriately explain his reasons for strongly preferring one of these modes of treatment over the others, but if all are within the range of what is acceptable to the dental profession at large, then Dr. Luban is required to explain that fact to Mrs. Kirchland as well so she has a clear understanding of all the alternatives available to her.

Third, if, under these constrained circumstances, Mrs. Kirchland chooses a mode of therapy inconsistent with Dr. Luban's philosophy of practice, the priority of the value of her autonomy over the value of his preferred patterns of practice requires him to provide this treatment if it is within his competence. (If it were not within his competence, of course, he should not indicate that it is available in his practice in the first place, although its availability under other, nonemergency circumstances from other dentists probably should be mentioned.) Dr. Luban may not refuse to provide this treatment (because of the higher ranking values of the patient's life and general health and the patient's oral health), and he may not require Mrs. Kirchland to accept the treatment he prefers if other professionally acceptable modes of treatment are available and she chooses one of them (because the value of the patient's autonomy, it is proposed here, ranks higher than the value of the dentist's preferred patterns of practice).

In this way, the hierarchy of central values does put constraints on the choices that a dentist can professionally make, although the circumstances in which these constraints will be felt are relatively rare for most dentists in our society. Of course, this discussion has not resolved the question of what counts as convenient accessibility of another dentist with a different philosophy of practice. If, for example, this scenario were carried out in a distant rural setting where the next dentist might be very far away, Dr. Luban's professional ethical deliberations would have to include a fair resolution of this accessibility question before he could determine whether or not professional ethics require him to perform a treatment contrary to his philosophy of practice.

Finally, it is important to note that conflicts can arise *within* the scope of each of these central values. All health professionals encounter situations in which different aspects of a person's general health are in conflict, and both cannot be satisfied at the same time or to the same degree. Conflicts of this sort commonly arise for dentists regarding patients' oral health as well. A partial or complete denture may well involve some loss of comfort and function, even compared with the natural teeth that need to be extracted because they are compromised in some other way, but this loss is necessary to maintain the most important aspects of function that the natural teeth can no longer provide or could provide only at the risk of systemic infection.

Thus it should not be surprising that conflicts will arise between different elements of other values in the hierarchy. For some patients, for example, a dentist may be able to preserve their range of clinical alternatives only by pressing very hard psychologically to get them to practice appropriate oral hygiene. One aspect of their autonomy, being free of psychological pressure about hygiene, is in conflict with another aspect, the opportunity to choose to keep their natural teeth functional.

The same could be true in regard to a dentist's philosophy of dental practice. Suppose Mrs. Kirchland was not a long-time patient of Dr. Luban's, but a patient never seen before who comes to his office because of her emergency. After he has relieved her pain, Dr. Luban's philosophy of practice may direct him to offer only endodontic therapy with a post and crown, with the indication that he will refer Mrs. Kirchland to another dentist if she chooses treatment that does not preserve the natural teeth. But his philosophy of practice may also include a strong preference for educating patients to practice effective self-care and to establish a continuing relationship with one dentist over years. Suppose Mrs. Kirchland indicates very quickly, while he is still addressing her pain and explaining her situation, that she would value a stable relationship with a dentist and that she in fact trusts Dr. Luban and hopes he would accept her as his regular patient. But suppose she also resists his recommendation of endodontic therapy.

In this situation, two elements of Dr. Luban's philosophy of practice are in conflict because of the particular facts of Mrs. Kirchland's situation and the particular stance that she, in the exercise of her autonomy, is taking. Dr. Luban can act on his commitment to preserve natural teeth and refer her, hoping that she will establish a relationship with that dentist or that she might return to his practice but recognizing that he is not presently working for that aspect of his philosophy. Or he can choose to work for a continuing relationship with this patient and, in doing so, perform a treatment that he would strongly prefer not to perform. Although neither of these choices is ideal, either of them is still professionally justifiable. As long as higher ranking values of dental practice are not violated in such choices, either element of the dentist's philosophy of practice may be chosen over the other.

There is no simple algorithm that can guide judgments in such matters. What is admirable about the dental profession is that it is committed to conduct in accord with certain norms and, among them, to a certain set of central values. The account of these values offered here is certainly not the last word about them. It is hoped only that this account will stimulate careful discussion, within the dental profession and in the larger community, that will lead to an increasingly clearer understanding of these values. But even the clearest account of dentistry's central values and of the other norms of dental practice will not eliminate the need for careful reflection and conscientious judgment in the face of each unique set of facts that daily practice provides.

CHAPTER 6

Ethical Decision-Making and Conflicting Obligations

Case: How Much Sacrifice?

When Dr. Sharon Sullivan returned from lunch around 1:00, she saw a new patient in Operatory 2. "Who's in Operatory 2?" she asked her hygienist, Elizabeth Minowski. "I checked the day-list and I don't recognize her."

"That's Edith Blake. She's an emergency. She says she's been in pain for 3 or 4 days, but she obviously hasn't seen a dentist in a long time. Every quadrant has caries and perio involvement. She lives at the Transition Home, and someone there sent her over here."

"Where's the pain?" asked Dr. Sullivan.

"Upper left. I saw a large lesion in #13, but there are several teeth with inflamed gingiva as well. She was squeezed in as an emergency before Mrs. Livingston at 1:00. I just got her in the chair and took a quick look when I heard you come in. Do you want me to examine her and do a full record before you look at her?" asked the hygienist.

"No, Liz," said Dr. Sullivan. "I might as well see her myself right now, since Mrs. Livingston isn't here yet. But what do you mean, that they sent her over from the Transition Home? What's that?"

"The Salvation Army runs a home for women who are trying to get out of prostitution over on Third Street. I thought you might have heard of it. Carolyn Elward was one of the supervisors there. She was a patient of ours before Dr. Bingley retired, although I don't remember seeing her since then. I don't know if she still works there or not. Anyway Ms. Blake is a resident at the Transition Home. She says that her hall leader told her she should see a dentist when aspirin wasn't strong enough to control her pain, and someone said she should come here because she could walk over from the Home."

"Okay. When Mrs. Livingston gets here, have Jane explain to her that it might be a little wait because of a patient with an emergency problem," said Dr. Sullivan. "She's better waiting in the waiting room than in a chair because she gets so anxious once she's in an operatory." Then she went to meet Edith Blake.

"Hello, I'm Dr. Sharon Sullivan," Sharon said to Edith. "Ms. Minowski tells me that you've been having quite a bit of pain in the top left part of your mouth. Is that correct?"

"Yes, it's been hurting for 3 or 4 days, but this morning it got so bad that even aspirin wouldn't help it."

"How long is it since you've seen a dentist?" she asked, beginning her examination.

"It's a long time," said Ms. Blake. "It's since I was in high school."

"How old are you now?" asked Dr. Sullivan.

"I'm 26, so it's almost 10 years, I guess."

"Well, I'm sorry to say that your teeth have some problems."

"I'm not surprised, I guess," said Edith. "I really didn't take good care of myself for quite a long time. I was on the street, if you know what I mean, and I didn't care very much about things like that. I really didn't care very much what happened to me at all, in fact, so taking care of my teeth wasn't much of a priority."

"I understand what you're saying," answered Sharon. "Ms. Minowski mentioned that you're staying at the Transition Home now. Has that helped you get a better hold of things?"

"Oh, yes," said Edith. "I feel safe there, and I'm even beginning to think it's worth taking care of myself. The counselling and the other girls who live there, and the girls who have completed the program and come back to help us, they have helped me a lot. They really understand what it's like to be on the street, and what it does to how you think about yourself. The Little Handbook they give you says the first goal for every girl is to restore your self-esteem, and I certainly need that."

"How long have you been living there?"

"I found out about it about 3 months ago and talked to them on the telephone. But it's not easy to get off the street; you can't just walk away. It took me until 5 weeks ago to get away. That's when I went there and they accepted me in their program," said Edith.

Meanwhile Dr. Sullivan had completed her examination. Besides the deep cavity in the upper left second bicuspid, which was the likely cause of Ms. Blake's pain, there were carious lesions in half a dozen other teeth and periodontal involvement at several sites as well, plus whatever else X-rays might show. At first look, it seemed likely that all of the teeth were salvageable, but Ms. Blake clearly needed a lot of dental work. Dr. Sullivan excused herself to see if Mrs. Livingston had arrived and to ask Elizabeth Minowski to take some X-rays.

"Excuse me for asking, Sharon," said Elizabeth. "But have you talked to her about paying for this?"

"Actually, no, Liz," said Sharon. "I was so focused on getting the exam done before Mrs. Livingston got here that I haven't mentioned money."

"That's why I made a point of telling you she was from the Transition Home. I doubt she has any money to pay for a lot of dental care," said the hygienist.

"And you were trying to clue me in by mentioning the Home without actually saying she can't pay?"

"Yes."

"Well, I appreciate the effort," said Sharon. "But I didn't get the hint. Mrs. Livingston still isn't here, so I'll talk to her about it. Would you take the X-rays in any case when I'm done speaking with her so we actually know what we are talking about?"

Sharon returned to the operatory and explained to Edith what she had found in her examination. "I've asked Ms. Minowski to take some X-rays of your mouth when we are done talking here to make sure there aren't any further problems that I can't see. But even if there aren't, it would take three or four visits to deal with the cavities you have and give your teeth a proper cleaning and scaling. And then we would have to decide how much additional treatment you would need for the periodontic problems, especially if they are more serious than they appear right now."

"I don't have that kind of money," said Edith. "I told the woman who brought me in here that I didn't know if I could pay for this, but she said you wouldn't send me away in pain so I should talk it over with you. But you were so nice and talking with me that I forgot to say anything. I'm sorry."

"Well, I enjoyed talking to you, too," said Sharon, "and that's why I forgot to mention it also. But you really should get these problems attended to or you will have more bouts of pain, and maybe much worse ones that this. Do you have a job at the Home or somewhere? We could certainly arrange a long-term payment plan so you wouldn't have to pay a lot of money right away. I do that with many of my patients."

"At the Home, the work I do helps pay for my room and board. I only get $20.00 a week for spending money from that. That's what I brought to pay for this appointment; I just got paid this morning. I hope it's enough. If I do well in the program, the Home will help me find a real job after 3 months. All the girls who have left the Home have left with real jobs, and the Home helps them find an apartment and they come back for counselling and to help the girls who are still there. But I won't be able to do that for 2 more months, or maybe more."

"I don't want to take your $20.00, Edith," said Sharon. "If you can stay for a while this afternoon, I will work around the other patients in my schedule and fill the big cavity in your upper second bicuspid because that is what is probably causing your pain. I don't have to charge you for that, if you will stay here so I can fit it in between my other patients."

"That is very kind of you, Doctor. You really should take some payment for that, even if it isn't close to enough. I really appreciate it," said Edith.

"But my concern is your other teeth," said Sharon. "You will be in here again in no time if they aren't attended to, and you need to have a good cleaning done, so you can begin taking proper care of them again."

"Well, I will start brushing them, like I am supposed to. But I really couldn't pay for a lot of appointments and it isn't fair for you to have to do all that work for nothing. I think it will just have to wait until I get on my feet."

"I really don't think that would be the best thing for you," said Sharon. "Let me think about it. My next patient is here now. I will be back to work on that cavity as soon as I can. In the meantime, Ms. Minowski will be taking some X-rays."

Dr. Sullivan has a lot to think about. First, there is the financial question. One obvious possibility would be for her to accept a major financial loss and do everything Edith Blake needs in the best way possible. Or she could find a way to help her some, but not provide the best possible care, using amalgam buildups instead of crowns, for example, so it would be less of a loss for her. Or maybe she could find a way to get Edith to pay for some of it, while taking the rest as a loss. Or she could just tell Edith what she needs and leave it up to her, whether she can afford it or not.

Besides that, Sharon has seen some marks on Edith's arms that suggest she might at some time have been an IV-drug user, probably during her days on the streets. Sharon wasn't comfortable raising that question with Edith in this first visit. But it means Edith could have been in contact with the HIV virus by sharing needles with infected users, and Edith is high-risk for HIV infection in any case because of her time as a prostitute. If she is HIV-positive, that would pose additional risks for Sharon and her staff if Sharon would treat her.

All in all, Dr. Sullivan has a lot of thinking to do. What is she professionally obligated to do for Edith Blake? Are there limits to her professional obligations in a case like this? Are there things she could do that would be above and beyond the call of her professional obligations, and should she do them even though it is beyond what is required of her? And, for each of these options, why or why not?

DIFFICULT PROFESSIONAL-ETHICAL JUDGMENTS

Many professional-ethical judgments are easy and straightforward and, like most actions in other areas of our lives, they are mostly relegated to good habits rather than having to be, each time, the work of conscious deliberation and choice. Of course, thoughtful people carefully examine their professional habits from time to time, as well as their other moral habits. As Chapter 1 indicated, it is precisely reflection of this sort that legitimates the claim that actions done from habit are still rational actions, even though they are not the product of explicit deliberation in the situation. In fact, although the examples used in this book focus on cases at hand and examine the deliberations required to judge how to act in each case, it is really careful reflection on professional habits of conduct and habits of moral reflection that the book hopes to stimulate.

Nevertheless, for all the centrality of habits in our moral and professional lives, there are still three sets of circumstances that can arise in which determining what one professionally ought to do requires explicit and careful deliberation on the alternatives at hand. These three circumstances are (1) when a situation requires a professional to think about the limits of his or her professional obligations and about the extent to which he or she is committed to sacrificing other things for the sake of a patient, (2) when one's professional obligations are themselves in conflict, and (3) when a person's professional obligations conflict with his or her other commitments and obligations to other people.

None of these circumstances has been discussed very carefully in the literature of professional ethics, even though the most difficult ethical dilemmas that professionals face ordinarily involve one or more of them. Discussing them here will not yield some tidy algorithm that readers can then apply to resolve such difficult questions. But careful reflection on the general structure of ethical thinking and then on the characteristics of each of these three sets of circumstances will shed some useful light on the dentist's most difficult ethical decisions.

A MODEL OF PROFESSIONAL-ETHICAL DECISION-MAKING

The first step will be to propose a model of the steps of professional-ethical decision-making. Any model of decision-making is necessarily an oversimplification. For it separates out reflective activities that we actually perform all mixed together, and identifies as separate "steps" of the decision-making process activities that are highly interdependent in actual ethical reflection. In addition, in our ordinary ethical reflection, we do not completely finish Step Two, for example, before beginning Step Three. Instead we move back and forth between the first four steps, learning from one of them that we haven't adequately answered another, and gathering data from one of them that proves informative for another, and so on. But it is still worthwhile to carefully separate and describe the several distinct sets of activities involved in ethical decision-making. When an ethical decision is particularly complex, then having a bit of a "road map" of the steps involved can often be useful. It is also valuable to ask in general terms how professional norms relate to other moral considerations within moral decision-making.

Step One: Identifying the Alternatives

The first step consists of <u>determining what courses of action are available for choice,</u> and identifying their most important features. Sometimes this is easily done, without the need to stop and think carefully about it. At other times it can be very difficult. Special circumstances about the situation or our own habitual ways of perceiving and acting can cloud our vision of our options. Our questions for this step include, but are not limited to, the following: What courses of action are available to us? What would be their likely outcomes? To what other choices for ourselves and for others are they likely to lead? Just how likely are such outcomes and such future choices? (It is taken for granted that both clinical and nonclinical aspects of our alternatives are considered here.)

Step Two: Determining What is Professionally at Stake

Once we know our alternatives, since we are professionals, we must examine them specifically from the point of view <u>of what ought and ought not be done *professionally.*</u> The details of this process will depend on one's general conception of what it means to say a group is a profession and what it means for a person to be a professional, and it will involve identification and careful consideration of all the specific professional obligations relevant to the situation that have been accepted by the professional group and the larger community in dialogue. Each of the identified alternatives must be examined from this point of view.

The criteria to be used in this step of the process are precisely the norms of one's profession, in other words, the content associated with each of the eight categories of <u>professional obligation identified in Chapter 3.</u> Obviously, the principal purpose of this book is to help readers come to a more detailed and more sophisticated understanding of these norms for dentistry so that readers can make these judgments of what is professionally at stake more precisely and with greater confidence.

Step Three: Determining What Else is Ethically at Stake

In addition, each alternative must be examined specifically from the point of view of the broader criteria of what ethically ought and ought not be done, <u>over and above the norms of the person's professional life.</u> For one's professional obligations never constitute the entire moral content of a person's life. Moreover, the professional norms themselves depend on *certain reasons* and are accepted for professional practice *for certain reasons.* If specific professional norms conflict, if they fail to adequately determine action in the situation at hand, or if other commitments conflict with one's professional commitments, then the more fundamental moral categories need even more careful consideration because they are the key to resolving such conflicts.

The details of this process will depend on the particular approach that a person takes to ethical reflection in its "largest" or "deepest" sense. Ordinarily, at the most general level, people do their moral reflection chiefly in terms of maximizing certain values for certain persons, conforming to certain fundamental moral rules, or actualizing certain human virtues. So the details of this process will ordinarily have one or the other of these structures, or it may combine several of them together.

Step Four: Determining What Ought to be Done (Ranking the Alternatives)

The process of determining what is ethically and professionally at stake will sometimes yield, without further effort, the conclusion that one of our alternatives is ethically and professionally better than all the rest. At other times, matters will be more complex because the various values, rules, virtues, and professional norms that are involved favor different courses of action. Then one's choice of action becomes also a choice between the alternative values, rules, virtues, and professional norms,

In addition, judgments about actions can sometimes leave a person with a choice between several equally superior alternatives, and sometimes one's leading alternatives are functionally equal because of an inability or lack of time to get all the information needed to judge more carefully between them. In such cases, one may morally choose either of the equal alternatives, provided that they are all superior to every other alternative considered.

When a person can successfully rank the leading alternatives, then the best of them is the one that ought to be done, and there may be others that we judge that ought not be done, no matter what. When a person judges several alternatives to be equal or functionally equal, then the person must choose between them, for the faculty of judgment will then have done the best it could under the circumstances.

Step Five: Choosing a Course of Action

Choice is considered to be distinct from judgment in this model of ethical decision-making. For after a person has come to a judgment about what ought and ought not be done ethically and professionally, he or she may still choose to act otherwise. So actually choosing to do (or not) whatever one judges to be the morally best or most required course of action deserves to be identified as a distinct "step" of the decision-making process. Thus the term *decision* is taken to include both activities, in other words, both *judging* and *choosing*.

SACRIFICE AND THE RELATIVE PRIORITY OF PATIENTS' WELL-BEING

Most sociologists' descriptions of the institution of profession mention "commitment to service" as one of the essential features of professions. Similarly, most health professions describe themselves, in their codes of ethics and elsewhere, as giving priority to patients' interests or being in the service of the patient. To cite one example, the first Principle in the American Dental Association's *Principles of Ethics and Code of Professional Conduct* begins: "The dentist's primary professional obligation shall be service to the public."

But expressions like "service to the public" and "priority of patients' interests" admit of many different interpretations with significantly different implications for actual practice. Four different interpretations of such expressions will be examined in this section in order to provide a framework for discussing the extent of dentists' professional-ethical obligations and the amount of sacrifice of other interests that a dental professional undertakes.

First, one could understand the dentist's commitment to service to mean that dental professionals have an obligation to consider the well-being of their patients to be *among the most important* of their concerns, but without its being the case that a patient's well-being has any specific priority over any other concerns that the dentist deems important. This has to be considered a *minimalist* interpretation of this commitment because if the dentist gave the patient any less consideration than this, we could not say that the patient's well-being had any special importance in the dentist's professional life at all.

In this minimalist interpretation, it would always be a complete judgment call whether or not a patient's well-being outweighed any other interest or obligation of the dental professional. In fact, only two things would clearly violate a commitment to "the priority of the patient's well-being," interpreted in this minimalist way: first, a dentist who *failed to consider at all* the well-being of a patient when the patient's well-being happened to be at stake in some choice that the dentist was making, and second, a dentist who *knowingly* chose an action detrimental to the well-being of the patient and did so *for the sake of* some value that the dentist truly considered *not* very important. If the dentist chose something detrimental to a patient for the sake of something the dentist considered important, there would be no violation of a minimalist commitment to the patient.

Given, however, what health professionals in general and dentists in particular say about themselves as well as what the larger community routinely thinks and says about health professionals' obligations, it is clear that dentists in our society are regularly understood to be committed to the patient's well-being in such a way that it has much more priority than the minimalist interpretation provides. The same conclusion is supported by sociologists' research into the health professions. Therefore we must set aside the minimalist interpretation and consider others.

At the opposite extreme is what can be called the *maximalist* interpretation. In this interpretation, the commitment to the priority of the patient's well-being would be understood to mean that dental professionals have undertaken an obligation to place the well-being of their patients *ahead of every other consideration*, not only all their own other interests, but also all other concerns and obligations they might have regarding any other individual or group. This is an extreme view of the professional's obligation to serve others, but it deserves examination, particularly because the rhetoric of the professions so often seems to be giving the public just this message.

But the maximalist interpretation is again too extreme a view of the dentists' professional obligations to patients. Few health professionals and few members of the larger community would claim that dentists or any other health professionals are obligated to place their patients' well-being ahead of literally everything else without qualification. In fact, the reason why we have questions about the kinds of sacrifices health professionals are obligated to make for their patients is that we understand, though often not articulately, that the maximalist interpretation is inadequate because it is too extreme. That is, we have questions because we know the answer is not simply, "You are obligated to make everything, absolutely everything, subordinate to the well-being of your patients." So this interpretation must be set aside as well, and we must examine some interpretations of the priority of the patient's well-being that fall between these two extremes.

One intermediate interpretation can be called the *parity* interpretation, where the word *parity* refers to the equal importance of the patient's well-being and the dentist's well-being. In this interpretation, the dentist is professionally obligated to consider the patient's well-being to be *at least equal in importance to his or her own well-being*. Thus the dentist would be obligated to choose the patient's well-being over any aspect of his or her own well-being that the dentist judges to be of *lesser* moral significance than the aspect of the patient's well-being that is at stake under the circumstances.

But, in this interpretation, the dental professional is also permitted to choose his or her own well-being over that of the patient in any circumstance in which the aspects of well-being at stake on the two sides are of equal moral importance. The rationale for this conclusion is that if the two aspects of well-being are of equal moral significance and if the dental professional is not obligated to accord greater significance to the patient's well-being than to his or her own, then in such a case the dentist is choosing between morally equal alternatives and may therefore morally choose either one.

For example, in the parity interpretation, provided other things are equal (which would include that informed consent has been properly accounted for if the patient is competent), then a dentist could ethically recommend, between two courses of treatment that are equally effective and involve equal risks, the one that yields the greater profit for the dentist. For the dentist's financial well-being and the patient's financial well-being are of equal moral significance. By the same token, a dentist could decline to care for a patient with a serious infectious disease in order to protect himself or herself from serious infection.

The evidence that this interpretation is not a correct interpretation of dentistry's commitment to service, as it is currently understood in American society, is more subtle than the evidence against the two extreme interpretations. But the way in which most members of the larger community react to dentists who act or who are thought to act along the lines of the two examples just given is indicative, and many dentists would react similarly. Dentists who act in these ways would be widely judged to be violating their professional commitments to their patients, to the community, and to their fellow professionals. First, dentists, and health care providers generally, are widely understood to have undertaken an obligation to accept more than ordinary risk of infection, even of life-threatening infection, if the patient's well-being requires it and if sufficiently important aspects of the patient's well-being are at stake in the matter. This view of dentistry and the other health professions will be examined in greater detail in Chapter 11.

Similarly, a dentist would ordinarily be considered to be acting unprofessionally if he or she recommended one professionally acceptable treatment over another simply in order to increase earnings. The issues associated with charges, profit, dentistry as a business, and patients' access to health care resources will be examined more fully in Chapters 13 and 14. The point to be made here is that these two examples, and many others that could be cited, strongly indicate that the parity interpretation is not an adequate account of the dentist's professional commitment to give some kind of priority to the patient's well-being.

A fourth interpretation of this professional commitment is also intermediate between the two extremes, but places the degree of the dentist's obligation somewhere between the parity interpretation and the maximalist interpretation. According to this interpretation, the dentist clearly is *not* obligated to sacrifice *every* aspect of his or her own interest and other commitments for the sake of the patient. But the dentist *is* obligated to assign *greater* importance to *certain aspects* of the patient's well-being than to his or her own, and also greater importance to the patient's well-being than to *some* of the dentist's other concerns and commitments regarding other persons. This might be called, rather clumsily, the *greater-than-self-but-within-limits* interpretation.

Can this rather vague idea be made any more precise? Not in any simple way. There is no simple formula for determining how much sacrifice a dentist is professionally obligated to bear for the sake of his or her patient. But as is often the case in moral matters, the range of professionally ethical and professionally unethical actions can be narrowed by considering some examples and looking for common threads. The two examples already identified above and one more like them will be discussed here.

In the United States, patients' access to needed dental care is ordinarily dependent either on their own ability to pay or on insurance arrangements, with some patients consequently having very little access to dental care. In such a society, a dentist who did no charity care and was unwilling to offer payment plans and other flexible financial arrangements for treatment would probably be acting unprofessionally. Only very special obligations to family or the like would justify so little sacrifice for the sake of meeting patients' dental needs when there are so many patients who cannot get their dental needs met without such assistance.

On the other hand, the larger community does not presume that a dentist must make extreme financial sacrifices to fulfill this obligation. A dentist in our society is not obligated, for example, to ask his or her family to live in poverty in order to meet more patients' unmet dental needs. Of course, a dentist's or other health professional's family might choose to make additional sacrifices in order to provide more needy people with treatment. But such actions would be above and beyond the dentist's professional duty, and the health professional could not justifiably claim that such sacrifices were required by his or her professional commitments.

As a second example, dentists are surely obligated to make their services reasonably available to their regular patients for routine care, and they are obligated to respond directly to the emergency dental needs of any patient either in person or through an effective referral mechanism. But they may surely close their practice to new patients when they choose to, and they are not obligated to be available at all times for routine care, even to regular patients, nor are they obligated to make no exceptions in their schedules for personal and family reasons, nor must they simply make themselves subject to the convenience and schedules of their patients. (There might be exceptions to some of these items if the frame of reference were a geographical area with very few other dentists or if other conditions transformed adequate dental care into a scarce resource. Under such circumstances, the special ethical considerations that apply to the rationing of scarce health care resources might supersede the ordinary requirements on health professionals. But this is a topic beyond the scope of this book.)

A third set of examples concerns dentists' risk of contracting infections through contact with their patients. This topic will be examined in detail in Chapter 11. But the same general pattern will be noted here that is evident in the two previous examples. Dentists in our society surely undertake a general obligation to face greater-than-ordinary risk of infection, even fatal infection such as HIV, if their patients' oral health requires it. Hence the dentist who refused to treat an HIV-positive patient simply to avoid risk of infection would be acting unprofessionally.

But this requirement presupposes two important things. The first is that dentists conscientiously employ "universal precautions" to protect themselves (and their patients) against HIV infection. The use of these precautions is not without its costs in both dollars and effort on the part of the dentist, and costs for the patient in dollars passed on in fees and to some degree in the quality of treatment, particularly, for example, in procedures requiring exceptional dexterity. But all these costs have been accepted by the larger community as necessary to limit dentists' risk of infection. The second fact is that when dentistry is practiced with universal precautions, the chances of a dentist becoming infected from an HIV-positive patient are extremely low. They are low enough that, as will be explained in Chapter 11, the community's on-going interest in not excessively risking the lives of its health care providers is still well met, even though that risk is increased somewhat when care is provided to HIV-positive patients.

This last mentioned interest of the community in limiting the risk to its health care providers means that, if the risk of fatal infection from some disease were much higher than it is in the case of HIV when universal precautions are practiced, then the larger community would surely begin to control the degree of contact between infected patients and health care providers. For the sake of the community, and not only for their own sake, dentists' obligation to face greater-than-ordinary risk of infection is a limited obligation, just like the rest of a dentist's obligations as a professional to accept sacrifice for the sake of his or her patients' well-being.

Every health profession's norms include guidance, like that articulated in part in the previous paragraphs, regarding the relative priority of the patient's well-being in comparison with the professional's other interests and the other obligations and concerns that the professional might have outside of his or her professional life. But few professions have made any attempt to make these norms explicit. One legitimate reason for this reticence is that these norms rarely can be expressed as precise rules for conduct; they must be stated more in the form of guidelines for ethical reflection, just as they have been discussed here. But even this brief discussion makes it clear that, with regard to dentistry, the dental professional has made a commitment not to place his or her well-being simply ahead of, or even only in parity with, the patient's well-being. Instead, the dentist's obligation is to accept significant sacrifices for the sake of the patient. But at the same time, this obligation is not unlimited or unqualified either.

CONFLICTING PROFESSIONAL OBLIGATIONS

The norms of a profession that guide the resolution of difficult ethical judgments by identifying the relative priority of the patient's well-being in comparison with the well-being of the dentist and other concerns will never be inclusive enough to resolve all conflicts between obligations that arise in professional practice. One set of conflicting obligations that these norms will rarely resolve involves conflicts between different elements of the dentist's professional commitment itself. For a dentist's professional obligations, as has been explained, can be differentiated into eight distinct categories, and there is nothing to guarantee that conflicts will not arise *between* a dentist's obligations from different categories.

Suppose, for example, a pediatric patient old enough to comprehend the need for care and the value of cooperation nevertheless behaves uncooperatively in the chair, and the reactions of the patient's parents worsen rather than improve the situation. A dentist's efforts to establish a relationship with the patient and with the patient's parents that is as close to the ideal interactive model as possible may be in sharp conflict with the dentist's efforts simply to practice within the norm of competence. Or a dentist's efforts to maintain appropriate relationships with other dentists, with the dentist's own staff, or with other health professionals, as will be discussed in Chapter 10, can conflict with the dentist's efforts to maintain an interactive relationship with a patient or even to maintain the proper priority of the patient's oral health in the face of other pressing considerations, and so on.

Similarly, there is no guarantee that there will not be conflicts between obligations within the same category. One category, the category of the central values of dental practice, includes a hierarchical ranking of the six central values, at least as it has been proposed here. So conflicts between different values in the hierarchy would frequently be resolved simply by reference to the hierarchy, as examples in the previous chapter were used to demonstrate. But even then there can be conflicts between different aspects of the same value in the hierarchy. Moreover, internal conflicts between different elements of the other seven categories of professional norms have no clear hierarchy to assist in their solution.

One way to read the case in Chapter 4, "The Dreaded Root Canal," for example, is as a conflict between two different elements of the patient's autonomy within the hierarchy of central values. For autonomy is actually a very complex feature of human experience, as the discussion in Chapter 7 will make clearer, and it is not uncommon for its elements to come into conflict such that not all can be maximized together. Dr. Clarke's choice in that case could easily be interpreted as a choice between respecting Mr. Vianni's consistent valuing (of the highest degree of dental health over the years), which is one aspect of Mr. Vianni's autonomy, and respecting Mr. Vianni's likely choice (not to have endodontic therapy), which is another aspect of his autonomy. Sometimes a profession's norms will provide guidance in such cases, for example, by providing an error-control rule that tells the professional to err, if erring is a serious risk, on the side of (something). But often conflicts that are internal to a category of professional norms, or even to a single norm like the central value of autonomy, will not be resolved by other norms of the profession. What is the thoughtful ethical thinker to do in such cases?

When there are conflicts between the elements of a set of norms that the norms in the set do not themselves provide a method for resolving, then one must ask a different kind of question about the norms of the professional group, a question about *why* the community has this profession and *why* it has accepted these particular norms to govern its practice in the first place. Every profession and every norm of every profession exist for certain *reasons*. That is, there are benefits to be gained and harms to be avoided that are the *reasons* why the profession and its particular norms for practice at any given time are maintained by those who are members of the profession itself, by those who interact with the profession as its clients (e.g., dentistry's patients), and by the whole larger community in its support of the profession and its norms by various means. It is these *reasons*, these benefits to be gained and harms to be avoided, to which the professional must turn to make an appropriate ethical judgment when faced with an internal conflict between elements of the profession's own accepted norms.

Thus in the example of the disruptive pediatric patient, the dentist will have to consider such factors as the possible harm to the patient and its likelihood because of the dentist's inability to practice with ideal attention to the procedure; the possible harm to the patient and its likelihood if the diagnostic and treatment interventions that the patient needs are not performed at this time or by this dentist; the relative value and likelihood of actually educating the patient to a different pattern of behavior and the impact of such education, or lack of it, on the patient's future health care; the relative value and likelihood of involving the parents in a more effective role regarding their child's dental care; and the impact of efforts to achieve these ends on the dentist's ability to serve other patients presently awaiting treatment, scheduled later in the day, and so on.

Although preventing certain serious harm to the patient in the chair may always take precedence over other considerations, yet as soon as the possible harm is not certain or not so serious, many conflicting ethical considerations will need to be considered. And when the profession's accepted norms do not provide clear guidance among conflicting considerations, the dentist must return to the most fundamental values and principles behind his or her commitment to becoming a dentist and to the values and principles behind the society's establishing this profession in the first place.

CONFLICTS BETWEEN PROFESSIONAL AND OTHER OBLIGATIONS

Some people live psychologically sound and happy lives focusing almost exclusively on the values and norms of a single role and set of relationships. But for most people, a broader range of values and norms of conduct is esteemed because participation in a broader range of communities and relationships, and therefore in a broader range of roles, is needed for happiness and psychological health. Thus most people make a commitment to another person as husband or wife. Most establish lasting relations of friendship with other adults. Most make the commitment of parenthood to children and accept the obligations of adult children to their parents, as well as commitments to other family members, and so on. All of these relationships and numerous other roles, with their values and norms, are part of the ordinary lives of most dentists.

Every dentist, and every professional in any field, has experienced conflict between his or her professional obligations and other obligations based on other commitments that he or she has made. One category of the accepted norms that the dental profession attempts to articulate is the relative priority that the well-being of a dentist's patient is supposed to take in comparison with other ethical considerations and commitments. But like the other categories of professional norms, this category cannot answer every question that might be asked of it. It cannot resolve every kind of conflict between professional and other obligations that can arise. In some cases, the norms that it contains, namely, the principle of *greater-than-self-but-within-limits* proposed above, provide not so much answers as useful questions for the thoughtful dentist to pose in trying to determine what he or she ought to do. As in the case of *internal* conflict between the elements of one's professional norms, so when professional obligations conflict with *other* obligations, one must look to the *reasons* behind the two sets of obligations, to the benefits they support and the harms they try to avoid, and to the most fundamental values, principles, and ideals that have motivated the larger community to establish this profession with these norms and that have motivated the individual to make his or her professional commitments to these norms in the first place.

Suppose an elderly patient of long standing calls around lunchtime on Friday afternoon to say that he is still feeling some tenderness in the quadrant where a large, old amalgam restoration that had fractured had been replaced 2 days earlier. He is not really in pain, he says; it's just tender and uncomfortable. But the dentist knows the patient and recognizes that he is very anxious that something has gone amiss with the treatment. Under ordinary circumstances, the dentist would invite the patient to drop in later that afternoon to have the area looked at. But that afternoon is the occasion of a prize music recital in which the dentist's 13-year-old daughter will perform. The dentist knows that his presence at his daughter's recital not only will be pleasing to him but is also an important moment in their relationship. Unfortunately, it is Friday afternoon, and seeing this worried patient on Saturday rather than putting him off till Monday would conflict with another commitment.

The accepted norms of a profession cannot provide clear answers to every such question. But that does not mean that they provide no guidance at all. At the very minimum, as was already mentioned, they identify important questions about the values, principles, and ideals at stake, and about their relative priority in more clear cut cases, to assist the thoughtful decision-maker in ethical deliberation.

CONSCIENTIOUS DISOBEDIENCE OF PROFESSIONAL OBLIGATIONS

The fact that professional obligations can conflict with obligations based on other commitments raises an important question whose answer must be stated clearly. For the rhetoric of the professions could easily be read to imply that when such conflicts arise, if responding to some other commitment would involve a clear violation of one's professional obligations, then one's professional obligations must always "win." In other words, it might seem that the only time that a member of a profession may morally favor obligations arising from other sources is if there is no clear violation of professional obligations.

But this claim is surely false. Situations will sometimes arise in the life of almost every professional in which the professional is certain, after careful deliberation, that acting according to some other moral commitment would involve violating a professional obligation, but that the *other* obligation is the weightier under the circumstances. In such a situation, something very important will be lost either way, but life is sometimes like that. If the other obligation is, on conscientious reflection, the weightier, then the moral action is the one that favors it rather than the professional obligation that conflicts with it.

What this fact about professional obligations reminds us of is that professional obligations are "made" obligations, made first in their being accepted through the ongoing dialogue of the expert group and the larger community that creates and defines the profession and its norms in the first place, and made significant in the life of each dentist by his or her commitment to abide by them. "Made" obligations are made, as has been said, for *reasons*. These reasons—which can be summarized in terms of the benefits to be secured and the harms to be avoided by establishing this particular profession with these particular norms of practice—are more important than the norms of the profession, and are the bases of those norms' importance. If a profession's accepted norms somehow came into conflict with these reasons, then obviously the norms would have to be set aside in that situation and would have to be changed if the situation were common. But another possibility occurs more often. It is the situation in which one's professional obligations are in conflict with *other* benefits and with the avoidance of *other* harms. In such a situation, morality requires the decision-maker to ask whether the other reasons, the other benefits and harms, the other principles and ideals at stake in the situation are weightier than the reasons behind the profession's norms. If they are, then the profession's requirements must take second place and the dentist must *conscientiously disobey* what is professionally required.

On the one hand, it may seem a very strange thing to say in a book on professional ethics in dental practice that sometimes one must conscientiously disobey one's professional obligations. Certainly such situations should not come up very often. Ordinarily, if a person found situations requiring conscientious disobedience to arise regularly, it would be time to ask whether he or she were in the right profession. But on the other hand, it should not be news that after careful and conscientious reflection, a person ought to do what he or she sincerely judges to be ethically required in the situation, even if this means violating professional obligations. Saying this does not demean and should not undermine professional commitment. Instead it affirms an essential element of professional obligations—that they are "made" obligations—and reminds us of what being responsible for acting ethically means, at the deepest level, in the first place.

HABITS, MORAL REASONING, AND CONSCIENCE

The point was made in Chapter 1 that the vast majority of our actions as human beings are the product not of careful, self-conscious deliberation, but of habits. These habits include not just habits of acting in certain ways, but also habitual ways of perceiving, of thinking about and conceptualizing what we perceive, of evaluating what we think about, and of ranking or prioritizing what we evaluate. Without habits of these sorts we would be functionally paralyzed because the task of deliberating about every one of the millions of alternative actions that we encounter each day could not possibly be completed. Being able to act from habit is so much a part of normal human functioning that persons who are unable, for some psychological reason, to trust their actions to habits and who therefore try to deliberate carefully about every set of alternatives they face are considered to suffer from a profound deficit, indeed from a form of psychological or mental illness.

But many of our habits, and especially the habits that affect our moral and professional lives, are not static. As a person grows more mature and incorporates more and more experience into his or her habitual patterns of perceiving and conceptualizing, the person grows capable of an increasingly sophisticated grasp of his or her circumstances. Consider the difference between a novice dentist who must attend very carefully and self-consciously to every step of the process of placing a restoration, and a more experienced dentist who can place the same restoration with very little conscious attention to the steps attended to by the novice. The attention of the more experienced dentist is thereby freed up to take note of more subtle and less obvious elements about the case, which the novice would likely miss because the novice has no attention left for them. A still more experienced practitioner, the true expert, will take in even these more subtle, less obvious factors without self-consciously noticing it, and will therefore have his or her conscious attention available to watch for truly unique and unusual circumstances about the case.

In a similar way in the professional-ethical realm, a dental student who wishes to practice ethically may have to focus his or her self-conscious attention on the essential elements of informed consent, for example, to be sure that this rock-bottom ethical criterion of relationships with capable adults is not violated. As a consequence, the student may not be able to notice the subtle variations in patients' ability to participate in treatment decisions that a more experienced dentist will observe, in part because the essential elements of informed consent can be attended to by this more ethically experienced practitioner without self-conscious attention. The most experienced dentist, the dentist who is "expert" in professional-ethical conduct, will take account of even very subtle variations in patients' ability to participate without having to focus on them and will have self-conscious attention available to notice the truly unique and unusual aspects of a particular patient-practitioner relationship.

What is it that enables the more experienced person to do, without self-conscious attention, things that the less experienced person must explicitly attend to? It is habituation, the formation through repeated experience, of habits of perceiving, thinking, and valuing. As the "lower level" (because they must be learned first) skills become part of a person's habitual repertoire, the person has awareness and energy released for "higher level" (because they come later and because they depend on a finer and finer reading of the data of the situation) matters.

It is not chiefly the fact that a person gets in the habit of acting in a certain way, the right way, that prompts us to say that such a person has good moral habits and is, to use the old-fashioned term, virtuous. Rather it is because a person can judge correctly how to act without apparent reflection, namely, on the basis of solidly habituated patterns of perceiving, conceptualizing, valuing, prioritizing, and acting, all of which make the person sensitive to and effective at employing more and more subtle data about the situations of his or her life. The virtuous person, the moral "expert," is imitable not so much because he or she habitually does the right thing—as if the rest of us could be assured of doing the right thing simply by doing whatever he or she does—but by reason of the virtuous person's ability to see, process, and act on morally significant features of life's situations that the rest of us do not see as well, do not know how to process as well, or do not know how to act on. It is his or her "expert" perceiving, conceptualizing, valuing, and prioritizing, and not so much his or her actions, that we can learn from the most.

Consequently, becoming professionally-ethically "expert" is a matter of developing more and more subtle *habits*, habits of perceiving, conceptualizing, valuing, and prioritizing about what is morally and professionally significant in one's life. A book like this can assist this process, not by creating habits in its readers of course, but by pointing to features of dental practice that the professionally-ethically "expert" dentist would perceive, by proposing sets of concepts to assist in their conceptualization, by noting key values and proposing ways of prioritizing them, and above all by providing thoughtful decision makers with sets of questions to ask as they go about their deliberations. By gathering together in one place discussions of many different elements of professional-ethical decision-making, this book tries to provide the reader with a streamlined set of themes to transform into questions that the reader then can use in moral and professional deliberation. In that respect, every claim about dental professional ethics that the authors make in this book is best viewed, as a famous law professor once put it, as "a question in the form of an answer."

The reader must form his or her own habitual patterns. But by drawing together in one place the fruits of many thoughtful, and even virtuous, dentists' reflections on professional-ethical conduct in dentistry, a book like this can facilitate the process.

Because moral decision-making is so complex, it is probably impossible in any short description of a case to mention all of the data that a virtuous dentist would take into account in coming to a professional-ethical decision about it. Thus the cases in this book are oversimplifications in a way not yet mentioned; namely, they are invariably too short. An ethical dentist who faced one of these cases would look for, either self-consciously or by habituated skills of perception, many additional items of data in the case before finally judging how he or she ought to act in regard to it. These might include additional clinical facts; they would certainly include many additional facts about the patient, for example, his or her values and goals, ability to participate, and many other matters. This is also the reason why, when we comment at the end of each chapter on that chapter's case, our reflections do not ordinarily include the claim that some particular course of action is what the dentist in the case ought to do. For ordinarily a final judgment about that would require data that the case as given, even when it is quite lengthy, does not provide.

In daily life, the complexity of professional-ethical decision-making, and moral decision-making generally, should not leave finite human decision-makers in despair. It should motivate them, rather, to keep working to develop their habitual capacities for perceiving, conceptualizing, valuing, and prioritizing more and more subtly in moral and professional-ethical matters. It is just such habits, such moral "expertise," such virtues that enable humans to meet the complexity of their moral and professional lives successfully.

THINKING ABOUT THE CASE

Moral decision-makers rarely follow the steps of the model proposed earlier in this chapter in the order presented. Instead, as was noted above, they move back and forth between the steps, finding in reflections on Step Three something crucial for completing Step Two, and so on. But in this commentary on this chapter's case, "How Much Sacrifice?," the steps of the model will be followed in order.

It turns out, however, that Dr. Sullivan actually has two very different sets of facts to deal with, and therefore two very different decisions to make. One of these concerns the fact that Edith Blake is at high risk for being HIV-positive, and Dr. Sullivan must determine if that fact should affect her decisions about Ms. Blake. Two points about this have already been made, though very briefly. The first is that dentists and other health professionals undertake to accept a greater-than-ordinary risk of infection, even fatal infection, when they become health professionals. The second is that the risk of HIV infection when universal precautions are being followed is low enough that it is within the range of risk that, from the point of view of the larger community, health professionals are obligated to accept. Each of these points, as well as many other important matters about HIV infection, deserve much more examination than this short commentary can provide, and they will be taken up in detail in Chapters 11 and 12. So this commentary will focus on the other decision that Dr. Sullivan has to make, namely, how to deal with Edith Blake's financial situation, given her need for extensive dental care.

Step One: Identifying the Alternatives

Theoretically, Dr. Sullivan could have just told Ms. Blake what she needs and left it up to her, whether she could afford it or not, including the restorative work on the upper left second bicuspid. In that case, perhaps Dr. Sullivan would simply have provided Ms. Blake with pain medication and referred her to someplace where she could get the emergency restoration on the upper left second bicuspid for free, or where her $20.00 would cover it, if there is such a place in town. But Dr. Sullivan has already foreclosed that option by telling Ms. Blake she will do the restoration and refusing her $20.00. So that possibility is gone.

But Dr. Sullivan still has quite a few options. She could simply accept a major financial loss and do everything Edith Blake needs in the best way possible. She could try to meet all of Ms. Blake's dental needs, but provide only the minimum acceptable level of treatment for each problem. As mentioned above, this might mean amalgam buildups instead of crowns, for example, and other minimum treatments for the other problems. In that way, Ms. Blake's needs would be met, but the work would involve less financial loss for Dr. Sullivan. Or Dr. Sullivan might only provide the emergency treatment that Ms. Blake needs today at a loss, namely, the restoration on the upper left second bicuspid, and then wait on additional treatment until Ms. Blake can pay for it, either as it is provided, or by some sort of payment plan. Or Dr. Sullivan might provide the emergency treatment and then wait until Ms. Blake can pay a certain part of the cost of remaining treatment, with Dr. Sullivan taking the rest as a loss. There are probably other alternatives, but these seem the most important ones.

Step Two: Determining What Is Professionally at Stake

Dr. Sullivan is certainly professionally required to address Ms. Blake's emergency condition, even at some sacrifice to herself. Because she has (1) responded with diagnostic procedures and X-rays that the patient has accepted, (2) proposed and the patient has accepted restorative treatment on the upper left second bicuspid, and (3) proposed not charging her usual fee for either of these, Dr. Sullivan is obviously both professionally and morally obligated to do what she has said. But since Ms. Blake has again offered her $20.00 in at least partial payment for the treatment, Dr. Sullivan could change her mind about taking it without fault, at least from the point of view of the commitments the two parties have made to each other. But these are not the issues that Dr. Sullivan most needs to address. The more important question is how she should deal with Ms. Blake's need for additional care when she has so little money to pay for it.

Since Dr. Sullivan already offers payment plans to her patients to help them get the dental care they need, we can assume that she believes that she has an obligation to assist patients in obtaining dental care. As was mentioned, this seems an unavoidable obligation of dentists who practice in a society that does not provide its citizens with secure universal access to needed dental treatment. But this obligation also has limits, as was noted. Thus the fact that Dr. Sullivan acknowledges this obligation and has responded by providing needy patients with payment plans does not tell us whether she is obligated to make additional and perhaps greater sacrifices for Ms. Blake. Some principle of consistency might suggest that Dr. Sullivan should at least provide a payment plan to Ms. Blake, and, in fact, Dr. Sullivan has already offered that. But even that might be above and beyond the call of professional duty if she is already carrying a lot of patients' unpaid accounts and accepting considerable financial loss as a result.

Our society's understanding of the extent of dentists' obligation to accept financial sacrifices to secure dental treatment for patients unable to obtain it in other ways is far from clear. Most assuredly, dentists are not obligated to risk the solvency of their practices (provided they are otherwise well managed). They surely would be acting wrongly if their efforts to provide care to the needy deprived their other patients of record of needed care, at least if those other patients had no convenient alternative for treatment (and maybe even if they did, since there are important values in an established dentist-patient relationship that the dentist is obligated to consider). Dentists are also not required to deprive themselves and their families of a decent standard of living. Our society's standards in this regard are hardly precise, but it certainly seems acceptable to the larger community at the present time that dentists have secure standards of living in the middle-to-upper middle class, so a dentist would not seem professionally obligated to sacrifice so much that this level of earning was placed at serious risk. Since dentists must also provide for their own savings for retirement in our system, they may also legitimately reserve some portion of their earnings for this purpose.

Nevertheless, in a society like ours, a dentist is still professionally obligated to make some sacrifices for patients who need care that they cannot pay for. Most dentists acknowledge this obligation and provide some degree of charity care, either free care or care provided at a loss, to needy patients. Of course most dentists provide some measure of charity care after the fact in the form of treatments that are not paid for, but this is certainly better viewed as a business loss than as the fulfillment of the dentist's professional obligation to assist needy patients with access to care. But awareness of all these facts about her professional obligations still does not automatically resolve Dr. Sullivan's ethical question about how to deal with Edith Blake's need for additional treatment.

One line of thought for Dr. Sullivan to pursue is the idea that Ms. Blake is not her only patient in need of charity care, and Ms. Blake's needs are considerably more extensive than most patients of this sort in her practice. Would she be fulfilling her professional obligation better if she declined to provide extensive treatment for Edith Blake in order to provide a greater quantity of less expensive charity care for a larger number of other patients? Or is there something professionally inappropriate about counting people and dollars in this way?

Suppose Dr. Sullivan were to follow out this line of thought, considering her charity care in terms of trade-offs among her charity patients. Since there is a limited amount of financial leeway in her practice, such trade-offs are actually very likely, if not inevitable. One reasonable approach would be for her to figure out a set amount of charity care that she would be able to provide per year or, more effectively, per quarter. In a well-managed practice, she would already have calculated her regular costs and what she needs to save to replace and improve equipment, for example. She would also have to determine what would be a just payment to herself for her services, which might also require some thinking about, and perhaps some consulting with, her family and other dependents. What is left after these matters are covered is profit, and one appropriate use of profit, it would seem, is for the fulfillment of a dentist's obligation to provide charity care. On the basis of such thinking, Dr. Sullivan could set the upper limit of the amount of charity care that she would be able to provide each quarter.

One benefit of planning for charity care in this way is that when a patient needs charity care, Dr. Sullivan would be able to quickly determine if the needed care was within the range of the sacrifices that she professionally owed her patients, or if doing the case for delayed payment or partial payment or no payment would be taking her beyond that amount. In addition, if she were over that amount for a given quarter, she could honestly say to a patient that she couldn't afford to help just now. She could be more forthright about it and more confident that what she said to patients about it had been carefully thought out. She might also be able to tell them that they could return in the next quarter, at least for treatment that could wait, since if she didn't borrow too much from future quarters, there would always be something there that a patient could come back for.

Of course, Dr. Sullivan would not have time to work all of this out as she raced back and forth between operatories, trying to finish Edith Blake's restoration while taking care of Mrs. Livingston and the other patients scheduled that afternoon. But these are the sorts of professional-ethical considerations that would be part of her thinking about the financial question when she had time to think it all out clearly.

There are, of course, may other aspects of Dr. Sullivan's obligations as a dental professional that might have bearing on this case. But only one other set of questions seems especially pressing: how Dr. Sullivan should act in order to respect and enhance Edith Blake's autonomy and bring their relationship as close the ideal of an interactive relationship as possible.

The conversations between Dr. Sullivan and Ms. Blake have been open and straightforward. There is no reason to think that Ms. Blake is not participating as fully as she can in the treatment decisions that are being made. But she is a person who has, only very recently, spent a long time thinking of her life as something out of her control and not worth controlling. Therefore Dr. Sullivan ought to pay special attention to the other aspects of their relationship, besides the decisions specifically focused on treatment, to see if she is helping or hindering Ms. Blake's now-growing sense of positively controlling her own life.

One important candidate concerns the decisions yet to be made about finances. Ms. Blake has already expressed fairly strong convictions about not wanting to take unfair advantage of Dr. Sullivan's generosity. It might not be very respectful of Ms. Blake's efforts to choose her own path now if Dr. Sullivan unilaterally determined how the financial arrangements should be handled. In this instance, because the case has certain distinctive characteristics, the dentist probably has a professional obligation to involve the patient not only in choosing whether or not to accept a particular payment plan that the dentist offers, but in the thought processes necessary to devise it. For by doing this, Dr. Sullivan will do the most to support and enhance her patient's autonomy and the possibility of them working together as interactively as possible, even on narrow treatment issues.

On the other hand, the reader may doubt that this last concern is properly part of the dentist's professional obligations in the situation. This will depend on how strongly one believes that the several areas of decision-making that go on between dentist and patient can be separated, and on how broadly one understands the reach of the dental professional's obligation to enhance autonomy and to work for the ideal of an interactive relationship. The authors submit that it is very difficult to separate the various kinds of decisions that dentist and patient must make together and that, under the special circumstances of such a case as this, the dentist's professional obligations do reach to such matters.

Step Three: Determining What Else Is Ethically at Stake

Even if the considerations discussed in the last two paragraphs are not properly part of the dentist's obligations as a professional, the values and moral principles at stake in them are still of unquestionable moral importance. For respecting and enhancing people's autonomy is an important standard of moral conduct in almost every modern culture and almost every theoretical description of morality. Perhaps even more important is a person's ability to see himself or herself as valuable and worth taking care of, which is a necessary condition of most other relationships and other achievements that make life worthwhile. Consequently, Dr. Sullivan cannot be satisfied that she has attended to everything that is morally significant in this case until she has asked herself how to best support Ms. Blake's autonomy and sense of self-worth whether doing so is, at least to some extent, part of her professional obligations in the case or not.

There are also other, broader moral principles, besides those deriving narrowly from her professional commitments, about whether Dr. Sullivan is obligated to make sacrifices for Ms. Blake, as a fellow citizen and fellow human being, when she is in significant need. These principles concern the justness of a society's systems for distributing its resources, especially in response to people's basic needs, and the extent to which Dr. Sullivan's (and her family's) resources are more than, less than, or equal to her (and their) fair share within those systems. It is possible that Dr. Sullivan gives far more than she is professionally obligated to in charity care, and yet falls short of what she ought to be doing for the needy of our world because good fortune, the gifts of parents or an inheritance, or even good investments or hard work have given her so much.

These are examples of the kinds of additional, and in truth more fundamental, ethical concerns that have bearing on a case of this sort. There could well be others, but these two are the most obvious. It is also important to emphasize here the point made earlier that sometimes the additional, not specifically professional, moral concerns will outweigh even clear cut professional requirements with which they conflict. In such cases, morality requires the dentist to act on the most significant of his or her obligations, even if this involves conscientiously disobeying professional norms. But the additional concerns in the case at hand do not seem to be in direct conflict with what Dr. Sullivan is professionally required to do. They either reinforce her professional obligations in the case, or they require her to go beyond what she is professionally required to do.

Step Four: Determining What Ought To Be Done

Even with this much detail about the case and about the professional and additional moral considerations that Dr. Sullivan ought to consider, we are not in a position to say without qualification that she ought to resolve the financial issue about Ms. Blake's future treatment in such-and-such a way. It has still not been specified how much charity care she already provides or the extent of her own and her family's financial resources. Nor is there any convenient way to provide this information here without writing a novel, or at least a sizable short story.

But the authors can say this much for sure. Both Dr. Sullivan's professional commitment to respect and enhance autonomy and to work for as interactive a relationship as possible and her obligations to Edith Blake as a fellow human being who is trying to find her way back to a life of self-respect and self-determination require Dr. Sullivan to find a way to work with Ms. Blake so that Ms. Blake can obtain the treatment she needs if she is willing to do that. Unless doing so would somehow be an extreme hardship for Dr. Sullivan or require her to break very important commitments or violate very important relationships of other sorts, we do not believe she may merely say to Edith Blake (in effect): "Here is what you need, and I will provide it if you can pay for it, period." Moreover, if working out a way with Ms. Blake for her to receive the needed treatment would involve such extreme "costs" for Dr. Sullivan, then we believe Dr. Sullivan is obligated—again by the importance of Ms. Blake's now growing potential for self-respect and self-determination and for related professional reasons as well—to explain enough of the relevant circumstances to Ms. Blake that she will understand that Dr. Sullivan is not rejecting *her*, even if Dr. Sullivan cannot offer her all the help that she needs.

Suppose, finally, that Dr. Sullivan and Ms. Blake have a careful conversation about a long-term care plan for her, including various possible financial arrangements. Let us say that Dr. Sullivan is not able to offer all the treatment that Ms. Blake needs at no cost, but offers it at a reduced rate, with a payment plan as a possibility or even the possibility of Ms. Blake paying for the treatment in work, either directly for Dr. Sullivan or for some charitable organization. But suppose Ms. Blake views this offer as too generous to be acceptable. Suppose she sees, in her growing sense of her own worth and ability to choose her own way, a need to refuse such generosity in order to take care of her needs by her own efforts, without special assistance. Suppose she thanks Dr. Sullivan sincerely and promises to come back once she has a real job, even though she knows that her teeth may be considerably the worse for it, because she is strong enough in her sense of caring for herself to see her self-determination as a priority at this point. How should Dr. Sullivan respond to this refusal?

This question obviously takes the case to a new point, with different alternatives and many additional facts in place. But it is worth posing because, first of all, it challenges the reader to ask whether the action we have attributed to Dr. Sullivan would now have to be thought of as a failure because the patient is choosing to delay needed treatment. Or should this offer and response be thought of as indicating two important truths about the dental profession that have already been stressed several other times in this chapter. First, the values that dentistry is committed to bringing about for its patients are clearly not the only values in human life, so sometimes they will be outweighed by other concerns. Second, dentistry exists for the sake of these values, not these values for the sake of dentistry. Or more broadly, the dental profession and the practice of dentistry exist for the sake of enhancing people's well-being, not the people or their well-being for the sake of the profession or its norms. It is important to stop and recall, from time to time, that this profession and its practice, honorable and worthy though it truly is, is only a part of a larger and considerably more important whole, as humans work individually and together, to live their lives the best they can.

Step Five: Choosing a Course of Action

Moral reflection concludes in a judgment about what ought to be done or not done. But after a person has come to such a judgment, there is always one more step before any course of action is carried out, and that step is *choosing*. Other persons can contribute to someone's moral reflection, by invitation or unbidden, directly or indirectly, in many ways. Other persons can also form judgments of the action that the person eventually chooses. But no one can choose for another. Dr. Sullivan is a fictional person, but if she were a real person, there is no one who could choose her actions but Dr. Sullivan herself.

Moreover, judgments about what ought to be done, even very carefully deliberated judgments, do not automatically determine choices. It is always possible for a person to choose a course of action different from what the person judged he or she ought to do. It is also possible for a person to choose a course of action when his or her judgment about what ought to be done is not fully formed, or when the best judgment that he or she can form is that two (or more) alternatives are superior to all others, but are themselves of equal moral significance. If Dr. Sullivan were a real person, the authors would hope, as they would about anyone they cared about, that she would choose the course of action she judged morally superior to the other possibilities.

But she could do otherwise.

Finally, if Dr. Sullivan were a real person, it would be important for her to recall often that when a human being chooses a course of action, choosing is not simply over and done with once the action has been carried out. Every act of choosing has an impact on the chooser, making it easier and more likely that he or she will perceive the situation the same way the next time, will conceive alternatives in the same way the next time, will value in the same way the next time, and will prioritize and act in the same way the next time. Choosing, in other words, habituates. Each choice sticks with us, predisposing us slightly each time to perceive, conceive, value, prioritize, and act similarly the next time. This is something to take account of as one chooses, and to keep track of as patterns of predisposition, and eventually habits, are built up over time.

CONCLUSION OF PART ONE

These first six chapters have offered a general framework for discussing professional ethics and have filled it out in a variety of ways with proposals about how dentistry and a dentist's professional obligations ought to be understood. With this material as background, Part Two will address a number of narrower, more focused sets of ethical issues in dental practice. The reader will quickly note that the resources of Part One cannot be used in the later chapters as a kind of formula to calculate the correct moral answer to each new issue under discussion. Once again, the task will rather be to draw lessons from what is fairly clear and widely agreed on within the dental community and the community at large, and then try to work from that to shed light on situations that are less clear. The business of moral reflection, as has often been said in this chapter, is not a matter of applying a formula to a set of facts. It is not a matter of looking up the answers in the back of the book. It depends far more on growing habitually sensitive to the right things and learning to routinely ask the right questions. As Part One has been, then, Part Two will also be, for the most part, a set of "questions in the form of answers."

ETHICAL ISSUES I
PRACTICE

CHAPTER 7

Patients With Compromised Capacity

Case: Mrs. Morris's Wonderful Teeth

Dr. John Benedict has agreed to provide dental services to the residents of Riverside Retirement Center and Nursing Home who do not have their own dentist. Prior to this, Riverside did not have a regular arrangement with a dentist, but changes in state law now require that every nursing home patient must be examined by a dentist at least once a year. One of his first patients in his new capacity is Martha Morris, a 78-year-old widow who has resided at Riverside for 8 years. She was previously a long-time patient of Dr. W. C. Elbinger, a dentist in the area who died 5 years ago at the age of 76. Mrs. Morris has not had a dental examination since Dr. Elbinger's death.

Mrs. Morris's 48-year-old son, who visits her regularly at Riverside, brings her to Dr. Benedict's office. He recalls enough about the previous dentist to say that Mrs. Morris liked the man and his work very much and that she took great pride in the fact that she still had all her natural teeth. The son remembers that Mrs. Morris had received periodontic scaling on several occasions since coming to Riverside because he remembers that, at least twice, she needed a repeat visit for Dr. Elbinger or his staff to complete the treatment. But since she did not mention going to a dentist after Dr. Elbinger died, and the nursing home people didn't mention it either, the son never thought about it. In addition, over the last 4 1/2 years, Mrs. Morris has suffered increasing memory loss and other mental deficits, probably as a consequence of a continuing series of TIAs (transient ischemic attacks) during that period.

When questioned by Dr. Benedict, Mrs. Morris recognizes that she is in a dentist's office and that Dr. Benedict is not her previous dentist. But she cannot remember Dr. Benedict's name, and she asks him what it is every few minutes. Her reports about her last trip to the dentist vary with each telling, both as to how long ago it was and on many other details. But her great satisfaction in having avoided every sort of prosthesis is repeatedly mentioned, with the work of her previous dentist and her own life-long efforts at oral hygiene receiving the credit.

Unfortunately, it is clear that Mrs. Morris has not practiced good oral hygiene for quite a while, perhaps since her level of mental functioning began to wane 4 1/2 years ago. Many nursing homes that are otherwise quite well run fail to adequately emphasize daily oral hygiene in the care of their patients. To judge from Mrs. Morris's oral condition, Riverside seems to be one of these, and Dr. Benedict makes a mental note to press this matter forcefully with Riverside's medical director at their next meeting.

But that will not help Mrs. Morris's current condition. There is such advanced periodontal involvement of both upper and lower posterior teeth, bilaterally, that Dr. Benedict sees no alternative to maxillary and mandibular partial dentures for Mrs. Morris. Even major periodontal treatment, including surgery and bone grafting, will not save the teeth, which are quite mobile in their sockets. It is a wonder that Mrs. Morris is not experiencing considerable pain from the condition.

After explaining his findings to Mrs. Morris and her son, Dr. Benedict asks her, "Does it ever hurt when you chew?"

"No, my teeth are in wonderful condition," she answers. "Dr. Elbinger and I made sure of that."

"Is she on a regular diet," he asks the son, "or on a soft diet that would place less strain on these affected teeth?"

"She started complaining a while ago that the dining room was serving tougher meat than they used to," says her son. "She may have been having a problem chewing, but institutional food is never terrific, so I didn't think about it being her teeth that were the problem."

"My teeth have never been a problem," says Mrs. Morris, "and I take good care of them. I intend to take every one of them to the grave."

"I'm afraid, Mrs. Morris," says Dr. Benedict once again, "that your back teeth are all very loose because the gums and bone have become diseased. There is no way that we can correct the problem without removing a number of those teeth and giving you a partial denture to wear, one for the top and one for the bottom."

"Do you mean false teeth?" asks Mrs. Morris in horror.

Dr. Benedict shows her samples up upper and lower partials and points out on a diagram which of her teeth cannot be salvaged.

"I don't want those things," she says adamantly. "I'll never ever wear false teeth! After all my years of taking care of them and all of Dr. Elbinger's good work, you're not going to take my good teeth out and give me false ones!"

What should Dr. Benedict do and why?

TREATMENT DECISIONS FOR PATIENTS WITH COMPROMISED CAPACITY

Two principles are widely accepted, within the health care community and in American society more broadly, as the best guidelines for ethically correct treatment decisions when a patient is not able to participate at all in a treatment decision. The first principle is to do whatever the patient would choose in the situation if he or she could choose. This is sometimes called the principle of "substituted judgment" because another person's decision substitutes for the patient's, but precisely in choosing what the patient would choose if he or she could do so.

Obviously, the judgment that a patient *would* choose a certain course of action if he or she could is not only a hypothetical judgment but a judgment based on a hypothesis that is contrary to the facts of the case. For the patient is, in fact, *not* able to choose his or her treatment. Therefore the judgment that a patient *would* choose a certain course of treatment if he or she could must be accompanied by another judgment about how dependable the first judgment is. That is, we must continually test the evidence on which the judgment about what the patient would do is based to make sure that this judgment is supported strongly enough that it is reasonable for treatment decisions to be guided by it.

It might seem that the moral reason for this principle of doing what the patient would choose is respect for autonomy. But that cannot be literally the case because we are talking here about a patient who is incapable of choosing autonomously. In such a case, there is no autonomy in the strict sense for us to respect. Instead, what is being respected in this principle is a different feature of human beings, the value that human beings associate with acting consistently over time, of acting on the basis of a fairly consistent set of values in one's life. One of the most important values for most human beings is achieving a sense of being one within oneself, of what in the 1960s was called "getting it together," of what might be quite accurately spoken of as *integrity*. The principle of choosing what the patient would choose if he or she were able tries to preserve for the patient the value of living consistently according to a consistent set of values over his or her lifetime.

In some instances, patients provide sufficiently detailed directions about their health care that, although they are incapable of decision-making when the decisions must be made, those who make the decisions can be fully confident that they are doing what the patient would have chosen if he or she were able. But directions this detailed and specific are not common. People's health care circumstances are too variable for this to be the usual situation. Much more often, decision-makers must interpolate what the patient would choose in the present situation from other sorts of data from other situations in the patient's past. For example, family members or friends, or perhaps the health care giver personally, may have had conversations with the patient about conditions the patient wants to avoid or treatments that the patient would never choose under any circumstances. Or these persons may at least have a fairly clear understanding of the values or principles or ideals of conduct that guided the patient during his or her past, and may be able to use this information to judge what the patient would choose in this situation if he or she could do so.

But obviously many patients will not have given indications as helpful as these. Even then, sometimes if enough data about a patient's previous choices or values is available, although none of the items is clearly indicative alone, a total picture will still emerge that can support a judgment that the patient would choose a certain course of action if he or she could. But often there is not enough data, the data available is not clear enough, or there is contradictory data from different sources, so that a dependable judgment about what the patient would choose is not possible. In such a case, when the judgment about what the patient would choose is not well supported or is doubtful for some other reason, then this first principle cannot guide treatment decisions, and a second principle must be used.

The second principle is to do whatever is in the patient's best interest, what maximizes the patient's well-being. This is the principle to follow when the first principle, doing whatever the patient would do if he or she could choose, cannot be followed because we do not have strong enough evidence of what the patient would choose. It is also the principle to follow with regard to patients who have never been able to make their own choices, for example, small children and persons who have had severe mental deficits from birth, because these patients have had no opportunity to exhibit the kind of evidence of commitment to certain values, ideals, and ways of life, that we need to look for to judge what they would do if they could.

Notice that it is the best *net* well-being of the patient that is to be sought according to this second principle because we know that every course of action involves both benefits and burdens, losses, costs, and pains for every patient. Notice also that what is in the patient's best interest is not necessarily what the patient would choose if he or she could choose in the situation. That is, the first principle preserves the patient's option to act in a way that is not in his or her own best interest, but for the sake of some other person or group or for some other reason. Consequently, the second principle will not necessarily pick out the same action to be done for a patient that the first principle would pick out, provided there is sufficient evidence that the first principle can be used at all. But when the second principle is used, the range of alternative actions to be considered narrows, because only courses of action that are arguably in the patient's best interest can be considered.

Sometimes, people are uneasy with a principle that tells them to do something in another person's best interest because, they say, they are not necessarily privy to what the patient would consider to be in his or her best interest. But the second principle does not say, "Do what the patient would consider to be in his or her best interest." If we had enough data that we could determine what the patient would judge to be in his or her best interest, we would most frequently have enough data to judge what the patient would choose in the present situation. In that circumstance, we should act according to the first principle because it is the principle that should be applied first if it can be applied at all. (In technical terms, these two principles are "lexically" ordered.) Because the second principle comes into play only when data about the patient's interests and values are not sufficiently available, the person or persons judging what would be in the patient's best interest must use their *own* best judgment, taking account of whatever information about the patient and about human beings generally is available to them. In the last analysis, they must simply make the best judgment about the patient's best interests that they can.

THE ROLE OF PARENTS AND LEGAL GUARDIANS

Every dentist knows that in the United States a minor child's parents have a legal right to choose dental treatments for their child, and court-appointed guardians have the same legal right to choose treatments for their wards. The moral justification for such legal structures presumably lies in the fact that a child's parents are ordinarily the parties most concerned about the child's best interests and are most likely to be the best judges of what will maximize the child's well-being overall. Presumably the sense of obligation accompanying the role of court-appointed guardian, plus the efforts of courts to select in each case the best person for this role, provide a similar likelihood that wards' best interests will be served by guardians' treatment decisions. But we also know of many cases in which both patterns have been violated, and both parents and legal guardians have made choices to the greater or lesser detriment of a child's or ward's health.

Many health care providers have wanted to argue that in matters of health care, dentists, physicians, nurses, and other professionals are at least as committed, by their role, to the well-being of the incapable patient as are parents or guardians, and they are almost always better informed about the child's or ward's best interest in health care matters. So instances of children or wards being ill-served by their parents or guardians make many health care professionals doubt the wisdom of the legal structures currently in place. Except in emergencies, however, health care providers' only recourse within the current legal system is to make their case in court when they believe that a particular child or ward is being harmed by parents' or guardians' treatment decisions.

From the point of view of the ethics of the health professions, however, as contrasted with health care law, the role of an incapable patient's parents or guardian is not that of final decision maker about treatment, but as a resource for the data needed to apply the two principles explained in the previous section. That is, the role of parents and guardians is to assist the health care provider in acting according to the principle of doing what the patient would choose if he or she could, assuming there are enough of the right kind of data to follow this principle, or if not, to do what is in the patient's best interest. It is simply a fact of dental practice, then, that dentists' obligations as health professionals sometimes point them toward a course of action different from what the law requires by its determination that parents and guardians are to make the final decisions about treatment.

In extreme cases, a dentist may be professionally obligated to use the courts to try to overcome the law's presupposition in favor of parents' and guardians' judgments of patients' best interest. Laws regarding the reporting of child abuse have grown stronger in recent years, and it might be argued that the presupposition in favor of parents and guardians is now weakening or becoming more qualified in American society. But so far these changes have not made dentists' choices between what is best for a patient and what is legally required any easier. In cases when matters are not extreme—for example, when the choice is between two treatments that both meet minimum acceptable standards, but one would be far better for the patient's health than the other—if the dentist's judgment about a child's or ward's best interest conflicts with a parent's or guardian's, it is still most often the case that the dentist will feel forced by the legal risks involved to act against his or her best professional judgment.

One of the questions of the sort asked in Chapter 6—about how much sacrifice a dentist's professional commitment requires—concerns the amount of legal risk that a dentist is professionally committed to facing for the sake of his or her patient's well-being. There are no clear statements on this matter anywhere in the ethical literature. But the larger community does continue to support the general presupposition expressed in the law in favor of parents and guardians, even when occasional bad judgments on their part are widely known to occur. This continuance of support can therefore also be taken as evidence that dentists and other health professionals are not considered to be obligated to face extreme legal risk when the risk to the incapable patient's health is not extreme. Dentists, in their commitment to their patients' dental and general health, will often feel quite guilty in such situations, concerned that the failure is theirs for not successfully educating the patient or guardian who makes a bad choice for a patient. But there are limits, both human and professional, in how much a dentist is required to try to change a parent's or guardian's choice, provided the risk to the patient is not one of extreme harm. When the risk of harm is extreme, however, as was stated above, the dentist may well be obligated to try to use the courts to prevent it, with all the sacrifices and legal risks that this might involve.

At the other end of the spectrum, there are many patients and guardians who would happily participate in an interactive decision-making process with the dentist regarding their child's or ward's dental care. Thus in addition to the two principles explained in the previous section, the dentist should also attend to the professional ideal of interactive decision-making when trying to make a treatment decision for a patient incapable of participating. The difference in this case is that the ideal interactive relationship would be with the patient's parent or guardian.

Of course, an interactive relationship with a parent or guardian does not fulfill the ideal of an interactive relationship with the patient. But when a patient is incapable of participating, then obviously such an interactive relationship with the patient is impossible. (Some patients, arguably a great many of them, are in fact capable of *partial* participation in treatment decisions; their situation will be discussed in detail in a later section.) Nevertheless, given the role of final decision-making assigned by the law to parents and guardians, and given the dependence of the dentist on parents and guardians for the information needed to act on the two principles discussed above, there are obviously excellent reasons for a dentist to employ his or her skills at developing an interactive decision-making process in dealing with incapable patients' parents and guardians as well.

THE CAPACITY FOR AUTONOMOUS DECISION-MAKING

Up to this point, the discussion in this chapter has focused on patients in the health care system who are wholly incapable of participating in treatment decisions. The most clear-cut examples of such patients are infants and patients who are unconscious. But dentists rarely treat patients of either of these types, and many patients in the larger health care system do not fall into the category of *incapable to participate* either, even though it would also be incorrect to describe all of them as *fully capable* of participating.

In other words, the simple division of patients into those who are fully capable and those who are wholly incapable is inadequate. It must be replaced with a more fine-tuned set of concepts. This section will identify five distinct sets of characteristics that we have in mind when we attribute the capacity for autonomous decision-making to someone. Along with these characteristics, it will also be possible to name some of the corresponding ways in which the capacity for autonomous decision-making can be diminished, that is, some of the ways in which a person might be only *partially* capable of autonomous decision-making. The next section of this chapter will address the ethical questions that arise when a patient is neither fully capable nor wholly incapable of autonomous decision-making. That is, how ought a dentist deal with patients who are only partially capable?

The components of the human capacity for autonomous decision-making fall into five fairly distinct categories:

1. The ability to understand the relationship of cause and effect
2. The ability to see alternative courses of action available for choice and to choose between them (As indicated in Chapter 6, we take for granted that the activity of choosing among alternative courses of action is dis-

tinct from the activity of reasoning and judging about alternatives, whether before or after choosing one of them.)

3. The ability of a person to conceive of herself or himself as one who can choose between the alternatives in a given situation

4. The ability to reason comparatively about the alternative courses of action to reach a moral judgment about them

5. The ability to form and choose values, principles of conduct, and personal ideals to guide one's moral judgments and to shape one's moral reflections and conduct accordingly

Two different perspectives can be useful in discussing the contents of each of these categories, although a detailed analysis of their contents from either perspective would be a major undertaking and is well beyond the scope of this book. One is to focus on what abilities a growing child must develop for adults to think of him or her as a fully capable decision-maker. The other is to focus on the kinds of deficits we observe in those who have developed a fuller capacity for autonomous decision-making, but who then experience some loss or diminishment in that capacity.

1. For the first category, consider the developing ability of a child to understand the relationship of cause and effect, both in general and also in relation to matters affecting the child's body and health, the oral cavity, and the child's oral health. At some point, a child begins to understand that there is a cause-effect connection between tooth brushing and healthy teeth, for example, or between the dentist's removal of a carious lesion and placement of a restoration and the cessation of pain in chewing.

There is developmental evidence, however, that up until about age 6, most children retain a "magical" view of the relation between their health and various other factors in their environment, rather than understanding even rudimentarily the cause-effect relations that are relevant. In fact, one well-known article on young children's understanding of their bodies and illness is called "There's a Demon in Your Belly." In a similar way, some developmentally disabled persons and those with certain neurological deficits—for example, persons with certain kinds of senile dementia or Alzheimer's disease—may be unable to understand the relationship between their own or a dentist's actions and the condition of their oral cavity, their oral comfort and functioning, and other aspects of their oral health.

2. The second component is the general ability to see alternative courses of action as being available for choice and to choose between them. The child learns that he or she may direct his or her actions in any of several different ways in each situation, according to his or her own choice. In the authors' observation, the general capacity for choice seems to develop some time between the ages of 4 and 6, but we have not located psychological research on this topic to support this or any alternative account of the matter.

Some persons whose development is retarded do not achieve this ability until later in their lives, and some developmentally disabled persons do not achieve it at all. In addition, certain neurological conditions can destroy the neurological structures on which the activity of choice depends, and certain severe forms of emotional or mental illness seem to render their victims generally unable to choose between different courses of action.

3. The third category concerns the ability of a person to see himself or her-

self as a chooser in a given situation, as contrasted with the general ability to conceive of alternatives and make choices at all. This is the ability that some psychologists call "locus of control." In the development of a child, the fact that a child has learned the general truth that he or she can make choices between alternative courses of action does not guarantee that the child will be aware that this ability is relevant in a particular situation or category of situations. The child may attribute the controlling power to some other party or to other circumstances beyond the reach of his or her own choices. That is, depending on the facts of a situation or type of situation, and the child's understanding of the situation and of his or her own abilities in relation to it, the child may or may not view himself or herself as a "locus of control" regarding that situation. The question is whether the child perceives that the matter at hand depends, at least partially, on her or his own choice rather than solely on the choices of other persons or on other kinds of factors that are not influenced by the child's choices and actions.

The developmental evidence is that in matters potentially controlled by adult authority figures, children's sense of themselves as effective choosers seems to wax and wane during various stages of late childhood. Many 9-to-11-year-olds, for example, are apparently more aware of their capacity to control matters affecting them than many 12-to-14-year-olds, who tend to consider adults in positions of authority to be more controlling of events affecting them than they are themselves. In addition, persons who are retarded in their development or are developmentally disabled, and persons suffering from neurological conditions and severe emotional and mental illness, may also lack an awareness of themselves as capable of choice in certain categories of circumstances that they face.

Once a person matures into adulthood, and the general sense of oneself as affecting events beyond oneself is fully in place, the principal deficits to a person's sense of self as an effective chooser are chiefly the particularized effects of other persons' actions. Other persons' actions may severely limit the range of a person's alternatives in a given situation, perhaps eliminating all of the alternatives that the person hoped to be able to choose from. In such circumstances, it is often difficult for even very independent individuals to retain a strong sense of being in control of their life and what happens in it in the relevant situations. (Natural conditions may have the same effect on the range of a person's available alternatives, but learning that one is an effective chooser ordinarily includes learning that there are many natural limits to effective choice, as well as many imaginable and desirable alternatives that are nevertheless not available at all. The realization that this fact is not truly a lessening of one's genuine capacity as an effective chooser but rather a limit on the alternatives available for a person to choose from is itself a mark of maturation.)

The most dramatic form of such influence by other persons is coercion, where a chooser's range of significant alternatives is narrowed drastically by another party's threat of harm. But people's emotional connections to one another are so powerful and so diverse that there are many ways to manipulate a person's emotions so as to diminish their sense of themselves as choosers without formally threatening them with harm. Children and others whose general awareness of themselves as choosers is either not fully developed or is precarious for other reasons are even more susceptible to the destruction of this awareness as a consequence of others' coercion and emotional manipulation.

One particular deficit that belongs under this heading, and which dentists are unfortunately all too familiar with, is excessive fear. Fear in its most extreme forms seems capable of rendering some persons completely incapable of choice in a given matter, most likely by preventing them from seeing themselves as capable of influencing their situation in any choosable way. But it would be a serious mistake to assume that fear routinely renders patients incapable of choice if they are capable of choice in other areas of their lives and are aware of themselves as choosers in the same or similar situations. For there are many situations in life in which some measure of fear and awareness of potential harm, for example, is not only reasonable but even a necessary source of data for judgment and action. In other words, the judgment that a given patient is so fearful that he or she is thereby rendered incapable of autonomous choice should be a very rare one, made only under the most extreme of circumstances.

4. The fourth category is a person's ability to reason comparatively about alternative courses of action to reach a comparative judgment among them. Neither of the first three abilities alone or in combination necessarily implies that a child also has the ability to *understand* complex cause-effect systems or *examine* alternative courses of action in detail, nor does it imply that he or she has the ability to *rationally compare* alternatives once they are understood and thus to form a *moral judgment* about them. These activities that are involved in forming judgments about alternatives, as was indicated in Chapter 6, are considered by the authors to constitute a category of human activity distinct from the activities and abilities discussed in the previous headings.

The exercise of these abilities requires, as a precondition, the development in the child of the ability to suspend judgment from a course of action presently under consideration in order to examine and compare additional alternatives. It also requires, for its fullest development, the development of the ability to compare alternatives in terms of more general standards, such as a set of values, principles of conduct, ideals, virtues, and so on. This component depends in turn, for its fullest exercise, on the child's having developed the ability to reason both inductively and deductively (and in other ways if, as some philosophers claim, these two categories of reasoning do not exhaust the field), to conceive of future states of affairs, to predict (or comprehend a prediction of) their likelihood, and to hypothesize. Some of these capacities have been closely associated with the emergence of what Piaget called the "formal operational stage" of cognitive development, which he saw typically appearing at about 12 years of age. But a more important point for present purposes is that the many component abilities that are requisite for the fullest exercise of moral judgment do not develop at the same rate.

The most obvious form of partial incapacity that falls under this heading is the inability of a patient to make an autonomous choice by reason of their having only incomplete information or understanding of the alternatives that are available for choice. Obviously this form of incapacity can come in varying degrees, for a person might have all the relevant information to make a judgment about some of the available alternatives, either more or fewer, but in any case not about all of the alternatives that are important. Or a person might know of the possibility of each of the most important alternatives, but lack key information about the nature of consequences or implications of some of them, either more or fewer.

Another form of incapacity falling under this heading is the condition of a person who is making a logical error in reasoning about the alternatives he or she is facing. Sometimes what appears to be an error in logical reasoning is more correctly described as a conceptual mistake or, perhaps, simply a conceptual misunderstanding. That is, the parties involved may not be reasoning with the same set of concepts, and the deficit can be corrected by establishing a consensus about the meanings of key terms and the implications of key ideas. Logical and conceptual errors can often be corrected with careful instruction.

A more radical kind of incapacity exists if the person's ability to reason logically is impaired for physiological reasons, including the effects of otherwise appropriate medications on the person, or by reason of the effects of emotional or mental illness. Determining the extent of a deficit in logical ability, if it extends beyond a particular piece of reasoning, can be a difficult task.

The fact that the reasoning involved in making a treatment decision is moral reasoning—that is, that it involves judgments involving a person's values, principles of conduct, ideals, and so on, as well as the obligations arising from the dentist's professional role and the other roles and commitments of the parties involved—is no reason to assume that standards of logical reasoning and conceptual clarity are less relevant than in other areas of human reflection. One obvious presupposition of this book is that conceptual clarity and logical reasoning can take a thoughtful moral reasoner a long way toward good moral judgments. So the dentist seeking to judge a patient's capability for making an autonomous choice, or to judge the effectiveness of his or her efforts to enhance a patient's autonomy in decision-making, should pay as much attention to logical reasoning and conceptual clarity in matters of value, principle, and ideals as in any other.

5. The fifth component of the capacity for autonomous decision-making is a person's ability to form and choose values, principles of conduct, and personal ideals to guide his or her moral judgments and to shape his or her moral reflections and conduct accordingly.

It might seem that as soon as a child is able to judge and compare alternative courses of action and to choose according to his or her judgments, the child is capable of the full exercise of autonomous choice. But autonomy implies more than judgment and control in the present instance, regarding only the present set of alternatives. It also implies that present judgments and choices are part of a pattern that extends across situations, that they are the work of a self who is not only making them in each instance, but who connects them and makes them repeatedly and coherently across (at least a part of) a lifetime. Consequently, the fullest exercise of autonomy requires a person to be aware that he or she is a self with a particular history and with a distinct identity shaped by that history, that he or she has a particular set of values that motivate actions consistent with them, that he or she is moving toward a future that will be significantly shaped by present values and choices both in external fact and in the contents of the self that he or she will then be.

Without these elements of awareness, the person cannot be said, in any strong sense, to be forming and choosing values, principles of conduct, and so on, nor can that person be said to be shaping moral reflection and conduct according to them.

The older child, who can exercise the abilities described under the first four headings, still has rarely had enough experience of their exercise that we could say he or she has already formed and chosen a set of values or principles of conduct or ideas. At best the process is just beginning, and even then only in an unusually mature older child or young teenager. But as a child approaches the end of his or her teens, we ordinarily expect to see signs of a chosen set of values, principles of conduct, and personal ideals. There will often be much naivete to such choices at this point, but if this process is not at least under way, we would consider a late teen to be morally immature and to lack any really important sense of who he or she is and of what should guide his or her actions. We would, in other words, not attribute a developmentally appropriate capacity for autonomous choice to such a person.

When this component of the capacity is more fully developed in adults, we often speak of it in terms of integrity or authenticity because what is developing is a person's sense of who he or she is over a lifetime, or in terms of virtue and character, because this capacity cannot be effectively exercised unless the key values, principles, ideals, and patterns of perception, reflection, judgment, and action become habituated so they can be operative in most situations without self-conscious attention. Another way to speak of this component is in terms of the notion of consistency in one's values and commitments that was mentioned in the previous discussion of the first principle guiding treatment decisions for patients wholly incapable of participating.

Mature adults who have developed this component of autonomous decision-making do not ordinarily lose it altogether except as a consequence either of a severe neurological deficit that attacks the parts of the brain on which its exercise depends or of an extreme psychological disruption of the personality. But persons who suffer from serious phobias, addictions, or compulsions do have the experience of performing actions or experiencing needs or desires that are profoundly alien to their formed and chosen values in the affected areas of their lives. This is why persons who suffer from such maladies are not held fully responsible for the experiences they have that are driven by their phobias, addictions, or compulsions because their chosen, choosing, self-forming self is somehow separated from these elements of their make-up.

Less dramatic and less broken are desires to act, and possibly actions as well, that are simply inconsistent with the person's own chosen values, principles of conduct and so on. Such desires are common in human experience, and their presence is not in itself a sign of any lessening of the capacity for autonomous decision-making. But if a person acts on such a desire, and does so knowingly (i.e., there is no deficit of understanding, as described under the fourth heading above), we may ask if the act was autonomous precisely because it is "out of character," in other words, it is in violation of the pattern of values and so on that the person lives by. But it is always possible that the person has now made a choice to live by a changed set of values and so on and that the unusual choice is a mark of this. Consequently, it is rarely possible to hold that an individual's capacity for autonomous decision-making is seriously impaired, much less destroyed, solely on the basis of a single judgment or choice on his or her part that is contrary to his or her usual pattern.

Finally, a deficit may be partial not just in the sense that only one or several component abilities is compromised, but also in the sense that only decisions regarding a particular subject matter, possibly only the subject matter at hand, are affected. A person may, for example, be able to conduct quite sophisticated business affairs with full understanding yet be unable to comprehend adequately enough for autonomous decision-making the relations between her oral structure and her oral function that determine her current treatment alternatives. Or a person may act with complete confidence and see himself as an appropriate "locus of control" in all other areas of his life, but find it psychologically difficult to see himself as a chooser in matters of dental treatment when drilling or other feared operations are involved.

The effort to identify the nature of a patient's partial deficits therefore involves two judgments, not just one. The dentist must first try to identify the specific abilities affected by the deficit, as well as the degree of shortfall from full functioning. Second, the dentist must also determine whether the aspects of the patient's experience that are affected by the deficit(s) include matters crucial to the decisions in which the dentist hopes the patient will participate. A partial deficit in another area of the patient's life may not make any significant difference in his or her ability to participate in a treatment decision about the matter at hand.

DEALING WITH PATIENTS WITH PARTIALLY COMPROMISED CAPACITY

The last point in the previous section is the first point to stress here. Before evidence of a partial deficit in decision-making capacity leads a dentist to take any particular action, he or she should make sure that it has bearing on the dental treatment decisions that must be made. If the deficit does not affect matters crucial to decisions about the patient's dental care, then the dentist should deal with the patient in regard to those decisions just as he or she would deal with any fully capable patient under the same circumstances.

Although many people have a tendency to assume that a deficit (or incomplete development) in one component of autonomous decision-making justifies dealing with a patient as if he or she were wholly incapable, this simply is not so. A dentist who acted in this way would be in violation of the norms of dentistry that make autonomy an important central value for dental practice and that identify an interactive relationship as the ideal relationship between dentist and patient. So whenever there is a suspicion of a partial deficit in the capacity for autonomous decision-making, the dentist must determine if it affects matters crucial to present dental treatment decisions or other important aspects of this dentist-patient relationship.

The dentist must also be on his or her guard not to move too hastily from one or two pieces of evidence that a patient is not fully capable to the conclusion that this is certainly the case and to actions based on this conclusion. While evidence of a patient's partial incapacity may, in some cases, be simply obvious and overwhelming, the importance of autonomy as a central value and of the ideal of an interactive relationship in dental practice place the burden of proof on one who would judge a patient partially or wholly incapable.

Admittedly, in some parts of the health care system, the burden of proof often seems to run the other way, at least when the patient is not choosing the provider's recommended course of treatment. That is, when the patient disagrees with the care giver's recommendation, the patient is often made to bear the burden of proof to show that he or she is nevertheless capable of autonomous decision-making in the matter at hand. Treating patients in this way, and placing the burden of proof on them to demonstrate they are fully capable if they are to play any role at all in the decision-making process, violates a number of the norms of professional dental practice that have been articulated here.

Now let us examine some of the specific sorts of deficits outlined in the previous section and ask, at least in general terms, how the dentist ought to respond to them.

It seems clear that if a person cannot grasp cause-effect relations at all or cannot grasp them specifically in regard to his or her health, we must consider that person simply incapable of participating in deciding about health care interventions, dental and every other sort. The same is true if the person in wholly incapable of choosing between alternatives or of recognizing that alternative courses of action are open, and if the person is wholly incapable of reasoning comparatively about alternatives and reaching a moral judgment about them. Such complete deficits render a person incapable of autonomous decision-making. The two principles explained previously articulate how the ethical dentist will make treatment decisions regarding patients who are so completely incapable of participating.

But there are many kinds and degrees of partial capacity for autonomous decision-making. The dentist cannot simply deal with a partially compromised, partially capable patient as if he or she were wholly incapable any more than such a patient could be rightly treated as fully capable. What then can we say about the obligations of dentists toward partially capable, partially compromised patients when it comes to treatment decisions affecting their oral health?

The short answer to this question comes from what has already been said about the hierarchy of central values and about the ideal of an interactive relationship between dentist and patient. Both norms of professional dental practice require that the dentist work to maximize the patient's exercise of autonomy, provided the patient is not choosing interventions contrary to his or her oral or general health. Because the patients currently under consideration have a compromised capacity for autonomous decision-making, the dentist is obligated to try to correct whatever it is that is lacking, to eliminate the deficit so that, together with the dentist, the patient can make a choice about treatment with full autonomy.

Exactly what a dentist is called upon to do to rectify a deficit in a patient's capacity for autonomous decision-making will depend on the nature of the deficit. So the dentist must first try to determine which component ability (or abilities) of the many diverse abilities that make up the capacity for autonomous decision-making is (are) affected. We can begin here with examples of some of the simplest deficits to correct.

If the patient lacks some understanding of what alternatives are available or of information about any of them, the dentist obviously must determine where the gap in understanding lies and then address it with relevant information or education. For example, a patient may have all the relevant information to make a judgment about some of the available alternatives but not about all of the alternatives that are important. Or a patient might understand the availability of each of the most important alternatives but lack key information about the nature or consequences or implications of some of them.

In a similar way, if the patient does not understand the cause-effect connections between the available treatments and the outcomes for his or her oral health, comfort, and function, the dentist needs to carefully explain these connections, perhaps drawing on analogous connections of cause and effect that the patient might already understand.

Such defects in understanding are generally the easiest deficits of autonomous decision-making to correct, provided the dentist can determine what is missing and then can either teach it to the patient who lacks it or guide the patient to learn it in some other way. But such deficits can also prove less corrigible. Those who try to communicate the missing information may be unable to do so because of a lack of ability to grasp it on the patient's part, because the patient is of a mind set that will not permit new learning on the subject, or possibly because of some other reason. The question how a dentist ought to proceed when a deficit proves uncorrectable will be addressed later in this section.

Dentists are also familiar with fearful patients. Many dentists have developed or learned special techniques—beyond just saying "These are the facts and the choice is yours," which treats this deficit as if it were a deficit of understanding— for comforting fearful patients and helping them make autonomous choices in spite of their fear. Sometimes, however, the patient's fear is not only seriously compromising his or her capacity for autonomous choice, but it is beyond the dentist's own ability to address. A referral may be indicated, unless emergency care is called for. Then the question of how a dentist should deal with an uncorrectable deficit arises again. For example, if the patient's fear of endodontic therapy in the case in Chapter 4 was interpreted to be seriously compromising of his capacity for autonomous decision-making, then unless Dr. Clarke has techniques for addressing it that she has not yet tried, she will be faced with exactly this question of possible referral for the nonemergency aspects of his treatment and how to deal ethically with the emergency aspects when his deficit proves to be uncorrectable.

Patients can also be affected by other powerful emotions or other psychological states such that they cannot accept the fact that they have certain alternatives and not others, or that their alternatives are limited in certain ways. This may seriously limit their ability to consider relevant treatment alternatives or to view themselves as choosers—as the locus of control—in the treatment decision situation. Patients might also have powerful feelings or other psychological states that make them unable to fully evaluate their alternatives in terms of their own values, principles of conduct, and so on.

Depending on the severity of the underlying cause of the deficit, a dentist may be able to correct the deficit with a friendly chat or a bit of friendly advice or by suggesting a bit of personal reflection in a certain direction. But more severe deficits might require the tools of psychotherapy and may be well beyond the dentist's ability to handle, even though the affected decision concerns dental treatment. Again the dentist might need to refer the patient, particularly if there seems to be a need for professional psychological treatment, and will be faced with how he or she ought to deal with emergency care for a partially compromised patient when the deficit there and then proves to be uncorrectable. But the dentist is obligated, nevertheless, as when the deficit is one of information and understanding, to take extra effort to bring the patient as much as possible to an affective state in which autonomous decision-making is possible. The dentist may not say, "This patient's problems are not my concern; I am only concerned about the functioning of the oral cavity."

The same conclusion is required when the focus is on a dentist's obligations toward children who are patients. Because of the importance of the dentist's commitment to patients' autonomy and to the ideal of an interactive relationship, the dentist is obligated to work proactively to assist the development of each child's capacity for autonomous decision-making. At whatever stage of development of the five component abilities a dentist finds a youthful patient, the dentist is obligated to work to enhance the child's growth in this regard. This is not the dentist's first obligation, for the child's oral health and general health and life take precedence. But the dentist may not say, "I am only concerned about the oral cavity; the development of this child as an autonomous decision-maker is not my concern."

It is also true that the dentist's obligation specifically to support and enhance every child's oral and general health has implications for how the dentist deals with children. For the relationship between a dentist and a child can have a powerful impact on the child's ability to deal cooperatively and without great fear with future health care providers, both within dentistry and in health care generally. The dentist must consider whether his or her actions toward a child might yield more negative health effects for the child in the long run by the impact these actions might have on the child's future ability to relate to health care providers than the specific oral benefit that is currently the focus of the dentist's attention. But the point being made in this section is that in addition to this concern with the child's reactions to future health care and thus the child's future health, the dentist is obligated to maximize the child's capacity for autonomous decision-making by enhancing the child's development of the relevant abilities whenever doing so does not compromise the child's oral or general health.

Circumstances nevertheless will arise, of course, when children sit in the chair who have sufficient developmental or other deficits that the dentist's efforts to enhance the child's autonomous decision-making will come up short. In addition, and most frequently, children will be in the chair who are well developed in autonomous decision-making for their age, but who are still only functioning partially in this regard. When either of these circumstances is the case, the question arises again about how to deal with patients with partially compromised, but uncorrectable, capacity for autonomous decision-making.

Before addressing that question, a comment is also in order about the amount of time and effort that a dentist is obligated to expend in trying to correct partially compromised patients' deficits. Dentists are certainly obligated, as was argued in Chapter 6, to sacrifice their own self-interest and their other commitments to some extent for the sake of their patients' well-being, and this chapter has argued that enhancement of partially compromised patients' capacity for autonomous decision-making counts as part of that well-being. But there certainly are no clear guidelines about this in the most obvious components of the on-going dialogue between the dental profession and the community at large about dental professional norms. The dentist must surely balance such efforts for each particular patient against the effort needed to provide adequately for that patient's oral and general health, since these outrank autonomy in the hierarchy of central values. A dentist must also balance efforts of this sort for each patient against the needs of other patients, in other operatories and the waiting room, and in the dentist's practice at large. But these considerations do not address the still harder question—of the sort raised in Chapter 6—of how much sacrifice of other considerations a dentist is professionally obligated to accept to assist patients in this way.

It seems clear that the attitude of Dr. Prentice, in the case in Chapter 2, is open to serious challenge. Dr. Prentice told Jack Williamson that if patients want education beyond what is essential information about proposed treatments, they can have it, but only "with the meter running," in other words, in return for additional charges to the patient. The discussion in this chapter supports the view that a dentist's ordinary dealings with a patient ought to include *some* additional assistance for a patient's partially compromised decision-making capacity if it is needed.

At the other end of the spectrum, a dentist is surely justified in limiting his or her efforts in this regard to what will not *seriously* jeopardize the dentist's own well-being and the dentist's other justifiable commitments in his or her non-professional life. Thus a dentist may be justified in telling a patient that additional assistance in dealing with the patient's fears or other difficulties in reaching treatment decisions is available, but that the extra time and effort involved on the part of the dentist will involve an additional charge. Similarly a dentist's special efforts to assist developmentally compromised patients may deserve an additional charge. Absent a more clearly formulated guideline, the most important point to stress is that assisting the partially compromised patient with a view to the patient making a fully autonomous treatment decision, in as fully interactive relationship with the dentist as possible, is most certainly an ordinary requirement of ethical dental practice.

Now, finally, let us consider the issue of treatment decisions for partially compromised patients whose deficit proves to be uncorrectable, given the limits of the dentist's ability to assist and appropriate limits, as just discussed, on the dentist's expenditure of time and effort in doing so. This is a very subtle matter that has not been widely discussed in the literature of health care ethics or anywhere else, and those who consider it carefully may well differ in their solutions. The authors' proposal is to follow the same two principles proposed previously in this chapter regarding patients who are wholly incapable of participation, but with an important modification of the first principle.

First, then, a dentist who concludes that a patient's partial incapacity for autonomous choice is uncorrectable must ask whether he or she has (or can obtain within appropriate limits of time and effort) enough understanding of this patient that, by taking account of those components of autonomous decision-making that the patient is still capable of carrying out effectively, the dentist can produce the choice that he or she can reasonably claim the patient *would have* produced if the patient did not presently lack this component. In other words, can the dentist "make up the difference" for the partial incapacity through the dentist's acquaintance with the other, properly functioning elements of the patient's autonomy, together with information about the patient's previously held values, principles of conduct, ideals, and so forth?

Answering this question will be difficult in almost every instance, especially because dentists often do not have detailed understanding of their patient's larger systems of value and so forth, even when these are long-term patients. But if a dentist can answer this question conscientiously in the affirmative, then the authors propose that the dentist act on the choice that he or she judges the patient would have made if the patient had not been partially incapacitated. Under such circumstances, the care giver enables the patient to function, if not autonomously in the strict sense, then at least in a manner consistent with his or her own values, principles of conduct, or personal ideals to the maximum degree possible. This is the closest conformity to the norms of the value of patient autonomy and the ideal of an interactive relationship that the patient's circumstances permit.

But if the dentist judges that he or she does *not* have—and cannot get with the appropriate help of others—enough understanding to "make up the difference" for the patient in this way, then the authors propose that the patient must be viewed as *functionally incapable* of autonomous decision-making, even if not actually incapable. For the patient's partial incapacity or incapacities cannot be "made up for" by any available means. In such a case, the patient should be cared for under the second moral principle that is appropriate in care of patients who are wholly incapable of autonomous choice, namely, to act in the patient's best interest, as was explained previously.

In some cases, as has been indicated, it may be possible to provide a partially compromised patient with assistance that the dentist can't personally offer, in the form of an appropriate referral. When this is possible, it is what a dentist ought to do, providing only emergency treatment—and using the two principles just explained to determine the nature of that treatment —until all appropriate efforts to bring the patient to full capacity have been made. But the patient may refuse this referral effort. If the patient refuses, wanting to proceed with treatment in spite of the dentist's judgment that the patient's decision-making capacity is impaired, the dentist should try to determine if there is any other way that a delay in nonemergency treatment might assist the patient in overcoming the deficit. If not, then the dentist is professionally justified in proceeding with treatment as determined in accord with the two principles just explained.

Finally, there is the situation in which the dentist is unable to determine with reasonable confidence whether the patient is functioning with partially (or completely) diminished capacity or not. Try as the dentist might with questions, visual aids, and other means, to determine whether the patient really understands the treatment alternatives, really sees himself or herself as a chooser in the matter, and so on, the dentist is still not confident that the patient is capable enough to participate in an interactive decision-making process. But at the same time, the dentist is not certain that the patient's capacity is significantly diminished either. How should the dentist proceed in a case like this?

Once again, if the dentist has any resources left to try and has not yet reached the appropriate limits of sacrifice of other interests for the sake of this patient's well-being, then clearly the dentist should try again or try something else to resolve the issue. For the differences between how a dentist deals properly with a capable patient and how a dentist deals properly with a patient with diminished capacity are morally significant, and the one approach should not be substituted for the other without good reason. But if the dentist is at the limit of his or her resources, and is justified in not trying further to determine the patient's condition in this respect, then he or she must treat the patient as if the patient were functionally one way or the other, since precisely what cannot be determined is how the patient actually is.

Some readers may take the view that, under such circumstances, the patient should be treated as if he or she were capable of autonomous decision-making out of respect for the value of autonomy. But the authors' judgment is that the alternate view is correct, that the dentist should deal with such a patient as the dentist would deal with one who is not capable of autonomous decision-making, applying the two principles already discussed above. The authors' reason for this judgment is the ranking of the patient's oral and general health above the patient's autonomy in the hierarchy of central values for dental practice.

THINKING ABOUT THE CASE

Mrs. Morris's inability to remember Dr. Benedict's name and the variations in her account of her last visit to Dr. Elbinger's office are strong evidence of memory deficits. But they do not point necessarily to any deficit in her ability to make a decision about the treatment proposed to her. This is a situation in which the dentist must be careful to ask, of each of the deficits in capacity that are present, whether that particular deficit is relevant to the treatment decision at hand.

But Mrs. Morris also seems to suffer from deficits that are relevant to this treatment decision. For she seems to believe that her posterior teeth and gums are actually in fine shape. While she still seems able to recognize that dental treatment can have beneficial effects on oral comfort and functioning, she seems unable to recognize the serious problems with her posterior teeth. Consequently, even though she has a long-standing value commitment to hygiene and proper dental care, she cannot apply these values and principles to the facts of her current situation and choose a course of action suitable to the present situation in accordance with them.

Dr. Benedict ought to pause mentally long enough to ask if the evidence he has of Mrs. Morris's partial deficit—her inability to affirm that her posterior teeth are seriously affected—is sufficiently strong to act on it. In the present case, however, the answer to this question seems clear. For even the brief conversation reported in the case contains at least four separate indications that Mrs. Morris does not understand the condition of her posterior teeth. One of these, her reported attribution of difficulty in chewing to tougher cuts of meat, is not implausible in an institutional setting, as her son reasonably concluded. But Dr. Benedict has observed mobile teeth and advanced periodontal disease in all four quadrants. While it is possible, if unlikely, that Mrs. Morris has experienced no serious pain or discomfort from her periodontal disease, the existence of the disease is a matter of demonstrable clinical fact in this case. Given what he has observed and Mrs. Morris's repeated claims that nothing is amiss, Dr. Benedict would be perfectly justified in concluding that she is suffering from a significant partial deficit in capacity. What then ought he do about it?

His first priority, in relation to the norms of respecting autonomy and striving to bring about as interactive a relationship with Mrs. Morris as possible, ought to be to try to correct the deficit. Dr. Benedict should therefore try again to explain to her that her posterior teeth are in serious trouble. Perhaps by using mirrors, he could help her see the affected gum tissue. Perhaps by gently manipulating the mobile teeth, or having Mrs. Morris do this herself, he can bring her to understand that there is a problem.

Here, unfortunately, he might face a difficult dilemma of competing values. For Mrs. Morris's conviction that her teeth are in excellent shape is clearly very important to her. It may be an important element of her self esteem at a time when she can sense that other faculties are weakening. Therefore Dr. Benedict needs to proceed cautiously in educating Mrs. Morris about her periodontal disease. At some point he may conclude that it would be better, in terms of her overall psychological health, not to press the reshaping of her understanding and imagination any further and to leave her with her deeply embedded view that her teeth are in excellent shape, treat her as one with an uncorrectable deficit, and apply the two principles explained above. This might be the best trade-off of valued elements of her well-being that the dentist can identify in the situation.

Let us assume that after a bit more conversation, Dr. Benedict justifiably concludes that Mrs. Morris is uncorrectable in her conviction that her teeth are in fine shape. She suffers, in other words, from an uncorrectable partial diminishment of her capacity for autonomous decision-making that is clearly crucial to participating in the treatment decisions that need to be made. The values of Mrs. Morris's oral and general health, not to mention the fact that Dr. Benedict has accepted Mrs. Morris as his patient, mean that Dr. Benedict cannot ethically just step aside from the case at this point. He must now determine how he ought to deal with this incorrigibly diminished patient.

The proposal made earlier was that the dentist first try to "make up" for the deficit from what he or she knows of the patient's other functioning capabilities. In this case, Mrs. Morris has a long and articulate history of valuing dental health and good dental treatment. It is quite reasonable to propose that *if* she could understand that her oral structures are severely impaired and she is at serious risk for deteriorating oral function, she would choose appropriate dental treatment to address the situation. Although such a choice would conflict with her conviction that her teeth are in excellent shape, it is precisely that conviction that is false and needs to be "made up for" by the dentist's interpolations. It is therefore reasonable to propose treating Mrs. Morris with extraction of the affected teeth and fabrication of removable partials to replace them.

This course of action also seems, from one point of view, to be supported by the second principle discussed earlier, namely to act in the patient's best interest. On the other hand, Mrs. Morris might be so resistant to using the partial dentures and so distraught that her "perfectly healthy" teeth have been extracted that her oral function, her psychological condition, or at the very least her nutritional situation might be affected negatively by this course of action. If the impact on her oral and general health were going to be great enough, concern for these values would take precedence over the effort to respect her autonomous decision-making capacity by following the principles proposed in this chapter.

So Dr. Benedict has a difficult judgment to make in this case. He may well need to get further information from the nursing home about Mrs. Morris's eating patterns, comfort in chewing in her present condition, and so on, before he can make a careful judgment about the likelihood of the possible negative effects of extraction and fabricating partial dentures. Only then can he weigh these effects against the positive effects for oral function and comfort, appropriate nutrition, and respect for her autonomy in its diminished degree that extraction and the dentures might produce. Unless Dr. Benedict has a fair amount of confidence about these matters, he may have to delay treatment of the posterior teeth until he can make a more confident judgment.

Patients with uncorrectable partial deficits in capacity that are crucial to the treatment decisions at hand can raise very difficult professional-ethical judgments for dentists. It is of the very nature of the case that the dentist does not have everything he or she needs to respect the patient's autonomy and to work for an interactive relationship with the patient, and, especially at the outset, the dentist also often lacks important information even for determining what course of action will be in the patient's best interest, including oral and general health as well as autonomy and the other central values. The best path for a dentist to take, both professionally and to reduce the anxiety and frustration that invariably accompany such cases, is to enhance his or her skills at facilitating autonomous decision-making and assisting patients in overcoming partial deficits in their capacity for it. This is also, obviously, the very path recommended by the ideal of making relationships with patients, whatever their abilities, as interactive as possible.

CHAPTER 8

Education and Cooperation

Case: Fear of Drowning

Jonathan Levinson is an 8-year-old patient of Dr. Nathan Silverman. From his first visit to the dentist at age 4 until 2 months ago, Jonathan's dentist was Dr. Edwin Samuels, his parents' general dentist. Jonathan's parents found Dr. Samuels considerate and caring, and assumed that Jonathan would like him as much as they did. But Jonathan claimed from the first visit that Dr. Samuels was "mean" and "doesn't like me." Every checkup was resisted, and it took major bullying by Jonathan's parents to get him to go. Routine diagnostic work and prophylaxis in the office were traumatic, and restorative work required one or both of Jonathan's parents to be at chairside restraining him. Eventually, his mother took a friend's advice and called Dr. Silverman, a pedodontist.

Mrs. Levinson mentioned to Dr. Silverman's receptionist that Jonathan's previous dentist had considered him a "problem patient." So before the first visit, Dr. Silverman telephoned her to ask about Jonathan's previous dental experiences. When he had heard her story, instead of sending the usual form letter to request his records, he called Dr. Samuels, whom he also knew, to talk about Jonathan.

"Both of Jonathan's parents have high dental anxiety, Nat," said Dr. Samuels. "I think they passed it on to Jonathan unconsciously before he ever set foot in my office. He was distrustful from the start. I talked to him a lot, as I do with all my patients, explaining the importance of good dental care and why the patient's cooperation is essential to receiving it. I really did try to get him to understand that I couldn't provide the best care if he wouldn't cooperate, but it didn't do any good. At each visit I would explain it again—give my little lecture—but I tell you, he had it in for me from day one.

"He would clamp his mouth shut, turn his head away, even push me away with his arms, just for routine probing and inspection of the dentition. Heaven help us when it came to cleaning! He wouldn't actually push Joyce away, maybe because she is a woman, but he would shout and scream out whenever he could feel her instruments touching tissue of any sort. And if I had to do restorative work, which I am grateful wasn't very often, I would always start all over explaining the procedure and the need for him to sit still so that it would go faster, be less uncomfortable, and so on, if only he'd cooperate. But he would resist and resist until finally I would give up and bring in his mother or father—once actually both of them—to hold him down and talk him into not resisting sufficiently that I could get the work done.

"I'm not proud of it, Nat, but I actually used hand-over-mouth on him once, on the very first visit. I just had one little pit to seal and after a lot of fidgeting and complaining, he finally just clamped his mouth shut when I had it nearly ready. I didn't want to bring his parents in—it was before I ever did that—so I covered his nose and told him to open his mouth. I have rarely done that, Nat; I really don't believe in it. But this time it just got my goat. I never said anything to the parents; I don't think he did either, and he never mentioned it to me afterwards. But after that happened, well, that's when I decided I had to bring his parents in because I don't think that's a good way to treat kids in the chair."

"I certainly agree with you, Ed," said Dr. Silverman, "we need to find other ways to get cooperation."

"Well, I wish you luck with Jonathan, Nat. Starting over with a new dentist is probably a good idea. Maybe you can get him to understand what I couldn't. He's a pretty smart kid, actually; I just couldn't get him to accept what I was saying."

At his first visit, Dr. Silverman met Jonathan in the waiting room, shook his hand and his father's, and invited Jonathan into his office. "These are more comfortable chairs for talking," he said, "and I'd like to get an idea of what you think of dentists before we talk about anything else."

Jonathan's opinion of dentists was not very high. Dr. Silverman asked him what he thought of regular dental self-care and whether he had ever had a toothache and what had happened about it.

Jonathan admitted that he once had a toothache and didn't like it, and that Dr. Samuels' intervention had ended the pain. He said that he knew that brushing his teeth would keep cavities from coming back, but he said he didn't like having anything in his mouth except food, so he only brushed his teeth when his mother or father were actually watching him.

"Does it hurt your mouth to have a toothbrush in it?" asked Dr. Silverman. "I only ask because a lot of people, even people with very small mouths, don't usually find it a problem. Do you have any idea why it bothers you?"

"When I was 4," said Jonathan, "I fell off a pier where I was playing with my friends at a lake, and I almost drowned. Whenever anything blocks up my mouth, I think about that and it scares me. I was really scared. I was under the water a long time, and I couldn't breath."

"That sounds terrible," said Dr. Silverman. "You must have been very frightened. How were you saved? Did someone dive in and pull you out, your parents or someone?"

"My parents never knew about it. I haven't told anyone about it before you because when I got out—I finally climbed up the logs that made up the pier— I was screaming that I almost drowned and my friends were laughing at me. They said that the water was only up to my waist, but I was so bent over that I just thought I was drowning, and all I had to do was stand up. They thought it was funny. So I never told anyone. I was really scared, but I thought anyone else would just laugh at me like they did."

"Well, I appreciate your telling me about it, Jonathan," said Dr. Silverman. "I certainly can understand how frightened you were, no matter how deep the water was. Not being able to breathe is one of the most terrifying things that can happen to a human being. I am very sorry that your friends laughed at you; they certainly wouldn't have laughed if the same thing had happened to them. It was mean of them to laugh at it."

"That's how I felt," said Jonathan. "But I couldn't tell anyone. If they had been there, maybe they would have understood, but I figured anyone else would just laugh at me."

"Would you be willing to try out some special, small sized toothbrushes that I've got? We could try them out here, where you can experiment without anyone knowing, and if we can find a brush that's comfortable for you, you can just take it home and use it, and no one will ever know that you were really concerned about suffocating. Would that be a good idea?"

Jonathan agreed, and followed Dr. Silverman into one of the operatories where Dr. Silverman pulled out a box of toothbrushes of different sizes and styles. Jonathan experimented with a couple of them and found one he was comfortable with. Dr. Silverman asked him if he would mind hopping into the chair so Dr. Silverman could take a quick look to see how hard he would need to brush, since he hadn't been doing it very regularly lately. "I won't put any instruments in your mouth, I promise; you just open wide and I'll take a look around." Jonathan got into the chair and opened his mouth.

"Well, everything I can see looks pretty good, Jonathan. Why don't you take a look." He gave Jonathan a mirror so he could look into his own wide-open mouth.

"Now I want to show you something, back here in my office." They returned to the more comfortable chairs. "What you saw in the mirror is just what I saw, looking in. It's pretty much what you can see if I hold this model of a set of teeth right in front of you, except this doesn't have any cheeks in the way. But let me ask you something, how would you go about looking at the back side of the teeth."

Jonathan reached out to turn the model around, and Dr. Silverman said with a laugh, "You're now looking through the back of this patient's head. I haven't had a patient yet that would let me do that. What do you think?"

"I don't know," said Jonathan.

"Do you think it would be good if a dentist could see the back sides of the teeth?"

"Sure," said Jonathan, "what if they have something wrong with them?"

"Right! Now let me show you something else," said Dr. Silverman, picking up a pediatric mouth mirror. "This mirror is actually smaller than that tooth brush you chose, but it is plenty big enough to let you see most of the back of the teeth. Here, try it."

Jonathan inspected the back of the model's teeth using the mirror. "Let me ask you something, Jonathan," said Dr. Silverman. "The next time you come in, could I use a mirror like this to look at the back sides of your teeth, to make sure there's nothing wrong with them?"

"You can look right now if you want," said Jonathan.

"Are you sure?"

"Yeah. But do I have to sit in that weird chair in the other room? It smells funny in there."

"If you wouldn't mind," said Dr. Silverman. "I know it's a strange chair and the room smells funny. The smell's because of what we have to clean it with, and the chair has a special light we can use to see into your mouth. Regular room lights don't light up the inside of your mouth enough."

They returned to the operatory and Dr. Silverman inspected Jonathan's teeth with the mirror, reporting in detail on what he saw, which was a mouth in need of cleaning, but otherwise in fairly good shape. "I have some more instruments here in this cabinet," said Dr. Silverman, "all of them smaller than that toothbrush. If it turns out that the toothbrush is okay to use, like you think it will be, then I would like to show you how some of these other instruments are useful for taking care of your teeth, too.

"Would you be willing to come back and see how I can use them? This one we use to give teeth a special cleaning. You probably saw one like it before. If you are comfortable with the idea when you come back, I think cleaning your teeth would be a very good idea, so you don't get any new cavities. But I promise you that I will not put any instrument or anything else in your mouth that you are uncomfortable with or that you don't understand what it's for and what job we're going to do with it. Would you be willing to come back for another visit in a few weeks and give that a try?"

Jonathan did not respond immediately. Instead, he carefully studied his new toothbrush for a moment. Then he agreed. "Okay," he said. "But can we talk in your regular office first, in the comfortable chairs?" he asked.

"Sure," said Dr. Silverman.

That was 2 months ago. Jonathan has now completed four visits to the dentist. He has received a complete prophylaxis, sealants, and small restorations on two deciduous molars. His oral hygiene is now very good, and he chats comfortably with Dr. Silverman at each visit about his many interests—school, sports, and stamp collecting—and also about his desire to learn to swim some day.

SUPPORTING PATIENT EDUCATION AND COOPERATION

Dentists caring for uncooperative pediatric patients rarely learn of a specific trauma that explains the child's lack of cooperation, and it is even rarer that the patient is the source of this information, carefully describing what happened and why it is relevant to the present situation. In that respect, this case is somewhat artificial. But the points it exaggerates are important aspects of the dentist's obligation to provide health care education and motivation at the patient's own level.

Like the case in Chapter 3, this is one in which everything turns out well. Situations in which everything turns out well are often the best teachers of how a person ought to act because they provide a positive line of action for a person to follow, as opposed to merely warning them away from something that is unprofessional or unethical in some other way. Of course, the young patient in this story makes a fresh start with his new dentist in a way that many children will not, and Dr. Silverman himself may seem to be more willing to spend more time talking at length with patients than is practical in most dentists' practices. So again the case may not seem so realistic.

On the other hand, guiding a patient to cooperate with dental diagnosis and treatment, and educating dental patients both about the care they receive in the dental office and about the self-care they should provide to themselves at home, are very important parts of dental practice. Many different categories of professional obligation support dentistry's commitment to patient education and to establishing the most collaborative relationship possible between dentist and patient. So it is important to reflect on ideal instances of collaboration and education, as well as defective ones, in order to conduct one's practice in the most professional and ethical way. In this case, the contrast between the two dentists is informative.

Dr. Samuels is not uncaring or lacking in sensitivity to his patients' fear and anxiety. In fact, he read Jonathan's anxiety and fear from his behavior as soon as Jonathan entered his care. Nor is there any hint in this case that Dr. Samuels lacks technical proficiency in diagnosis or restorative treatments.

But he approaches the fearful and anxious boy only with ideas rather than reaching out to him at the place where he is most in need: his feelings.

Sometimes changing a person's ideas can change their feelings. So the general approach of explaining and reasoning with a person is certainly not a mistake. But subtle connections between understanding and feelings are more common in mature adults than in small children, and even among mature adults, reasons and explanations alone are only likely to be effective when the person's level of anxiety at the moment is relatively low. So Dr. Samuels, though he may well have tried to facilitate Jonathan's cooperation to the best of his ability, was working with a very low percentage technique for the situation.

Dr. Silverman, by contrast, responds to feelings in kind, with first of all an affirmation of the feelings' importance, whatever their particular contents, and then with sympathy and concern. Unwittingly, Dr. Samuels had informed Jonathan that his fear of suffocating was not important, by trying to reason him out of it when he didn't yet know what it was or what had caused it. This response established a gap between Jonathan and Dr. Samuels that the dentist was unable to bridge from then on. But Dr. Silverman communicated, even while still ignorant of the story behind the fear, that Jonathan's feelings about dental care and dentists were important to him, and thus that Jonathan was important. He communicated this effectively enough that Jonathan was able to share his deep, fear-filled secret with the dentist, and the dentist was then able to build on that bond between them and develop a gradual plan to address the underlying problem of Jonathan's fear of suffocating.

This way of interpreting the two dentists' approaches to Jonathan represents just one of many ways in which the various educational techniques, communication tools, and human relations skills that are available to the dental community might interpret it. The authors are not proposing one of these approaches as opposed to any other. The point is that Dr. Samuels's mastery of any of these tools would probably have enabled him to deal more effectively with his young patient's fears and anxiety. He would not have lost a patient, to put the issue in economic terms, but more importantly, he would have responded more effectively, and more professionally and ethically, to his patient's needs.

Jonathan's needs are unusual in his having suffered a specific traumatic experience that is directly linked with his fear of dental treatment and even of regular self-care. Most children's dental anxieties do not have so dramatic an origin as Jonathan's. But the obligation of the dentist to educate and to work toward as interactive a relationship as possible with each patient remains.

Nor, obviously, are the challenges of education and patient cooperation limited to children or to chairside. For many dentists, the most challenging patients in terms of cooperation are adults who do not do the after-care they have been instructed to do, or who fail to appear for follow-up appointments, or who do not follow the regimen of daily self-care that their oral health requires. Here again, a dentist may try to achieve compliance with reasons and explanations. But often, it is not understanding per se that is lacking; the key factor is rather the patient's feelings and motivation. So the dentist whose skills are limited to giving reasons and explanations, as Dr. Samuels' are, has only a very low percentage technique to apply to these difficult patients.

Are we claiming that every dentist has an obligation not only to conscientiously use whatever techniques he or she has available to assist patient education and cooperation but also to acquire other, more effective tools when the dentist is not effectively assisting education and cooperation in a significant percentage of patients? The answer to this question is, yes. Just as dentists are obligated, by the norm of professional competence, to obtain and maintain the clinical skills necessary to correctly diagnose and treat the dental needs of their patients (with referral to specialists playing an important, but limited, role in each dentist's practice) so a dentist is obligated to obtain and maintain the skills the dentist needs to educate patients and prompt them to the levels of cooperation needed to maintain their oral and general health (with referral to those who are more skilled in these matters as another option if the dentist's own skills are too limited).

This obligation can be considered a further implication of the norm of competence. It is also strongly supported by the norms pertaining to the ideal relationship between dentist and patient and the norm of the central values of dental practice. But the most important support of this obligation derives from a normative category of professional obligation that is often overlooked, the category labelled in Chapter 3 "Integrity and Education."

THE IDEAL RELATIONSHIP, RESPECTING AUTONOMY, AND EDUCATION

The dentist's obligation to work for as interactive a relationship with the patient as is possible, on the view that an interactive relationship between dentist and patient is the ideal relationship to which all dentists are obligated to strive, has been examined in detail in Chapter 4, and again in Chapter 7 in connection with patients with partially diminished capacity. The dentist's obligation to respect and to try to enhance the patient's autonomy, as one of the central values of dental practice, has been discussed in detail in Chapter 5 and also again in Chapter 7. It is not necessary to reiterate the points made in those chapters.

But it is important to note that patients make choices regarding their dental health and function at least as much away from the chair as in it. Enhancing a patient's autonomy in regard to his or her dental health and establishing a long-term collaborative relationship with that patient is not just a matter of getting as interactive a relationship with the patient as is possible *when the patient is in the chair*. It also involves the patient's *self-care*, including regular visits for evaluation, prophylaxis, and treatment and, as needed, appropriate after-care and follow-up. These aspects of dental care depend principally on educating and motivating the patient not only about the need for them but especially about how to carry them out.

Dental hygienists are specifically trained to be effective dental educators, particularly regarding self-care and the regular use of dental services. Many dentists fulfill much of their professional obligation to educate their patients and to motivate them for long-term cooperation through their collaboration with dental hygienists. Dentists who cannot offer their patients the professional skills of a dental hygienist certainly have a lot more work to do to fulfill this aspect of their professional obligation than those who do offer them. But no dentist can simply leave this task to the hygienists. Every dentist must at the very minimum work closely with the hygienist to support and enhance

lly required to
ection. But even
tist must accept in
this norm and the
he dentist's profes-

ional efforts with the patient and to
th the patient in this regard. Conse-
of effective education, communica-
nstrumentality for every dentist to
for an ideal relationship with every
atient's autonomy.

e for the sake of the
ient away, either to
operation. The den-
of extra effort and
as well as the burden
company a patient's

ceived very little explicit attention
sions and in the professions' own
ns the subtle component of con-
to his or her clients, and to the
for as a member of that profes-
obligation was called the norm

efforts to modify the
is significantly inter-
etently. Then the den-
the patient's oral and
at the dentist refer the
better. If no such den-
ealth, the dentist has a
o try to overcome the
s oral or general health
ent may be justifiably
igated to provide treat-
nt. (Situations in which
s at all or dentists who
vailable, raise additional
ok to explore in detail.)
ggravation he or she will
reatment elsewhere (if it
tist sets this limit at the
ificantly affects the den-
ot only may but is oblig-
lso made that if this limit
her commitment to the
s of situations, which are
e current state of the dia-
community does not pro-

ands for certain central values,
communicate a very different
us implication of the norm of
ork to be effective educators
ely in the chair and to estab-
se of dental services, and so
ling the ideal dentist-patient
onomy as one of dentistry's
n requires these efforts.
nore. Are dentists obligated
y living that are consonant
who smokes or who uses
essionally in that respect?
or who abuses alcohol or
behavior's impact on the
sts may argue that these
nent as dentists. But the
values of his or her pro-
n to questions like this.
community, and what it
his or her profession.
notivated to place his
s in her daily patterns
patient thought that
ommitted himself or
cipline necessary to
d to make changes
are not making the
own lives. Conse-
ivate patients for
which they con-
the fulfillment of

her preferred patterns of
he would employ to try to
ive relationship, a limit in
. How would such a dentist
ical-professional practice?
d only be justified in adopt-
ern of practice or philosophy
eving that adopting this limit

ain. How much

sacrifice of other considerations is the dentist profess
undertake. This question will be examined in the next
though there are limits to the extent of sacrifice that a den
order to conform to the norm of integrity and education,
obligations to which it leads are unmistakably part of t
sional commitment.

HOW MUCH SACRIFICE IS REQUIRED?

The dentist's obligation to accept some measure of sacrific
patient certainly requires that the dentist not send a pat
another dentist or simply away, <u>at the first sign of nonco</u>
tist must accept, to some significant extent, the burden
<u>attention needed to work with a noncooperative patient,</u>
of feelings of frustration or rejection that will often ac
refusal to cooperate.

On the other hand, suppose that a dentist fails in
patient's uncooperative behavior and that this behavior
fering with the dentist's ability to treat the patient comp
tist's obligation to practice competently and to place
general health ahead of other values clearly requires th
patient to another dentist who can handle the situation
tist is available, then in the interest of the patient's he
difficult judgment to make about how much more t
patient's lack of cooperation. If the risk to the patient'
is great, some real risk of not fully competent treatr
accepted by the dentist. But the dentist is never obl
ment that <u>he or she believes is likely to be incompete</u>
dental care is a scarce resource, in which any dentis
are competent in the matter at hand are simply not a
ethical questions that are beyond the scope of this bo

May a dentist set a limit to how much effort and a
bear before telling an uncooperative patient to seek
is available)? The claim was just made that if a der
point at which the patient's uncooperativeness sig
tist's ability to treat competently, then the dentist r
ated to send the patient elsewhere. The claim was a
is set too low, the dentist will be violating his o
patient's well-being. But in between these two kin
fairly clear cut, lie many situations about which th
logue between the dental profession and the large
vide any clear guidance.

Suppose a dentist did adopt, as part of his o
practice, a limit to the amount of effort he or s
bring an uncooperative patient into a collabora
between the two kinds of situations already note
determine if this limit was within the range of eth

The first point to make is that the dentist wou
ing some limit as part of his or her preferred patt
of dental practice if there is some reason for beli

will enable the dentist to practice better over the long run, when the pattern of acting according to this limit is fully habituated in his or her practice. For it was this connection to long-term habits of practice that justified placing the value of preferred pattern in the hierarchy of values in the first place. But suppose a dentist sincerely sees not going beyond a certain limit of effort and aggravation as necessary to avoiding "burn out" in dental practice. Then having such a limit would not, of itself, be a violation of the priority of the patient's well-being. (Note also that a dentist's situation can change, for example, with age and other variables in dentist's life, so that the contents of a dentist's philosophy of practice or a dentist's preferred patterns of practice—and so his or her limits regarding efforts to help noncooperative patients—could also justifiably change as these other factors do over a period of time.)

Second, although some sacrifice of comfort and convenience by the dentist for the sake of the patient's well-being is part of the dentist's professional commitment, it is not required that these sacrifices be extreme. Imagine a very skilled and very thick skinned dentist who *could* treat extremely uncooperative patients competently, with only a great deal of wear and tear on his or her psyche as a byproduct. Does professional commitment require this dentist to bear so great a burden? It seems certain that he or she would not be required to endure *every* case of noncooperation to the very end, but it seems reasonable to say that such a dentist, because of his or her unusual abilities, would be required to bear *some* of the burden of extremely noncooperative patients, particularly those referred from less sturdy or less gifted dentists who had to tell patients of this sort to look elsewhere. But even if competent practice is not affected, extreme sacrifices are still not required to be borne without limit. (At some point, of course, persistent noncooperation will begin to be indistinguishable from incapacity to participate in rational decision-making about treatment, and the principles and proposals of Chapter 7 would then become relevant.)

FIRING THE EXTREMELY NONCOOPERATIVE PATIENT

Suppose Jack Jones, an intelligent, 40-year-old lawyer in excellent health, is a patient of Dr. Clara Lewis. Jack has a deteriorating tooth for which the treatment of choice is endodontic therapy with a post and crown restoration. In repeated conversations with Jack, Dr. Lewis has explained why this is the treatment of choice for a man of Jack's age and with his other health characteristics. But Jack has repeatedly refused endodontic therapy, though not out of any evident pattern of excessive fear, such as was observed in Roger Vianni in the Case in Chapter 4. Jack claims instead that he is opposed to having "dead things" in his mouth. If the tooth needs to be devitalized, he claims, then it should be removed. It should be replaced by an implant or with a fixed bridge, both of which he describes as "proper artifacts, not dead tissue."

Dr. Lewis could perform an extraction and either of the requested procedures to fill the space. But she would consider it a serious violation of her philosophy of practice to do so under these circumstances. If there were serious financial reasons for refusing endodontic therapy, Dr. Lewis would at least consider a clinically less appropriate alternative that was within the patient's means. Or if there were some other benefit to be gained by the patient, for example, the establishment of a long-term treatment relationship for a patient who previously had none (as was mentioned in Chapter 5), then Dr. Lewis might choose to violate one element of her philosophy of practice for the sake of another. But in the circumstances at hand, Dr. Lewis is being asked to violate her philosophy of dental practice for no good reason at all.

Here the patient's noncooperation does not involve obnoxious behavior. It is of the sort that one would expect would be changeable through simple education. But in the case at hand, education does not change the patient's stance. May Dr. Lewis "fire" this patient, decline to treat him further in her practice, in order to preserve the integrity of her commitment to her own carefully considered philosophy of dental practice?

It is essential that Dr. Lewis provide Mr. Jones with whatever emergency treatment he needs. If he is in pain, for example, Dr. Lewis must provide pain relief and other appropriate temporizing treatment if Mr. Jones will accept it independently of the extraction he wants. But with the proviso that emergency treatment must always be provided for, we believe that Dr. Lewis would be professionally-ethically justified in sending Mr. Jones away from her practice. Since Mr. Jones will need treatment soon in any case, Dr. Lewis should provide him with the names of other practitioners whom she respects, perhaps in this example the names of several oral surgeons and prosthodontists. By doing this she fulfills her obligation to preserve this patient's oral and general health, even as she preserves the integrity of her commitment to her own professional philosophy.

Suppose Mr. Jones' lack of cooperation was of a different sort. Suppose that, after a year of careful instruction by Dr. Lewis about how to care properly for dentition at increasing risk of severe periodontal involvement, Mr. Jones still demonstrated no sign whatsoever of even minimally adequate self-care. Here again, it is important that Dr. Lewis would have made extensive efforts at education and at motivating Mr. Jones to act on what was being taught. For it is by doing so that she fulfills her obligation to try to preserve this patient's oral and general health. Doing so may involve some sacrifice of comfort and convenience, as has been noted, but that may be necessary to fulfill Dr. Lewis' basic obligation to attend to Mr. Jones oral and general health.

But with the proviso of Dr. Lewis having made such efforts at educating and motivating Mr. Jones, and the proviso again that any emergency treatment needed by Mr. Jones be offered, we believe that Dr. Lewis would not be acting unprofessionally to ask Mr. Jones to seek treatment elsewhere. In this sort of case, Dr. Lewis' philosophy of dental practice is implicitly involved, insofar as she is a dentist who far prefers to practice in an interactive and collaborative relationship with her patients. But the burden on Dr. Lewis in this version of Mr. Jones' case is more the burden of additional effort and the affective burden of frustration and other negative feelings associated with one's careful professional advice being simply ignored. When the dentist has made appropriate sacrifices for the sake of the patient's well-being, even burdens of this sort may be sufficiently heavy to justify severing the relationship.

It is worth noting, by the way, that dentists dealing with uncooperative patients are often tempted to *threaten* to sever the relationship when they believe it is a relationship that the patient values as a way of motivating the patient to cooperate. Such threats may sometimes be useful educationally in bringing a patient to see that this valued relationship is at stake in the matter at hand. But threats are very often difficult to justify morally, even under the best of circumstances, because they are often coercive and would ordinarily not be thought of as likely to be effective unless they were coercive. They are thus almost always in direct conflict with respect for patients' autonomy and with efforts to develop as interactive a relationship with each patient as is possible. Thus within dental professional morality and within morality in the larger sense, threats should always be viewed as morally suspect.

In addition, a dentist should not threaten to sever a relationship with a patient that he or she cannot professionally-ethically sever if the patient does persist in being noncooperative. To do otherwise is to say to the patient that the dentist is willing to preserve his or her philosophy of professional practice or else to avoid the burden of excessive sacrifice for the sake of the patient. The first of these positions is incoherent, and neither of them is professionally defensible. Patients should be fired, if at all, only for ethically sound reasons, and not because a patient failed to respond to an ill-conceived threat.

THINKING ABOUT THE CASE

It seems clear that Dr. Silverman did well. But does that mean that Dr. Samuels acted unethically in the way he dealt with Jonathan Levinson before referring him to Dr. Silverman? The answer to this question is complex, and some parts of it depend on facts not available in the present case, especially facts about Dr. Samuels' previous efforts to develop his skills for dealing with difficult patients.

First, if Dr. Samuels had not acted conscientiously and to the best of his ability to apply whatever skills he had for establishing a cooperative relationship with Jonathan, that would have been professionally unethical. But let us suppose that Dr. Samuels did act conscientiously and to the best of his ability. Then the question is whether his skills were up to the task. Was he making enough progress toward establishing such a relationship with this patient, or were his skills falling short? If the former, then he could justifiably continue to pursue the relationship. If the latter, then he would be obligated to propose that Jonathan (and his parents) consider a different care giver.

As Dr. Samuels tells the story, it seems clear that he had plenty of time and data, over the course of 4 years, to recognize that he was not making much progress in establishing an appropriate relationship with Jonathan. He could conceivably have thought that Jonathan was the sort of patient that no dentist could bring into a cooperative relationship, so referral would be pointless. But reaching that conclusion would require that Dr. Samuels believe that his own skills in such matters were of the highest caliber, a judgment that would most certainly be unjustified and would raise questions about Dr. Samuels' willingness to obtain adequate information about such skills in the first place.

That is, Dr. Samuels ought to have proposed referral to a more skilled dentist long before Jonathan's parents took the initiative on their own. He is to be commended for sincerely supporting the change and providing a detailed history of his relationship with Jonathan to Dr. Silverman in a balanced and caring manner. But he ought to have referred this case to someone like Dr. Silverman long before. (Or, alternately, his ability to judge when a situation exceeds his skill level in such matters has become unacceptably inept, and he is at professional fault for not making, or not being able to make, the judgments that would have led to a more timely referral.)

Jonathan's current oral and general health do not seem to have suffered from Dr. Samuels' lapse. In addition, Dr. Silverman's skills seem up to correcting most of the damage that Dr. Samuels' failures might have done to Jonathan's long-term ability to trust and relate collaboratively to health care providers, as well as his developing ability to take personal charge of his health and other matters, that is, his developing capacity for autonomy. But Dr. Samuels deserves no credit for Dr. Silverman's skills, since Dr. Samuels did not initiate the referral. It appears, in fact, that Dr. Samuels would have allowed the unacceptable relationship to continue, in spite of the risk to Jonathan's long-term relationships to the health care community and in spite of the potential damage to, or at least his failure to actively support, Jonathan's developing capacity for autonomy.

Thus Dr. Samuels is guilty of placing Jonathan at some risk regarding his future health and of not supporting Jonathan's growth in autonomy in the present. But assuming Dr. Samuels' ability to practice competently was not impaired by Jonathan's behavior, he did not place Jonathan at present risk with regard to the highest ranking central values of oral and general health. In sum, he was professionally at fault for continuing a relationship that he did not have the skill to handle and for some negative impact of that action on Jonathan. But he acted properly in treating the young man in a technically competent manner throughout and in supporting the referral when it was initiated.

Second, a question must be asked about Dr. Samuels' skill level itself. One reading of the case would be that he has acted unprofessionally in not developing a better set of skills for dealing with uncooperative patients, especially pediatric patients. Responding to fear and anxiety with explanations and lectures is of uncertain effectiveness with the average uncooperative adult; it is obviously the wrong approach with a 4- or 5-year-old. So one might find Dr. Samuels at serious professional fault for not enhancing his skills in this arena, at least so long as he intends to take pediatric patients into his general dentistry practice.

While we agree that Dr. Samuels has a professional obligation to improve his skills for communicating with and responding to the fears and anxieties of his patients, especially his pediatric patients, there is a subtle point about this case that deserves attention and that might lessen the degree of Dr. Samuels' failure when it is taken into account. This concerns the diverse range of backgrounds of dental patients in the culture of contemporary America. Most elderly patients and many adult patients in their middle years were raised to simply trust and follow the directions of health professionals. Even when they find it difficult to be cooperative, they view such behavior as unacceptable and are often eager to be guided toward an alternative relationship. Many of these patients are also still very much in awe of the position of health professionals, entrusted as they are with fiduciary responsibilities that pertain to life, health, freedom from pain, and other important human values.

But there have been important shifts in the health care system as a whole and within dental care in particular in the last two decades, shifts toward a much greater emphasis on patients' participation in treatment decisions, and toward viewing the ideal relationship between patient and provider to be an interactive one. This has affected many adult patients, and especially younger adults and children, to a significant degree. The adults seek to participate in treatment decisions, to be adequately informed so that they may do so, and to be treated as peers of the dentist, not in understanding of dental care, but as moral peers and coequal partners in the decision-making process. The perspectives of pediatric patients are not the same as those of adults, but they have been materially affected by these and other social changes as well.

In addition, as the American economy has shifted from being a production-oriented economy to a service-oriented economy, a much larger percentage of the population than in previous generations occupy positions of fiduciary responsibility that pertain to important human values and activities. It is unlikely that patients will hold health professionals in great awe because of their special fiduciary role when the patients have similar roles themselves. This shift in many adults' view of health care professionals has also affected relationships with pediatric patients. Both shifts have had their impact on how a dentist can most effectively deal with a patient who is uncooperative.

These factors mean that many dentists, trained to provide dental care for a population that does not exist in the same form any longer, need to change their approach to patients and develop new communication and negotiation skills to deal with a changed population. One could easily conceive that Dr. Samuels' skill level was quite adequate for children of a different era, and that he has only fairly recently found himself at a loss about how to deal with today's adults and especially their children. Under such circumstances, Dr. Samuels might not be so seriously at fault for not yet undertaking the retraining that he needs, provided he learns from patients like Jonathan Levinson that he must undertake it now.

It might well be that if you go back 30 or 40 years, you would have to say that patients' autonomy was not even one of dentistry's central values in those days and that the ideal relationship between dentist and patient was not an interactive relationship, but one much closer to the Guild Model described—and rejected—in Chapter 4. It might well be that if you examined the ongoing dialogue between the dental profession and the larger community 30 or 40 years ago, the norm of integrity and education required above all that a dentist communicate to patients that dentists have the answers to their health care needs and that the community need only cooperate passively with their direction to receive the benefits of their dedication to people's health.

We have proposed, however, that examination of the contents of that dialogue today reveals that autonomy *is* one of the central values of dental practice today and that the ideal relationship toward which all dentists ought to strive today is an *interactive* relationship between dentist and patient. Today what the norm of integrity and education requires is that dentists demonstrate, in their words and in their conduct, a commitment to all the central values, including patient autonomy, and to the ideal of an interactive relationship and to educating and motivating patients at the affective level to learn enough about their dentition for effective self-care and to take initiative both in self-care and in working collaboratively with the dentist at chairside. This norm also requires that, whatever special skills a dentist needs to guide patients effectively in these respects, every dentist is obligated to acquire them and to regularly examine their adequacy.

CHAPTER 9

Bad Outcomes and Bad Work

Case: Dr. Singer's Vacation

Sandra Stuart, a 36-year-old corporate loan officer for a large bank, is experiencing discomfort in the area of a three-unit bridge placed 8 weeks ago by Dr. Frances Singer. Ms. Stuart calls Dr. Singer's office and learns from a recorded message that Dr. Singer is on vacation and that her calls are being taken by another dentist whose phone number is provided. But there is no answer at that number, and no recorded message either, so Sandra opens the telephone book and calls the first female dentist she finds, Maria Alverez, DMD.

On examination, Dr. Alverez finds that the bridge is loose, as Ms. Stuart had said over the telephone, and that it also has open margins. The gingiva are inflamed both in the area of the abutment teeth and in the pontic area, but there is no inflammation anywhere else in the mouth. She asks Ms. Stuart, "Was this bridge permanently or temporarily cemented? Do you know?"

"I had a temporary bridge in there while this was being made," says Ms. Stuart. "When Dr. Singer put it in, it was my understanding that I did not need to come back about it unless it gave me problems, and up until a week ago it didn't. She certainly didn't tell me it was temporary, and I've paid for it completely."

"Then she almost certainly intended it to be permanent," says Dr. Alverez.

"Is that a problem?" asks Ms. Stuart.

"Sometimes a dentist will cement a new bridge in temporarily to see if there are any problems with it before cementing it permanently. It depends on how the dentist wants to handle it, and both approaches are acceptable. So there is no problem in Dr. Singer's having cemented it permanently. That is one of the standard ways of proceeding."

"But why is it moving around? If she intended it to be permanent, why is it loose?" asks Ms. Stuart. "And why am I feeling soreness right in the same spot?"

"The gum tissue is inflamed along that whole section," says Dr. Alverez. "It's very possible that it's the bridge that is causing the inflammation, especially since you do not have any gum inflammation elsewhere in your mouth. I would like to remove the bridge to see if I can figure out what is going on there, if that would be acceptable. I can recement it, permanently or temporarily, depending on what I find when I am done. Would that be all right?"

"Yes, please do whatever you think will help," says Ms. Stuart. "I have been avoiding chewing on that side for nearly a week and I really want it fixed. Does it look like it was incorrectly made?"

"A lot goes into making a three-unit bridge," says Dr. Alverez. "At first look, I think some adjustment of the bridge may help avoid the inflammation. I think it would be better if it fit snugger under the gum tissue. That may seem strange, but the gums actually get irritated when there is a gap between the bottom of the bridge and the gum tissue, and they are much happier when there is no gap. It is possible that I may be able to adjust that for you right here this afternoon; it is also possible that I may not. First, I need to remove the bridge and see how it is fitted onto the teeth that are holding it in place, in case the irritation or mobility are coming from some cause I haven't seen yet."

"That's fine," says Ms. Stuart, "go right ahead."

Dr. Alverez removes the bridge and quickly determines that the preparations are nonretentive, conical instead of parallel, possibly over-prepared, and the anterior abutment seems too short. It seems very likely that Dr. Singer did not do a very good job on this bridge. It was probably fabricated at a lab rather than in Dr. Singer's office. But even if the fault is in the laboratory fabrication, still if Dr. Singer cemented in an inadequate bridge, the responsibility is hers, and there's certainly no blaming the lab for inadequate preparations. What should Dr. Alverez do about it? Should she tell Ms. Stuart outright that Dr. Singer made a bad bridge? And what should she do clinically, regardless of what she says about Dr. Singer? Dr. Alverez decides to first find out if Ms. Stuart has been told anything more about the bridge than what she has already said. "Did Dr. Singer say anything more or give you any special instructions about the bridge?" asks Dr. Alverez.

"Well, she did talk to me about brushing carefully in that area and flossing regularly. I didn't use floss before, but I've been brushing faithfully since I was a kid. So I started brushing in that area more carefully and flossing, too. I don't think I did anything to disturb the bridge though; it just started feeling like it was moving around one day, and pretty soon it started feeling sore there, too. Could I have done something to cause the problem?" asks Ms. Stuart.

This is as good an opening as Dr. Alverez is likely to get if she wants to get Dr. Singer off the hook. Should she take it, finding some way to make the problem appear to be with Ms. Stuart's self-care? Should she just recement the bridge temporarily and tell Ms. Stuart to chew carefully for another 10 days until Dr. Singer returns? Should she try to reach Dr. Singer to discuss the case before taking action? What ought Dr. Alverez do?

APPLYING PROFESSIONAL NORMS TO BAD OUTCOMES

Just as everything about a profession depends on its ethical commitments, so everything about a profession depends on its expertise, which is demonstrated in the ability of its members to dependably produce good outcomes. As a consequence, when a bad outcome occurs, determining what ought to be done about it can be very difficult. It is difficult enough when a dentist's own work has a bad outcome. It is even more difficult when the bad outcome is of another dentist's work.

All eight categories of the norms of the dental profession are relevant to determining how dentists ought to act when they are faced with another dentist's bad outcome. The most obvious category for such a situation might seem to be *ideal relationships between professionals* because two practitioners are involved, and the bad outcome complicates their relationship to each other and to the patient. But because a patient is also involved, the categories of the *central values* and the *ideal relationship between dentist and patient* are just as significant. The most important of the central values in such a case will be the patient's *oral and general health,* followed by the patient's *autonomy.* The patient's oral health is important in terms of the seriousness of the bad outcome and its correction. It is also important insofar as the "second dentist"—that is, the one who concludes that another dentist, the "first dentist," has had a bad outcome—may need to provide the patient with emergency treatment, specialty treatment, or continuing treatment as the patient's general dentist, depending on the circumstances. The patient's autonomy is important because both dentists must figure out how to deal with the patient in a manner properly respectful of his or her autonomy in a difficult situation. In a similar way, both dentists are obligated to develop as interactive a relationship with the patient as possible, an effort complicated by the fact that two dentist-patient relationships are involved.

The category of *relationship between dentistry and the larger community* is involved in such a situation because of the dental profession's commitment to the larger community that it will supervise its members' practice so that the profession's expertise is not used in such a way as to harm patients. The profession fulfills this obligation partly by making sure that dental school programs graduate well-trained practitioners, by requiring practitioners to maintain and improve their skills through continuing education, and to some extent by educating the public about good practitioners. But when a bad outcome occurs, another side of the profession's supervisory role comes into play. For the second dentist, and then possibly appropriate bodies within dental organizations, must determine whether the bad outcome is the result of bad work by the first dentist and, if so, whether the bad work is symptomatic of a potentially harmful pattern on the part of the first dentist, and what sort of response is then appropriate. The larger community would certainly judge the dental profession to have failed in its obligations if the dental profession and its individual members did not raise these questions and then follow through with appropriate action if a bad outcome has occurred.

Obviously, the norm of *competence* is involved. It applies to the first dentist, who may have tried to practice beyond his or her competence, or who may have been competent to practice in the manner appropriate to the patient's clinical situation, but who failed to carry it out, or who may have practiced in a fully competent manner but had a bad outcome occur in spite of this. The norm of competence also applies to the second dentist, who will have to determine whether the bad outcome is the result of the first dentist's failure to practice competently, how serious the bad outcome is, whether it is part of a pattern of bad work, and so on. In addition, the second dentist must provide competent treatment of whatever sort the circumstances of the case indicate. This may be emergency care, specialty treatment if the second dentist is a specialist receiving the patient for that purpose, temporary care for the condition resulting from the bad outcome, continuing general dental care, or ongoing care if the second dentist is the patient's new general dentist of choice.

The norm of the *chief client* is relevant here because cases of this sort remind the dental community that no patient is simply a patient of one dentist. Every patient is, in a certain way, a patient of every dentist and of the whole dental profession, not only because of public health and public education considerations and the potential need to provide emergency care to those who need it but also in exercising the supervisory role of the whole profession by noting and responding correctly to bad outcomes and especially to serious or continual bad work.

The relevance of the norm of *integrity and education* is difficult to summarize, but will play an important role in several of the discussions that follow. The norm of the *relative priority of the patient's well-being*, or the norm of how much sacrifice of other interests is required, is involved insofar as the second dentist must determine how much of his or her time and effort are owed to the patient with the bad outcome, how much are owed to the first dentist, and at the sacrifice of what other interests. This norm is also involved for the first dentist, who must determine what, if anything, he or she owes the patient who has experienced the bad outcome.

WHEN THE PATIENT IS ANOTHER DENTIST'S PATIENT

The situations in which a dentist observes another dentist's bad outcome can be divided into two groups: (1) those in which the patient is chiefly another dentist's patient, and (2) those in which the patient is either returning to a general dentist after emergency or specialty care or is visiting a new dentist for the first time, presenting the work of previous dentists to him or her for examination. In the latter group, the second dentist—the one identifying the bad outcome—is the patient's regular dentist or is being considered for that role by the patient. In the first group, the patient's chief relationship is with the first dentist rather than the second dentist, or the one who determines the bad outcome. This raises even more complex professional-ethical issues than we find in the other group. For in the first group, the second dentist must treat the patient as the *first* dentist's patient in every respect except the patient's need for emergency care or for specialty care. This and the next four sections will focus on this situation. Situations in the second group will be examined after that.

Most dentists see other dentists' patients when the patients present for emergency treatment they think they need, or when patients present to a specialist for specialty treatment. In both cases, there is an accepted set of obligations regarding the relationship between the three parties. The ADA's *Principles of Ethics and Code of Professional Conduct* expresses one part of this obligation very well: "If [emergency] treatment is provided, the dentist, upon completion of such treatment, is obliged to return the patient to his or her regular dentist unless the patient expressly reveals a different preference." (1-D) "....The specialist or consulting dentists upon completion of their care shall return the patient, unless the patient expressly reveals a different preference, to the referring dentist, or if none, to the dentist of record for future care." (1-E).

The second dentist is to treat the patient as the first dentist's patient in other respects as well. He or she must not only return the patient to the first dentist when emergency or specialty care is concluded, unless the patient expresses a different intention. The second dentist must also actively work to support the relationship between the patient and the first dentist. A subsequent comment in the ADA's *Principles*, that the second dentist should not make "disparaging comments about prior services" (1-G), identifies the bare minimum of such support. The second dentist should also encourage the patient to visit the first dentist for needed follow-up care and to communicate with the first dentist about the contact with the second dentist. The second dentist should also encourage the patient to develop appropriate programs of self-care and to schedule regular visits to the first dentist. The second dentist also ordinarily reports to the first about treatment given, conditions observed, and so on.

This obligation of the second dentist to support the patient's relationship with the first dentist is not just a bit of mutually self-serving professional etiquette. There are sound professional-ethical reasons for this requirement. First, the central values of the patient's oral and general health are better served through continuity of care by a single general dentist. Second, the central value of autonomy is respected by supporting the patient's choice of a primary dental care-giver and the plan of care that the patient and the primary dentist have worked out. Third, the goal of achieving as interactive a relationship as possible is supported by efforts to maintain and strengthen the patient's established relationship with his or her general dentist, as well as making the relationship with the second dentist as interactive as possible within its limited scope.

But the presence of a bad outcome complicates this situation because the achievement of each of these three benefits for the patient is put into question. First, we would not consider an outcome bad if it did not involve the absence or failure of a needed dental treatment or put the patient's oral or general health at some risk. Second, the patient's choice of a plan of care surely would not include choosing a bad outcome, as such. Of course, in such a situation the patient may have been fully informed of the possibility of bad outcomes by the first dentist and may have consciously chosen the treatment with this risk in mind. A few moments of conversation with the patient will usually reveal if this is the case. When it is, the bad outcome involves no direct conflict with respect for the patient's autonomy. But when it is not, then something has happened that the patient has not chosen, and a subtle question arises about how each dentist is to properly respect the patient's autonomy in what follows. Concern with supporting and enhancing interactive relationships with the patient, both for the second dentist and for the first, raises the same questions. The point is not that the occurrence of an unchosen bad outcome automatically terminates the patient's relationship with the first dentist. That is not the case. But the occurrence of the bad outcome complicates the effort to properly respect the patient's autonomy and work for interactive relationships.

The second dentist's first effort should be to maintain and strengthen the patient's relationship with the first dentist, for the reasons given, unless doing so is in fact in serious conflict with achieving these benefits for the patient. To determine whether this is so, the second dentist must determine early on, as clearly as he or she can, whether the bad outcome is also an instance of the first dentist's bad work and, if it is, then determine how serious this bad work is.

Some dentists will immediately say: "You never know for sure; you never have all the facts." They conclude, therefore, that the second dentist is never able to legitimately judge that the first dentist did bad work.

It is true that absolute certainty about the causes of things is rarer than might first appear, sometimes even for eye witnesses, but especially when time has passed and one of the crucial players is not available. But it is also true that many situations of life provide us with enough evidence about the causes of things, even at a distance and with some points of view not represented, that a reasonable person is justified in forming a judgment about the matter on the evidence available and then in taking action on the basis of that judgment. Even though other explanations are conceivable, sometimes the evidence available is strong enough to render those explanations too unlikely and to lead a reasonable person to judge that an error in judgment or technique or communication on the part of the another person has taken place. While there are good reasons, as will be explained, for giving the first dentist some benefit of the doubt, it would be intellectually dishonest to hold that the evidence of bad work can never outweigh it. In sum, while you may never know all the facts, sometimes you know enough that you must judge that a bad outcome is the result of another dentist's bad work.

It is unfortunate that the two phrases *bad outcome* and *bad work* sound so much alike. The word *bad* in the first phrase refers to the well-being of the patient. A bad outcome is an outcome that fails to accomplish some benefit of treatment for the patient or possibly involves some harm or risk of harm to the patient's oral or general health. The same word, *bad*, in the second phrase refers to the minimal standards of dental care. Bad work is a diagnosis or treatment or communication with the patient that falls below the standards developed and practiced within the dental profession.

It is important to stress that not all bad outcomes are bad work, because the standard of judgment is different. But in contemporary society and in many dentists' conversations with patients, the distinction between the two ideas is often overlooked. Most dentists prefer to speak very little to their patients about the possibility of bad outcomes because they do not want their patients to think they do bad work.

The conflation of these two ideas is a serious malady of contemporary culture. A widely accepted myth of contemporary society holds that the techniques and technologies of contemporary health care are as infallible as the science that has developed them. (It is part of this myth to ignore the fact that all our techniques and technologies, and even "infallible" science itself, are the work of fallible scientists and other fallible human beings, rather than coming from some truly infallible source.) This myth has enhanced the status of physicians and dentists who employ these techniques and technologies to address patients' ills. But it has also shaped patients' trust and expectations to accept the dubious corollary of the myth, namely, that all bad outcomes must be the product of human error, that is, they must be bad work. In such an environment, it is not surprising that dentists don't talk to their patients very much about bad outcomes.

But every dentist knows that even the most expert dentist practicing the most carefully on a textbook mouth of a fully cooperative patient can still have a bad outcome. The myth and its corollary are false. A bad outcome is not necessarily a sign of bad work.

To judge whether a particular bad outcome is an instance of bad work, the second dentist needs information. In some instances, the bad outcome

involves dental work that is physically defective, like the nonretentive preparations and the poor marginal fit of the bridge in the case at the beginning of
this chapter. But often the second dentist will have to make a judgment on
the basis of physical evidence that is less clear. When a patient presents with
significant periodontal disease, for example, the patient may state that the first
dentist never informed the patient first of incipient, and then continuing, periodontal involvement. This may be a defect in the patient's memory, or in the
patient's attention to the dentist's words, or in the patient's comprehension of
those words, and so on. In addition, some bad outcomes occur without anyone
being at fault because of the limits of human knowledge and human technology in the face of complicated natural processes.

The second dentist cannot justifiably conclude that a bad outcome probably is, or is not, the result of bad work without careful consideration of the
clinical facts, the patient's comments about the situation, and the evidence
available that the patient understood the first dentist's comments correctly.
Even then, however, the most that the second dentist will ordinarily be able
to conclude without obtaining information from the first dentist about the
clinical circumstances in which he or she operated is that the bad outcome
probably is, or *probably* is not, an instance of bad work. The separate question
whether the second dentist may, or ought to, communicate such a judgment
to the patient will be examined shortly.

Most dentists ordinarily give another dentist the benefit of the doubt even
when there is considerable evidence that a bad outcome is the result of bad
work. This may appear to be mere professional face-saving or an example of
inappropriate loyalty. For giving the benefit of the doubt in such a matter
may appear contrary to the dental profession's obligation to the larger community to watch for and eliminate avoidable bad work as much as possible.

But, in fact, there are two good reasons for presuming that another dentist
has attempted to do good work, in spite of the bad outcome that has resulted.
First, there are many possible explanations for most bad outcomes that do
not involve errors by the first dentist. If there is not very strong evidence of
bad work in the clinical facts and the patient's reports, it is more likely than
not that no bad work was involved. Second, the dental profession's training
programs are fairly carefully monitored to assure the larger community that
when new dentists are licensed, they have the knowledge and skills they need
to practice capably, and continual practice ordinarily enhances dental expertise rather than weakening it. So, other things being equal, it is far more likely
than not that a given dentist will respond correctly to any given situation.

Nevertheless, situations will arise in which the second dentist must conclude that a bad outcome is probably the result of the first dentist's errors in
judgment, technique, or communication with the patient. Other situations
will arise in which the evidence in this direction is not conclusive but is still
strong enough to outweigh the benefit of the doubt in favor of the first dentist.
About such a case, the dentist would have to conclude that bad work might be
involved, but the evidence does not resolve the question either way.

THREE SITUATIONS

How should a dentist respond to the following three kinds of situations: (1)
situations in which the second dentist judges bad work probably is not

involved, (2) situations in which the question of bad work cannot be resolved from the evidence available in the clinical facts and the patient's reports, and (3) situations in which the dentist judges on the basis of this evidence that bad work probably is involved?

The dentist is clearly obligated, in all of these situations, as the ADA's *Principles* puts it, to inform the patient of his or her "present oral health status" (1-G). This obligation derives from the central values of oral and general health, and from the value of autonomy, and also from the ideal of an interactive relationship between dentist (either of them) and patient. For all these bases of professional obligation require that capable patients receive sufficient accurate information about their oral condition that they can make appropriate—and, it is hoped, interactive—decisions about it. (This chapter will limit its discussion to patients who are capable of participating in treatment decisions. See Chapter 7 for the discussion of dental care of persons not capable of participating or having only diminished capacity. Obviously, bad outcomes and instances of bad work are likely to raise even more complex questions in the care of these patients than they do for patients who are capable.)

Describing a patient's "present oral health status" necessarily includes describing the facts of the bad outcome, and the dentist's professional obligations clearly require the second dentist to do this. In addition, there are no reasons based in the dentist's professional commitments that could override this requirement. The second dentist does have obligations to the first dentist as a co-professional. But even if these include an obligation to protect the co-professional from certain kinds of harm, the values at stake for the patient take priority over those at stake for the co-professional in this situation.

To consider another possible argument, if the second dentist is obligated to act in ways that support the first dentist's relationship with the patient, might not the second dentist sometimes do this most effectively by not mentioning the bad outcome at all, when the patient is not aware of it, or by leading the patient to believe that it is less important to oral health and function than it is, in order to let the first dentist deal with the bad outcome within his or her own relationship to the patient? Would not this be a legitimate way, and sometimes the best way, of supporting the patient's relationship with the first dentist?

Here the ethical complexity of the second dentist's situation becomes clear. For the second dentist is not simply the agent of the first dentist; the second dentist has a relationship with the patient as well. So the dental profession's requirement to respect the patient's autonomy applies to the second dentist, as does the obligation to work for as interactive a relationship as possible with the patient regarding those matters that the second dentist and the patient decide together. Consequently, the second dentist may not violate the patient's autonomy or accept an alternate kind of relationship with the patient for the sake of the first dentist's relationship. This is another way in which the norm of the *relative priority of the patient's well-being* applies here. The patient's autonomy and the present dentist's relationship to the patient take precedence over the first dentist's relationship when these come in conflict, even though the second dentist is obligated to support the first dentist's relationship with the patient in every way in which no such conflict occurs.

In a former era, in which the Guild Model of dentist-patient relationship seems to have had much more normative force in U.S. society, it might not have been professionally inappropriate to refrain from fully informing a patient about a bad outcome so that the first dentist could do so in the context of that dentist-patient relationship. But, as has been stressed at several points, there is no question that the understanding of dental professionals' obligations in today's on-going dialogue between the dental community and the community at large is that the patient's autonomy and working for an interactive relationship with the patient take precedence over all other competing considerations except direct risk to the patient's oral and general health.

In all three situations, then, the dentist is obligated to inform the patient about the condition of his or her mouth, including an accurate description of the facts of the bad outcome. But this conclusion does not imply anything yet about what more the second dentist may or may not say or ought or ought not say about the role of the first dentist in regard to the bad outcome.

There are two different sets of circumstances and several different ethical questions to be distinguished here. First, the patient may ask the second dentist whether the bad outcome is the result of the first dentist's bad work. Under what conditions is the second dentist professionally obligated to respond to this question by saying that the bad outcome probably is the result of the first dentist's bad work? Are there any other circumstances in which the second dentist *may* ethically say this, even if not professionally obligated to do so?

Second, even though provided with accurate information about the condition of his or her mouth, the patient still might not ask about the role of the first dentist. Are there any circumstances in which the second dentist is nevertheless required to broach the subject and offer a judgment about the first dentist's role? Are there any other circumstances in which the second dentist *may* do so even if it is not professionally required? This last pair of questions will be examined below in the section entitled "When the Patient Doesn't Ask."

Let us suppose that the patient directly asks the second dentist for his or her judgment about the first dentist's role regarding the bad outcome. How ought the second dentist deal with this question? We begin with the third kind of situation because it is the most difficult.

IF THE PATIENT ASKS IN THE THIRD SITUATION

The third situation is the one in which the second dentist judges on the basis of the clinical evidence and the patient's reports that bad work probably is involved. It will shortly prove necessary to make two further distinctions about this situation that will divide it into four subcategories. But we should first examine the strongest reasons for holding that the dentist in this situation should always answer the patient's question truthfully and accurately according to his or her best judgment.

First, as has already been noted, the central values of the patient's general and oral health and the patient's autonomy, and the obligation to work for as interactive a relationship with the patient as possible all argue for the dentist to inform the patient fully of the facts that the patient needs for treatment decisions. The second dentist's judgment regarding the role of the first dentist in relation to the bad outcome would seem to be one of these facts, so a judgment by the second dentist about the role of the first dentist would seem to be required.

Second, every dentist has an obligation to carry out the dental profession's commitments to the larger community that the actions of individual dentists, though regulated and supervised only by members of the profession, will nevertheless serve patients' well-being, both technically and ethically. A dentist who refrains from accurately answering patients' questions about a first dentist's role in a bad outcome, when that bad outcome is judged to be a probable instance of bad work, seems to fail in this obligation, both personally and in the name of the whole profession and thus, in some measure, to place the profession's privilege of self-regulation at risk.

Third, the norm of integrity and education requires that dentists' actions be guided by the values that the profession professes. As an expert group, the dental profession professes that its members both always act in accord with clinical facts, and place the well-being of patients ahead of their own (though within certain limits, as noted previously). A dentist who does not accurately answer patients' questions about the causes of a bad outcome, when these are judged to be probable instances of bad work, seems to misrepresent the profession in both respects by setting aside fact and by placing co-professionals' well-being above patients' and thus miseducates the community about what the dental profession stands for.

But these normative considerations apply to different subcategories of this third situation in different ways and lead to different ethical conclusions about them, rather than the generic conclusions that have appeared to follow from them so far. The first distinction to make is between instances of bad work that involve significant potential for future bad work and possibly worse harm to the patient by the first dentist, on the one hand, and instances of bad work that are merely the minor, occasional errors to which all expert practice is inevitably victim, because humans are fallible beings, on the other.

The ADA *Principles* identify the relevant distinction. The dentist must determine whether the first dentist's bad work is an instance of "gross or continual faulty treatment" (1-G) or whether it is only an instance of the occasional and isolated technical errors that the best of professionals inevitably make now and then. Obviously, concluding that a bad outcome is an instance of "continual faulty work" requires evidence from other occasions, and almost always from other patients of the same dentist as well. The judgment that an instance of faulty treatment is "gross" does not require such a body of comparative evidence and is therefore less difficult to make in practice than the judgment of "continual" faulty treatment. The judgment that a bad outcome is probably the result of "gross" faulty treatment is the judgment that the error is so serious or harmful that it must be considered potentially symptomatic of a serious lack of caution or some other deeper problem that the first dentist is not addressing. In both instances, in judging that the bad work is an instance of "gross or continual faulty treatment," the second dentist is also judging that the patient is at some risk of further bad work and possibly longer-term harm if he or she returns to the first dentist.

On the other hand, the dentist who never makes an error in clinical judgment, especially on a close call, and who shapes every restoration, makes every preparation, takes every impression utterly flawlessly is extremely rare, if such a practitioner could be found at all. Most such shortcomings from the theoretical ideal of perfect technical practice do not cause discomfort or harm to patients, or else are brought for adjustment or redoing to the same dentist who was responsible for them. Thus when they occur, they are mostly resolved within a single dentist-patient relationship without the involvement of a second dentist.

Few dentists would fault a dentist who makes an occasional error of this sort, unless the dentist is unconcerned about it, or the error is so serious or harmful that it seems symptomatic of a serious lack of caution or some other deeper problem that the dentist is not addressing ("gross" faulty treatment), or the error is part of a pattern of such errors that the dentist is not address-ing ("continual" faulty treatment), or the dentist fails to deal properly with the patient regarding it. (The question of how a dentist should deal with his or her own bad outcomes and bad work will be discussed later in this chap-ter.) The chief reason that dentists do not fault one another for such a mistake is that patients are not placed at risk of future bad work or possible harm by them. They are truly minor (vs. "gross") and truly occasional (vs. "continual").

The view that dentists rightly take of each other's occasional mistakes is unfortunately countercultural. Just as many people apparently accept the myth of infallible health care technology and technique, so many also seem to assume that flawless human technical behavior is invariably possible. For such people, the only ethical alternative to flawless technical performance by a professional is for the practitioner to withdraw, presumably in favor of a technical performer who is flawless. Such people also assume that the deter-mination whether one can perform flawlessly in a given situation is always clear-cut. Consequently, the distinction between occasional, minor bad work and gross or continual bad work is not widely accepted. But this distinction is crucial to understanding a dentist's professional obligations when he or she judges that another's bad outcome is probably an instance of bad work.

The second distinction needed here operates in the culture of the United States at large, but is most evident in certain kinds of legal settings. It con-cerns the amount of evidence that is needed for a person to proceed reason-ably to action, compared with the amount of evidence needed for a person to publicly offer a negative judgment of another person's conduct, especially in a setting in which relevant expertise appears to be involved. The way in which U.S. society deals with people's negative public judgments of others' conduct, especially in suits for defamation of character and the like, but also in ordi-nary discourse, indicates that, as a society, we believe a great deal of evidence is needed to support a negative public judgment of another's conduct, espe-cially when relevant expertise appears to be involved (rather than the judg-ment appearing to be casual, uninformed, or purely gossip, for example). The amount of evidence required to support such a negative public judgment is considerably greater than is needed to justify a person's course of action of some other sort.

Therefore it is necessary to distinguish situations in which the second den-tist justifiably judges in his or her own mind that the bad outcome is probably an instance of bad work (based on evidence of clinical facts and the patient's reports) from situations in which the evidence is strong enough to support a public negative judgment of the first dentist by the second dentist, for instance, by communicating to the patient that the first dentist probably per-formed bad work. For this communication must indeed be considered a *public* one. Communications from patient to dentist are private and therefore subject to the restrictions of professional confidentiality. But communications from the dentist to the patient may ordinarily be repeated by the patient at will without violation of their relationship to the dentist, so they must be considered public judgments, and it is obvious that professional expertise is involved in them.

Consequently, a greater measure of evidence is needed for the second dentist to tell the patient that the bad outcome has probably resulted from the first dentist's bad work than is necessary for the dentist to conclude privately that this is probably the case. (The authors are not claiming that dentists are under a legal obligation in this regard, but rather that a widely applicable social rule about the amount of evidence needed to publicly judge another's conduct negatively—a rule that is seen most clearly in certain legal contexts, but applies more broadly—is directly relevant to the professional-ethical issue under discussion here.)

The point was argued above that situations do arise in which the second dentist privately judges that bad work probably has occurred, even though some dentists sometimes protest that there is never enough evidence. But the evidence needed for this private judgment is often not sufficient evidence that the dentist would also be justified in communicating *to the patient* that it probably is bad work, because this is a public judgment. In fact, a dentist will frequently lack sufficient evidence to meet this burden of proof unless he or she has communicated about the circumstances of the work with the first dentist, and might lack sufficient data even then unless the communication was careful and detailed. Since most dentists who observe another dentist's bad outcome do not have the opportunity to communicate with the first dentist before speaking about the bad work with the patient, dentists are frequently not in a position to answer a patient's question about whether—in other words, they do not have enough evidence to make a public statement that—in their judgment, the bad outcome is probably the result of the first dentist's bad work.

There is one notable exception to the social rule about the degree of evidence needed for a public negative judgment, especially where expertise is involved, in U.S. society. If a person is called to testify in court, he or she not only may publicly state his or her negative judgment there, but is required to state it, together with the evidence for it, just as it is and without first determining whether the evidence meets the standard under consideration here. The restriction about speaking without sufficient evidence is lifted in this special setting because the judge, jury, and other participants are not only considered capable of evaluating the evidence offered for the witness's judgments for themselves, but are required to do so by their special roles in the court.

Now let us return to the question of how the second dentist ought to deal with a patient's question about the role of the first dentist in relation to a bad outcome when the second dentist's private judgment, justified by the clinical evidence and the patient's reports, is that this probably *is* an instance of bad work. We need to examine each of four subcategories of this situation, one at a time.

In the first subcategory are circumstances in which two things are true: (1)

the evidence available to the dentist is strong enough to support the dentist's private judgment that this is probably bad work, but *not* strong enough to justify a statement to the patient, which is here viewed as a public statement, to this effect because the standard of evidence just discussed is not met, and (2) the dentist's personal judgment is that the bad work probably is *not* an instance of gross or continual faulty treatment. Under these circumstances, if the patient asks, the dentist is *not obligated* to communicate his or her private judgment on the role of the first dentist to the patient. The dentist may instead respond that there is not enough evidence for him or her to judge the matter. This is a truthful and accurate answer, given the standard of evidence relevant to the question, and it therefore conforms to the requirements of the norm of identity and education, as summarized a few paragraphs back. In addition, this answer is consistent with the dentist's obligation to respect the patient's autonomy and work for as interactive a relationship as possible, because the relevant social standard of evidence qualifies the extent of the dentist's obligations under these norms, which are themselves socially constructed, conventional norms.

If the dentist answers in this way, he or she should inform the patient that the standard of evidence required for such a judgment is fairly stringent in order not to mislead the patient into thinking that some lower standard of evidence has not been met, especially the standard one would apply in forming a private judgment of the matter. Moreover, the dentist would certainly be acting unethically if he or she tried to intimate that the inadequacy of the evidence somehow suggests that the first dentist acted properly, since the second dentist's private judgment is that the bad outcome is probably an instance of bad work. Misleading the patient in this way would violate professional integrity and also the second dentist's commitment to an interactive relationship with the patient. But since the patient is not judged to be at risk of continued bad treatment or possible harm from the first dentist, the values of the patient's oral and general health and autonomy, and the requirement that the profession guard against harmful practice are not compromised by such an answer.

A typical answer of this sort, in response to a patient's question under the circumstances of the first subcategory, might sound like this: "That is a very reasonable question, Mr. Jones. Unfortunately, there are many factors involved in a bad outcome of this sort, and a judgment on my part would require fairly strong evidence for me to tell you that the outcome was probably the result of some error on Dr. Smith's part." (As subsequent discussion in this chapter and the next will indicate, we believe that the best resolution of such situations occur when the second dentist can also say, "I would like to call Dr. Smith to tell him what I have seen, and I would recommend that you contact him yourself, at your earliest convenience, so the two of you can work together to deal with what has happened.")

But if the second dentist is not *obligated*, under the circumstances of the first subcategory, to communicate his or her private judgment of probable bad work to the patient, *may* the second dentist do so? Or would that be a violation of professional obligation in some way?

The existence of the social standard of evidence, discussed above, argues against any public negative judgment of the first dentist when that standard of evidence has not been met. There is one professional consideration, however, that might justify telling the patient of one's private judgment about probable bad work even if the evidence did not meet this standard. Suppose the second dentist had good reason to believe that doing so would significantly enhance the patient's well-being, either by producing a significantly better relationship between the patient and the first dentist, or by bringing about a significantly greater realization of the central values for the patient, or something similar. Then the benefits to the patient might justify the second dentist in communicating his or her private judgment to the patient. Under such circumstances, when the second dentist *may* answer the patient's question, even though not obligated, the second dentist would be obligated to make it clear to the patient that the ordinary measure of evidence required for this communication is not available and that the second dentist's judgment is, for that reason, less certain than it would be if the ordinary standard for evidence had been met. The point to stress here, the authors propose, is that the only consideration that can justify a dentist's communicating his or her private judgment to the patient under the circumstances of the first subcategory is a significant contribution to the well-being of the patient. It is hard to imagine any other justifiable reason for such an action.

In the second subcategory are circumstances in which (1) the evidence available to the dentist is again *not* strong enough to justify a public judgment (in other words, communication to the patient) that the bad outcome is probably an instance of bad work, but (2) the dentist's judgment is that the bad work probably *is* an instance of "gross or continual faulty treatment." Under these circumstances, if the patient asks, the dentist's answer must again communicate that the evidence available does not pass the threshold ordinarily required for him or her to make a public judgment on the matter. But in this situation, we propose, because of the risk to the patient, the dentist must do two additional things.

First, the dentist must indicate to the patient that, although the evidence is limited, what it suggests is that the patient may be at risk of future bad work or harm. It will be a very subtle matter to communicate to a patient both that the outcome is a serious matter ("gross or continual") and that the evidence is very limited, so that this is only a "possible" or at most "probable" conclusion, rather than something that the second dentist is sure of. (Remember that in the second subcategory, the dentist does not have enough evidence to meet the standard of evidence for a public negative judgment, especially since expertise is clearly involved.) But the genuine risk of future bad work or harm for the patient (evidenced by the probable presence of "gross or continual faulty treatment") requires that the second dentist inform the patient about this risk, and in fact inform the patient about it whether he or she asks about it or not. To fail to do so would be a violation of the dentist's professional obligations to preserve and enhance the patient's oral and general health, to play a part in the dental profession's supervisory activity to prevent inadequate practice, and to respect patient autonomy.

Second, as the ADA *Principles* indicate, the dentist must report the probable instance of gross or continual faulty treatment "to the appropriate reviewing agency as determined by the local component or constituent [dental] society" (1-G). For if something is probably an instance of gross or continual bad work, then the patient is at risk of further bad work and possibly harm in the hands of the first dentist, and other patients of the first dentist are at potential risk as well. The dentist reports the matter to the dental organization because that group is collectively more capable both of determining conclusively if bad work and specifically gross or continual faulty treatment did take place and of taking action, if any is needed, to protect this and other patients of the first dentist from harm.

Occasionally, an individual dentist will have a close enough personal and professional relationship with the first dentist that his or her personal contact with the first dentist will be more effective in protecting this and other patients than reporting to a reviewing agency would be. When this is the case, the dentist may be justified in working for this end without reporting the matter to the appropriate dental organization. For the goal is enhancing and protecting patients' well-being rather than punitive action toward dentists. But feelings of colleagueship and friendship may weaken a dentist's judgment on this matter, so dentists motivated to forego reporting a colleague should test their reasons very carefully before doing so. Failure to act effectively to protect patients from future bad work and possible harm under such circumstances is a serious individual professional wrong and a violation of the profession's commitment to the larger community to make sure that its expertise is properly used.

In the third subcategory are circumstances in which (1) the evidence available to the dentist *is* strong enough to justify a statement to the patient that the bad outcome is an instance of bad work, but (2) the dentist's judgment is that the bad work probably is *not* an instance of "gross or continual" faulty treatment. Under these circumstances, if the patient asks, the dentist cannot justifiably answer that there is not sufficient evidence for him or her to offer a judgment, for this is not true. Professional integrity and the commitment to an interactive relationship with the patient require the second dentist, in these particular circumstances, to explain his or her judgment to the patient, along with the evidence that supports it.

It is important to recall the point made above, however, that a dentist will not often be faced with this decision unless he or she has already communicated with the first dentist about the circumstances of the bad outcome. On those occasions when this set of circumstances does prevail, then, the second dentist will ordinarily have maintained his or her judgment that bad work has occurred either because the first dentist has concurred in that judgment or because the second dentist has concluded, after hearing the comments of the first dentist and concluding contrary to the first dentist's view of his work, that bad work has occurred. In either case, the degree of evidence required for offering his or her judgment to the patient is so great that the ordinary objection of some dentists to telling the patient—namely, that "you never have enough evidence"—will not apply. In addition, if the first dentist concurs in the second dentist's judgment, then the two dentists can work collaboratively with the patient to deal with the situation and determine what should come after it. The general importance of contact between the two dentists when bad outcomes are involved will be discussed below.

It is important to note that since it is *not* probable in this situation that the patient is at risk of additional bad work or possible harm at the hands of the first dentist, the second dentist's obligations to return the patient to the first dentist and to support the first dentist's relationship with the patient remain intact. This may seem an ironic point to make, since a patient who has been informed that the bad outcome is probably the result of the first dentist's bad work might seem more likely to sue the first dentist, or at least leave his or her practice than to enjoy the benefits of a continuing interactive relationship there. But if there has been a good relationship and good communication with the first dentist, then it may still be possible for that relationship to continue productively.

In this connection, there is something else that the second dentist might do, although at some risk because of the cultural environment in which dentistry is practiced in the United States today. The second dentist might try to educate the patient about the difference between bad outcomes and bad work, with special attention to the difference between the occasional, minor bad work that is inevitable in the professional practice of fallible humans and the gross or continual bad work, which is not an element of this subcategory of circumstances, that puts patients at risk. Thus the second dentist might try to inculcate in the patient the same appropriate leniency of judgment regarding occasional, minor mistakes that dentists ordinarily have toward one another. Of course the risk is that the second dentist may then be judged by the patient to be less expert, less dependable, and less professional for having said such things. Yet these are precisely the truths about professional dental practice that could support the relationship between a patient who has experienced a minor, isolated instance of bad work and the conscientious, professional care giver who has made a minor, isolated mistake.

Far better than merely asking individual dentists in difficult circumstances to do this educating would be a strong initiative in this direction by the dental community as a whole. Like the dentist just described, dentistry as a whole would run a risk if it chose to challenge head-on the myth of infallible technology and technique and the myth of infallible performers, and the corollary that all bad outcomes must be the result of bad work. It is doubtful, in fact, that dentistry can undermine these myths alone, but it could take the lead in establishing a broad coalition of health professions to try to undo them.

Until these myths are undone, they will continue to fuel an environment of mutual suspicion between health care providers and their patients, increasing malpractice costs because juries continue to believe these myths, and all the groundless pressures that their sequellae produce for dentists, physicians, and others. If these myths are undone, of course, it is not likely that health professionals' expertise will be held so much in awe as it presently is in this society, with some loss of social status as a likely result and perhaps some change in dentists' (and physicians') level of rewards. It is an interesting question for the health professions whether they would be willing to accept this trade-off.

But such cost-benefit thinking aside, the dental profession's norms of competence and especially integrity and education require it to challenge these myths and to reeducate the society that accepts them. This profession's practice is based on facts, not myths, and these facts include the fallibility of the technologies and techniques its members employ and the fallibility of the members who employ them. The larger community's ability to depend with certainty on the members of this profession does not rest on infallible technologies or infallible performers but on the enduring *ethical* commitment of its members to use its (fallible) expertise for patients' benefit, without exception.

Realistic relationships between dentists and patients ought to be founded on these facts rather than on myths. Within relationships so founded, dentists could inform patients honestly of another dentist's incidental, minor mistake without fear that the latter would suffer grave losses as a result. In that environment, it would not be a source of relief to dentists that the circumstances of this third subcategory are uncommon because the standard of evidence needed for a dentist to tell a patient that another dentist's bad work is involved is not often met. In fact, in that environment, dentists might wish to change the social rules about evidence that govern their communications to patients so that the simple truths about fallible technologies and techniques, and more importantly the simple truths about the relationships of fallible humans working for one another's good, might be more directly communicated and supported.

In the fourth subcategory are circumstances in which (1) the evidence available to the dentist *is* strong enough to justify a statement to the patient that the bad outcome is probably an instance of bad work, and (2) the dentist's judgment is that the bad work probably is an instance of *gross or continual faulty treatment*. Under these circumstances, the dentist again must explain his or her judgment to the patient, along with the evidence that supports it, and must do so whether the patient asks or not because of the probable risk to the patient. The dentist must also report the probable instance of gross or continual faulty treatment to the appropriate reviewing agency.

The reasons for these two actions have already been explained. The likelihood that the first condition will occur is, as has been said, not great. The likelihood that it will occur in conjunction with the second condition, which is also uncommon, is even less. But if these two conditions should ever occur in tandem, the norms of the dental profession require that the actions indicated be taken.

THE FIRST AND SECOND SITUATIONS REVISITED

Now we can return to the first and second situations to ask how the second dentist in each of them should deal with the patient who asks directly about the role of the first dentist in relation to a bad outcome. In the first situation, the second dentist privately judges that the bad outcome probably did *not* result from the first dentist's bad work.

In this situation, the dentist may welcome the patient's question to make the point that the first dentist is probably without fault and to explain his or her reasons for this conclusion. Since our society's rules about evidence do not require evidence for *positive* public judgments of others' actions to meet the same standard as evidence for public negative judgments, the dentist would not be violating standards of evidence to offer his or her positive judgment, even though the forum is still a public one in the sense used above and even though the judgment is likely based on no stronger evidence than would support any other private judgment. In other words, because of the positive content of the judgment, the dentist does not violate professional integrity or other social rules to offer a judgment on only this measure of evidence, although it should be part of the dentist's communication to indicate the measure of evidence that supports his or her judgment and not to intimate that it is more substantial than it is.

In the second situation, the second dentist is not able to determine from the evidence available whether the bad outcome is the result of the first dentist's bad work or not. In this situation, if the patient asks, the dentist is obligated to answer truthfully that he or she is unable to determine the matter. The dentist may be tempted to make this uncertainty sound like evidence that the first dentist probably did not do bad work, but doing so would be a violation of professional integrity and of the dentist's commitment to work for as interactive a relationship with the patient as possible. If the dentist wishes this were an ethical option because the dentist fears that the patient will interpret such uncertainty in the opposite way, for example, as evidence that the first dentist certainly did bad work, the second dentist may ethically counter these mistakes in the patient's judgment, but not by trying to lead the patient to draw incorrect conclusions in the opposite direction.

This moment, if it should arise, might in fact be a good point to try to take up the educational task described above, leading the patient to challenge the myths of infallible technologies and techniques and infallible performers. There is always a minor risk here, however, since the patient may then judge the second dentist less competent, dependable, and professional because of this effort. As was noted, however, the profession's norm of integrity and education, as well as the second dentist's commitment to support the first dentist's relationship with the patient and to strengthen his or her own relationship, support and perhaps even require this educational effort if it has any prospect of success with the patient under the circumstances at hand.

The ethical issue of "what to tell the patient when there is a bad outcome" is widely known to be very complex. At the end of such a lengthy analysis covering three situations and four subcategories of one of them, it may appear strange that the answer to the question can now be summarized rather simply. The second dentist is obligated to answer the patient's question truthfully and accurately, according to his or her best judgment and in accord with the relevant standards of evidence that are accepted within the larger community for various kinds of questions about other people's conduct. But this general statement includes very different ethical actions depending on the particular circumstances, hence the need to divide the question into so many parts to address it.

After so much detailed analysis, the reader may also be surprised at the authors' position that it is uncommon that a dentist has sufficient evidence to justify telling an inquiring patient that a bad outcome is probably an instance of bad work. For so much detailed analysis might have been expected to have been undertaken only in order to disagree with the common opinion. But the fact that an opinion is common within dentistry neither demonstrates nor disproves its correctness. It is only careful analysis and argument that can do that, which is what we have tried to accomplish here.

It is most important to stress, however, that this is not the only conclusion of the arguments offered here. Equally important, although it takes far less reasoning to support it, is the claim that the dentist is always required to truthfully and accurately inform the capable patient about the condition of his or her mouth, including the facts of the bad outcome. There is no exception to this obligation, regardless of what else about the situation the dentist may or may not, ought or ought not say. Nor is there an exception to this requirement when, as may often be the case, the second dentist fears that the patient will draw unwarranted negative conclusions about the first dentist's work from the facts about the bad outcome. The second dentist may try to counter these conclusions in ethically appropriate ways if he or she chooses. But the capable patient must always be truthfully and accurately informed about the condition of his or her mouth, including the bad outcome.

WHEN THE PATIENT DOESN'T ASK

But what about the patient who does not ask? Is the second dentist professionally required to inform the patient even if the patient does not raise the question? And *may* the dentist inform the patient who does not ask, even when not required?

First of all, as has been said, the second dentist is obligated to inform every capable patient accurately and completely about the condition of his or her mouth, including the bad outcome. This information may not be ethically omitted in any case, whether the patient asks for it or not. But suppose the patient accepts this information with understanding, but does not ask the second dentist to offer a judgment about the first dentist's role regarding the bad outcome. Is the second dentist obligated to introduce the subject and offer his or her judgment? Or may the dentist ethically do so if not obligated? Each of the three situations distinguished above needs examination.

In the third situation, in which the second dentist's own judgment is that the bad outcome probably is the result of bad work, a strong burden of evidence is ordinarily required for public negative judgments of others' conduct. So under the circumstances of the first subcategory, the second dentist will not ordinarily be justified in volunteering his or her judgment about the first dentist's role. Nevertheless, as has been indicated, significant likely benefit to the patient might be a sufficient reason to outweigh this social requirement and justify offering one's judgment even when the evidence does not meet that standard.

In the second and fourth subcategories, the patient is at risk of future bad work or harm because of evidence of "gross or continual faulty treatment." Therefore the patient must certainly be told of this, for the reasons explained earlier in this chapter, whether the patient asks about the matter or not.

What about the exceptional third situation case—in the third subcategory—in which the second dentist does have enough evidence of the first dentist's bad work that if the patient were to ask, the second dentist's truthful and accurate answer would have to be that the bad outcome is probably the result of bad work? Suppose that the second dentist knew that the evidence was this strong, but still the patient did not ask about the first dentist's role. Ought the second dentist volunteer this judgment in this unusual situation?

The basis of an obligation to inform the patient would be to protect the patient from harm. Therefore the authors propose that as long as the patient is not judged to be at potential risk of future bad work or harm from the first dentist—that is, as long as the bad work is judged not gross or continual—the second dentist is not professionally obligated to inform the patient that the bad outcome is probably the result of bad work.

Is the second dentist professionally *allowed* to inform the patient in this situation, even if the patient does not ask? Here the second dentist would have to reflect carefully on why he or she would want to inform the patient and what doing so might accomplish. The goal of enhancing the patient's relationship with the first dentist is excellent, but the second dentist's informing the patient will not often be the most effective means to this goal. Given the prevalence of the myths of infallible technology and infallible practitioners in the current culture, there is a significant likelihood that the information might lead to a misjudgment by the patient and undeserved risk of loss for the first dentist, who has at most committed a minor, incidental mistake. We submit that it is far better that the discussion of the bad outcome and of the bad work, if it is such, take place between the patient and the first dentist. In that connection, it will ordinarily be preferable if the second dentist contacts the first dentist than if the second dentist informs the patient. In any case, the most important ethical question will be which course of action most serves the benefit of the patient within his or her relationship with the first dentist.

Finally, what about the first situation, in which the second dentist judges that the bad outcome probably is not the result of the first dentist? Here the second dentist has an obligation to inform the patient of this fact insofar as doing so will support and strengthen the relationship between the first dentist and the patient. In addition, if no harm to the patient was involved, it is hard to imagine a justifiable reason for remaining silent, especially when, in the current cultural environment, educating patients about the difference between bad outcomes and bad work is so important.

CALLING THE OTHER DENTIST

Frequently the question whether the patient should be informed that a bad outcome is an instance of bad work is discussed only in terms of the two alternatives that were the focus of previous sections: that the second dentist inform the patient of the first dentist's role or that the second dentist say nothing at all about it. But these are not the only two courses of action available.

Precisely for the sake of the relationship between the patient and the first dentist, the best environment for communicating with the patient about the first dentist's role regarding the bad outcome is *within that relationship*. It would also be better that the treatment decisions now needed because of the bad outcome be made by the patient and the first dentist, as interactively as possible, and locating communication about the first dentist's role regarding the bad outcomes within that relationship will ordinarily enhance this possibility as well. There is, in other words, a third course of action that dentists could routinely take in such situations. The second dentist could inform the first dentist of the bad outcome and of the strength of the evidence that bad work is involved, so that the first dentist could then communicate with the patient about the bad outcome and his or her role regarding it and deal with the sequellae of this communication accordingly.

To this point in the discussion, contacting the first dentist has been mentioned only in passing, especially in connection with the kind of evidence ordinarily needed to justify a public negative comment—i.e., to the patient—about the first dentist's role regarding the bad outcome. But there are good professional-ethical reasons for proposing that in every instance in which a dentist providing care to another dentist's patient identifies a bad outcome of the patient's own dentist's work, the second dentist should contact the first dentist to inform him or her of this fact. Such communication will ordinarily be one of the most effective actions the second dentist can take to support the first dentist's relationship with the patient and to preserve and support the patient's oral and general health and autonomy.

If this were the path routinely followed, then in every instance of a bad outcome the second dentist would inform the patient of his or her intention to contact the first dentist regarding the bad outcome. The dentist would also make it clear that the patient should expect the first dentist to get in touch with the patient or that the patient could choose to initiate the contact for further examination or treatment by the first dentist regarding the bad outcome. But to be effective, this communication must be made and received in a collegial, collaborative spirit, with the benefit of the patient and the enhancement of the dentist-patient relationship as its clear goals in the eyes of both dentists.

Unfortunately, many factors in the environment of contemporary dental practice in the United States make this difficult. Following this path would probably require an adjustment in dentists' willingness to talk with one another frankly about bad outcomes and about the evidence that bad outcomes are the result of bad work. In today's dental culture, most dentists would probably hesitate to tell any dentist but a close friend that they not only saw a bad outcome, but observed evidence that it is an instance of bad work. They would seem to be judging that dentist negatively, and because they would not want to be judged negatively by others, it might seem best not to appear judgmental themselves.

But suppose the facts that dentists all know—that many bad outcomes occur without anyone's bad work, and that some occasional bad work that involves no long-term harm to anyone is inevitable in every dentist's practice—were allowed to shape dentists' conversations about these matters. Then the phone call in which the second dentist informs the first dentist of a bad outcome, or even of the evidence of bad work, would not be an insult that puts their future communication and collaboration at risk but an effort by a colleague to enhance the first dentist's relationship with his or her patient and hence an act of positive colleagueship based on mutual understanding of the challenges of dental practice.

Of course, this communication between dentists would not have a supportive effect on the relationship between the first dentist and the patient and would not be an effective support of the patient's oral and general health if the first dentist did not respond by contacting the patient. The first dentist must be willing to discuss the bad outcome with the patient and, if appropriate, also the possibility that bad work, one of the occasional mistakes that all professionals experience, was involved. The first dentist must also be willing to work with the patient to make such treatment decisions and relationship decisions as are then needed. The next section will discuss the dentist's obligations to the patient when the bad outcome or the bad work is his or her own.

There is admittedly an aura of suspicion between professionals and their lay clients in the current cultural situation in the United States. The larger community fears that dentists and other professionals are more interested in protecting one another than in respecting the norms of their professions. Professionals fear that their clients will take advantage of bad outcomes, and especially of bad work, to profit, through law suits and other legal maneuvers, from the public's acceptance of the myth of infallible technologies. The media draw on this environment of suspicion to create audiences willing to listen to isolated examples on each side, with each side then believing that what it feared is even more widespread than before. Two important facts—that the vast majority of professionals practice conscientiously according to their profession's norms and standards of practice and that most people respect and trust the professionals who personally serve them—are widely ignored, and the environment of suspicion worsens.

In such an environment, establishing the third course of action recommended here as the standard pattern of response in the face of bad outcomes is not easy. But attempting to do so, even if the attempt initially begins only with private agreements among dentists within referral networks and coverage networks as a start, is more likely to lessen suspicion and persuade the larger community that dentists are not simply trying to protect one another than any other tactic that the dental profession might try. For it is this third course of action that most achieves the values and supports the norms of the dental profession in the face of bad outcomes, whether the second dentist judges that the bad outcome is not the result of bad work, or the second dentist cannot resolve that issue, or the second dentist judges that bad work probably was involved. That is, all three of the situations discussed above are best resolved by taking this third path.

WHEN MY PATIENT HAS ANOTHER DENTIST'S BAD OUTCOME

The other large category of situations in which a dentist sees another dentist's bad outcomes consists of the situations in which the patient is—or is beginning to be—chiefly the patient of the dentist who identifies the bad outcome of another dentist's work. Into this category fall situations in which patients return to their general dentist with a bad outcome after seeing a specialist or having emergency treatment by another dentist, and situations in which patients present to a general dentist for an initial visit, presumably as the beginning of a relationship with that dentist, but with a previous dentist's bad outcome in their mouth. (One additional category in which dentists see other dentists' work, the peer review, will be examined in Chapter 10.)

Here the patient's chief relationship is with—or is beginning with—not the dentist whose work yielded the bad outcome (the first dentist), but with the dentist identifying the bad outcome (the second dentist). Because of this difference in relationships, cases in this category differ from those examined in the previous sections in that the dentist identifying the bad work does not have the same strong obligation to support the other dentist's relationship with the patient because the latter either has been a transient relationship or is past and done with. Accordingly, the value of contacting the other dentist to strengthen the other dentist's relationship with the patient is also much lessened, though it will often be important for other reasons. The dentist who identifies the bad work should rather be investing effort in enhancing his or her own relationship with the patient because this is the chief dentist-patient relationship for this patient.

To accomplish this more effectively, the dentist may be tempted to overemphasize the bad outcome or to offer judgments about the other dentist's responsibility for the bad outcome that the available evidence cannot support. In fact, with regard to this dentist's judgments about the other dentist's role in relation to the bad outcome, all of the claims made and argued for in the previous sections apply to this category of situations as well. The dentist is obligated to fully inform the patient about the condition of his or her mouth, including the bad outcome, and is obligated to answer truthfully and accurately, to the best of his or her judgment and in accord with accepted standards of evidence, the patient's questions about the role of the other dentist in relation to the bad outcome. The second dentist is also obligated to report gross or continual faulty treatment to the appropriate reviewing body, as above. In neither matter may the dentist ethically lead the patient to a lower opinion of the other dentist than the evidence will bear, keeping in mind the points about standards of evidence made earlier.

However, what complicates this situation is the possibility that the patient will want to continue to work with the dentist whose work produced the bad outcome, especially if the bad outcome is an instance of bad work, in order to seek correction of it or some other form of compensation for the failed work. Thus the patient will often expect his or her regular (or new) dentist to assist in this effort. There are no clear professional-ethical guidelines about how a dentist ought to proceed in such a circumstance, particularly if the dentist privately judges that the other dentist has probably done bad work, but does not have sufficient evidence to meet the standard required for a negative statement to the patient.

It is certain that a collaborative effort by both dentists to try to resolve the patient's needs will most effectively support the professional values and norms that have been discussed elsewhere in this chapter. But the pressures pushing the parties in such a situation toward a conflictual relationship are very strong, particularly in the current environment where the myths discussed earlier are so prevalent. The ethical challenges that dentists face in such conflictual settings will be discussed further in Chapter 10.

WHEN THE BAD OUTCOME OR BAD WORK IS MY OWN

All such situations come out better, and collaboration between professionals becomes most productive, when the dentist whose work yielded the bad outcome responds properly to the conclusion that a bad outcome, and possibly bad work, have occurred. One aspect of this proper response certainly is to work collaboratively with the other dentist(s) involved to try to reach a shared understanding of what happened and why it happened. For, as has been noted, the norm of integrity and education, and other professional norms as well, commit dentists to basing their decisions on shared understandings of the facts and of the value of dental interventions. The central values and the ideal of achieving an interactive relationship with the patient also remain very important. But what is less clear, at first look, is what the dentist whose work yielded the bad outcome is professionally obligated to do for and to say to the patient who has experienced it. Let us begin with the situation in which the dentist judges that the bad outcome is the result of his or her own bad work, but is an occasional, minor mistake, not an instance of gross or continual faulty treatment.

When a dentist and a capable patient mutually choose some form of treatment, the dentist is committed by that choice to performing the treatment within the dental profession's accepted standards of performance. Therefore if a dentist in fact performs at a level that falls short of this standard, the dentist has not yet fulfilled his or her part of the mutual choice. There is not only a contractual obligation yet to be fulfilled, as would be affirmed in almost any system of ethical norms, but there is also a specifically professional obligation of competence that is relevant here, as well as a further professional requirement to carry out the contractual commitment because failure to do so would ordinarily violate the dentist's obligations to respect and support the patient's autonomy and to work for as interactive a relationship as possible. The only exception to this professional requirement to respect the patient's autonomy by carrying out the contract would be a situation in which fulfilling the contractual commitment would violate the dentist's commitment to serve the higher ranking central values of the patient's general and oral health. In the ordinary situation, however, the dentist who has done bad work is obligated, both contractually and professionally, to do the work he or she committed to do, or else to do work that achieves a comparable end for the patient if intervening events have made the work originally committed to not appropriate for the patient's well-being and purposes, or to find someone else to do one or the other.

The dentist may be able to fulfill this obligation simply by doing the work over, or doing the work that now takes its place, at no charge, if that is the patient's choice. Or the dentist may cover the costs of its being done over—or appropriate alternate work being done—by another practitioner. There may be fiscal and other business reasons for a dentist to prefer to do this work personally, but from the contractual and professional-ethical point of view, the ethical requirement is only that the work (or appropriate alternate work) be competently done.

Nevertheless, the dentist obligated to do the work is also obligated to consider how various ways of fulfilling this obligation do or do not support the patient's relationship with his or her primary dentist and how they fit in with the patient's total program for oral and general health. For respecting and supporting the patient's autonomy ranks below the patient's oral and general health on the hierarchy of central values and is of no greater importance than working for an interactive relationship with the patient's chief dentist. So other adjustments in the work done as restitution for the bad work, including possibly some additional sacrifices on the dentist's part, may be necessary to assure that this work does not detract from or interfere with other aspects of the patient's overall dental care and relationship with his or her primary dentist.

Another aspect of a dentist's obligations regarding his or her own bad work is the obligation that every dentist has to answer patients' questions about bad work truthfully and accurately, according to his or her best judgment and in accord with relevant standards of evidence. But a dentist who is examining his or her own bad outcomes will ordinarily have much better access to evidence about what happened than any other dentist. This means that this dentist will be much more likely than the other dentists considered in this chapter to meet whatever the relevant accepted standard of evidence is for a public judgment —a statement to the patient—about the bad work. It also seems likely that the standard of evidence for a public judgment about one's own work as a professional is greater than for a private judgment of one's own or another's work but less than is required for the kind of negative public judgment of another's work that was discussed above. Consequently, when it is one's own work that is under consideration, a dentist's obligation to respond truthfully and accurately to patient's questions about bad work will require acknowledgement of one's own bad work much more often than available evidence would justify a judgment about another dentist's bad outcomes being the result of bad work.

What if the patient doesn't ask? The dentist is obligated, as has been argued, to redo the work, do alternate work, or make other arrangements for the fulfillment of his or her contractual and professional commitments regarding the work, and the dentist is also obligated to provide the patient with accurate information about the condition of his or her mouth. The dentist's conscientious fulfillment of these obligations would ordinarily prompt an express question about the dentist's responsibility for the problem. But if no such question from the patient were forthcoming, would the dentist be obligated to broach the subject of his or her responsibility for the bad outcome anyway? (Remember that, in the situation under consideration, the dentist does judge that the bad outcome was probably the result of his or her own bad work.)

The answer to this question, as to so many others, depends on whether doing so will benefit the relationship between dentist and patient. Self-criticism is not easy, but if carefully and intelligently done, it can often strengthen a relationship, sometimes very much so. But if the dentist sincerely judges that broaching the subject will not help the relationship, then there is no professional obligation to raise the matter if the patient does not ask, provided all the other required actions and communication discussed here have been completed. At the same time, of course, the permissibility of the dentist not raising the subject under these circumstances does not justify him or her in trying to mislead the patient into thinking the opposite of what the dentist judges to be the case.

What if a dentist believed that his or her bad work was in fact an instance of gross or continual faulty treatment and that patients were at risk of continued bad work or possible harm in this dentist's practice? Obviously, such a dentist must immediately seek the assistance of appropriate organizational units, of friends and of other respected colleagues to first determine if such is the case and then to take measures to correct the situation. This dentist's obligations to patients would be no different from those already described unless his or her work truly was placing patients at risk. In that case, the dentist would be professionally obligated to refrain from practice—or from certain kinds of practice if the defects are localized—until the situation has been corrected. This obligation is obviously supported in the strongest manner by almost every category of professional norms.

Ordinarily, however, a dentist whose bad work points to gross or continual faulty treatment is not aware that he or she has such a serious problem and will often be slow to believe other dentists and reviewing groups that propose it. From an ethical point of view, however, how ought a dentist respond to such a proposal? Clearly, the dentist must take it seriously, seek assistance from colleagues he or she respects to examine it carefully, and work collaboratively to take appropriate action to correct the problem. Here the dentist is called upon to make one of the most painful sacrifices that a person can make for the sake of the well-being of his or her own and the whole profession's patients, namely, to take seriously and respond carefully to a challenge by dental colleagues of one's ability to practice competently. Yet, clearly, the dental profession is obligated to supervise the practice of its members and to take steps to identify and correct members who, for whatever reasons, have demonstrated a significant potential to do bad work and possibly to harm their patients.

What, finally, are the obligations of a dentist whose work has led to a bad outcome, but after considering the matter carefully, the dentist does not judge that the bad outcome was a result of bad work on the dentist's part? First, of course, the patient must be accurately informed about the condition of his or her mouth, including the bad outcome. Regarding the role of the dentist in relation to the bad work, the dentist is again obligated to explain his or her judgment about it if the patient asks. But in this instance the dentist will ordinarily be eager to raise the issue to explain why the bad outcome should not be considered the result of his or her bad work.

In this situation, the dentist has not failed to do the professionally appropriate work that he or she contracted to do, and hence neither the standards of professional competence, nor the patient's autonomy, nor the proper relationship to the patient have been compromised by the dentist's actions. From a professional ethical standpoint, the dentist has done exactly what he or she committed to do. The patient is presumably still in need of treatment—the work must either be redone or alternate work must be done in its place; otherwise the result would not have been considered a bad outcome in the first place. But, we propose, the dentist has no professional obligation to do this work at no charge, as the dentist would have if the bad outcome were the result of his or her bad work.

Other ethical standards are more ambiguous about what the dentist owes the patient. One position that might be taken is that the contract between dentist and patient is a contract for an *outcome*, rather than for only a particular set of interventions by the dentist. If this were so, then the dentist would not have fulfilled the contract in the case at hand because the outcome has not come about. But few dentists would agree that they are contracting for outcomes precisely because they know that it is interventions, not outcomes, that are within their control. On the other hand, patients who accept the myth of infallible technologies and infallible performers presume that proper performance of the proper intervention yields the outcome in every instance. Their view often seems to be that contracting for the intervention *is* contracting for the outcome, and therefore that all bad outcomes are the result of bad work. Dentists who do not make their actual contractual commitments very clear to patients, particularly in the matter of possible bad outcomes, obviously put themselves at risk for serious misunderstandings or worse. Dentists

are professionally required, of course, to explain the possibility of bad outcomes prior to treatment as part of the process leading to at least informed
consent and, ideally, to an interactive, shared choice about treatment. They
would also be wise to define with the patient at the same time (prior to treatment) their respective responsibilities in the event of a bad outcome.

However, another position that might be taken is that because the bad outcome is no one's fault (the presumption of the present discussion is that the
patient is not at fault either), then the burden of redoing the work should be
shared equally. Neither the dentist nor the patient should bear the burden
alone because they are equally innocent of the bad outcome. But the patient
has already paid for the first work, and the dentist has borne the burden of
doing it, so the two parties are now equals in the face of nature's or fate's
impersonal events. As equals, the ethical thing for the two parties to do is
share the cost equally.

The authors know no clear ethical resolution for this issue except to
strongly advise that these possibilities all be discussed and resolved between
patient and dentist in advance and that they then honor their agreements. In
practice, to retain patients, many dentists make a business decision to redo
the work at no charge or at cost. This is not because they judge that they have
an obligation to do so, professionally or otherwise, but because, when other
things are equal, retaining a long-term client is better than losing one. There
is nothing professionally or ethically wrong with doing this. But there is some
risk. Unless the patient is carefully informed, the patient may look on this
course of action by the dentist as either acknowledgement that bad work was
in fact involved—thus reinforcing the myth of infallible technologies and infallible performers—or as evidence that the dentist is professionally obligated to
make sacrifices of precisely this sort for patients' well-being. The authors submit that neither of these conclusions is valid and that a dentist who makes
such a business decision should pay serious attention to what the patient is led
to learn from it. The best course is to discuss such eventualities in advance.

Finally, there is the dentist who is unable to form a judgment either way
about his or her role in relation to a bad outcome. This dentist cannot find
enough evidence to answer the question. The obligations of this dentist seem
to be very similar to the obligations of the dentist just studied whose bad outcome is not the result of bad work. This dentist, like the preceding one, can
claim that the evidence does not support the view that the bad outcome
resulted from his or her bad work. Consequently, this dentist may similarly
have no strict obligation to redo the work. But this dentist's situation is even
more ambiguous that the previous dentist's because the evidence does not
support the judgment that this dentist did *not* perform bad work either.

In practice, the dentist in this situation is probably even more readily
drawn to the business solution of simply doing the work without charge or at
cost because his or her responsibility as not been ruled out. If so, the cautions
just mentioned above bear repeating. The dentist should try to be as clear as
possible about what conclusions the patient is drawing from the dentist's
actions, lest those actions, although otherwise morally defensible, inadver-
tently reinforce the myths that have made dental practice so much more complex in contemporary culture.

THINKING ABOUT THE CASE

Dr. Alverez's first obligations to Ms. Stuart are to provide her with complete and accurate information about the condition of her mouth, including the bad outcome, and to provide whatever emergency treatment the clinical circumstances call for. She has already explained all of the facts about Ms. Stuart's mouth that she could observe before removing the bridge. She has now determined that the problem with the bridge and the preparation require that the bridge be redone. Clearly she needs to tell Ms. Stuart this information because it is factual information that may not be ethically omitted from their conversation. In every version of the bad outcome case that can occur, the dentist must fully and accurately inform the patient of the facts about his or her mouth and dentition.

Even granting her fellow dentist some benefit of the doubt, Dr. Alverez is pretty certain that Dr. Singer has not done a good job on the preparations, since the length and shape of the preparations are ordinarily completely within the preparing dentist's control, unless the carious lesions originally were quite sizable. Admittedly, she does not know the circumstances of Dr. Singer's preparation for the bridge. Perhaps Ms. Stuart was hurrying Dr. Singer to finish, or was unusually active in the chair, or in some other way hindered Dr. Singer's preparation work. Perhaps, as does happen, something went amiss with the impressions or the lab miscast the bridge. Even so, however, the inadequate bridge should not have been placed.

Suppose, contrary to present appearances, Ms. Stuart was actually a very pushy, controlling patient and she is presently telling only half of the story. Suppose Dr. Singer had tried to place the bridge, had seen that it was inadequate, and had told Ms. Stuart it would have to be recast, but Ms. Stuart had wanted the work to be completed at that visit and so demanded that Dr. Singer place the bridge. Even in that case, Dr. Singer should not have cemented the inadequate bridge in place, regardless of the patient's wishes.

What should Dr. Alverez say? First of all, she does not have any evidence that Ms. Stuart has done anything to cause the problem, so she cannot ethically take advantage of Ms. Stuart's uncertainty about having done some sort of damage while brushing and flossing. Second, Dr. Alverez cannot ethically say or try to lead Ms. Stuart to believe that the bad outcome had nothing to do with Dr. Singer's work. For that is in conflict with her own judgment that Dr. Singer probably made an error, possibly several errors, in this case. Third, a point not mentioned before this is that Dr. Alverez must be careful to distinguish between differences in dentists' judgments about treatment that are grounded in differing philosophies of dental practice within the range of professionally acceptable treatment and the judgment that another dentist's work is outside that range and therefore an instance of bad work. That is, she may not ethically judge Dr. Singer's work to be bad work solely because the two practitioners have different philosophies as long as Dr. Singer's work meets the dental profession's standards of minimally acceptable practice. The facts of this case, however, point to a genuine issue of appropriate care rather than only a difference in dental philosophies.

Regarding what she is obligated to say, it is necessary to distinguish the question of how the bridge came to be inadequate from the question whether

Dr. Singer should have cemented the inadequate bridge. (Dr. Alverez correctly presumes that Dr. Singer should have recognized that it is inadequate. If Dr. Alverez subsequently learned that Dr. Singer did not recognize its inadequacy, that would raise another, even more serious issue.) Dr. Alverez actually has different amounts of evidence about her answers to these two questions, and therefore, because a standard of evidence is relevant to what she ought to say, she may have different obligations concerning her communicating her answers to these two questions to Ms. Stuart.

If Ms. Stuart asks about Dr. Singer's responsibility for the bad outcome, Dr. Alverez will ordinarily have to say that she does not have enough evidence to say exactly how things went wrong, that is, how the bridge came to be inadequate or why the preparations have been done as they have. At the minimum, she would need to talk to Dr. Singer to get more information about these matters because a number of different explanations—including the role of the lab and the possibility that carious lesions at the preparation site were considered—are possible. But with regard to Dr. Singer's placing of the bridge, Dr. Alverez clearly has enough evidence to say that the bridge is inadequate, that such an inadequate bridge should not have been placed, and that Dr. Singer did place it. Therefore Dr. Alverez must answer Ms. Stuart's question about Dr. Singer's responsibility for the bad work by finding some way to say clearly, "I think Dr. Singer should not have cemented this bridge in place."

To make the same point more abstractly, regarding the question of responsibility for the inadequacy of the bridge and the preparations, Dr. Alverez may justifiably conclude that her evidence does not pass the relevant standard for a public statement. She is, in other words, in the first subcategory regarding this matter. Only significant benefit to the patient, as was noted earlier, would justify Dr. Alverez in making an exception to the ordinary standard of evidence for public negative judgments and sharing her private judgment about the probability that bad work was involved with Ms. Stuart.

But with regard to Dr. Singer's placement of an inadequate bridge, Dr. Alverez's evidence is much stronger and does meet this standard. She is, in other words, in the third subcategory regarding statements to Ms. Stuart about this. In the face of Ms. Stuart's direct question, Dr. Alverez may not ethically remain silent about her judgment that Dr. Singer should not have cemented the inadequate bridge if Ms. Stuart asks the question.

On the other hand, three-unit bridges can go wrong, even for the best of dentists. There is no basis in the case as presented for considering the bad outcome and work here a probable instance of gross or continual faulty treatment (assuming Dr. Alverez has not seen a lot of faulty bridgework or worse from Dr. Singer's hands lately). There is therefore no justification in the case as presented for Dr. Alverez to contact the local dental society's review committee, much less to suggest to Ms. Stuart that the bad outcome raises a question about whether she should continue as Dr. Singer's patient. (Obviously, Dr. Alverez also may not ethically try to lower Ms. Stuart's opinion of Dr. Singer simply for the purpose of attracting her to Dr. Alverez's practice.)

What emergency treatment should she provide? This depends in part on how seriously irritated the gum tissue is. Simply replacing the bridge without taking other measures is too dangerous; the gingiva are already involved, and Dr. Singer is not due back for another 10 days. There may even be reason to

Dental E

ng 1.

Ms. Stuart wa
se. Suppose she most effe eventive
on learning Dr. Alve temp
nted the bridge. Suppose in she
would testify about what she
d Dr. Alverez respond?

y not wish to get further involve
his, although her statement will b
r reasons for this wish. She might
needs to follow her own conscie
ng to manipulate Ms. Stuart one
d professionally responsible answe
. Stuart further in the difference bet
oss or continual bad work. While Ms.
mfort and risk of harm from the bad wo.
has she been harmed in any lasting way.
se as Dr. Alverez has seen it to fear that Dr.
or harm Ms. Stuart or other patients in the t.
could most profitably try to communicate at this
. Alverez may be concerned that Ms. Stuart will t
e brush she appears to be readying for Dr. Singer.
aboration between professionals that the next chapte
ully requires Dr. Alverez to take some risks and make s
o save and strengthen the relationship between Dr. Sing
dentist's obligations regarding testifying in court cases wil
in Chapter 10.

second dentist, Dr. Alverez in this case, in the face of a bad
probability of bad work by the first dentist is above all to
draw on the strengths of their existing relationship if this is
ase, Dr. Alverez does this by being complete and straightfor-
information so that the patient and her regular dentist can
the bad outcome, and possible bad work, on even ground.
proposing to address the most immediate problems in a car-
d way, even though this is not her regular patient and she
onnections to Dr. Singer either. Thus the patient doe
lar dentist angry at inconsiderate care or harmed
Alverez does this, finally, if she affirms a
essionally appropriate relationship be
st.

y how dentists can help th
actions. It is also ho
gies and techniques
l the dental professi

rela
to m

Sup
appears
Singer i
should not
Dr. Alverez
mouth. How s

Dr. Alverez n
tainly may say t
can articulate he
that Ms. Stuart
appear to be tryi
most valuable an
try to educate M
bad work and gr
fered some disco
fered greatly nor
reason in the ca
similar bad work
what Dr. Alverez

Of course, Dr
her with the sam
obligation of col
articulate more f
sacrifices to try
and Ms. Stuart. A
also be discussed

The role of the
outcome and the
help both parties
possible. In this
ward with factua
begin discussing
She does this by
ing and concern
has no special c
return to her reg
by lack of it. Dr
established, prof
her regular denti

This is not on
vent malpractice
human technolo
being and to fulf
nity.

e pron
d de with
ide
er it due t
ide emegen
usual fes for
If Dr. Snger v
ell to contact h
emergency care
Ms. Stuart soon
cation between l
and Ms. Stuart's
cumstances, Dr.
inform Dr. Sing
done about it. Sl
Dr. Singer on he
and she should r
after her return.

It is a more di
tist covering for
erage relationshi
call. If the cover
number suggests
sense of collabor
sense if Dr. Alver
care.

Finally, what
Singer?

This book is a
and detailed cor
place. But this m
where the bad w
dental malpracti
mutual respect, l
be remote and in
technical matters
Whether Ms. S
se. But her wil
blem, though
as a joint w
hen this
nd com
bad

CHAPTER 10

Working Together

Case: Two Sets of Gums

Dr. Jesse Watkins was a soft-spoken, personable man who did not push his intelligence or technical skill on others. But few dentists who met him failed to notice them, and his patients recommended him warmly, for his skill, but especially for his gentleness and compassion.

He was the first African-American graduate of State University's graduate program in periodontics. It had been a gutsy choice on his part to enter the program, giving up a solid, 5-year-old African-American middle-class practice of general dentistry and knowing that he would be dependent as a periodontist on referrals from dentists from many ethnic backgrounds. But in addition to his own desire to meet the intellectual and technical challenges of specialized practice, he also chose this path to bear witness to the ability of African Americans to excel in highly technical, intellectual occupations. It was his way of repaying a part of his personal debt to all those who had given him the opportunity for education in a society where many young men and women of talent do not get it.

He located his specialty practice in a near suburb of the state's largest city, close enough to the city's middle-class minority neighborhoods that he might get referrals from the little group of minority general dentists who served them. But he knew that he needed referrals from majority dentists in the city and the suburbs if his practice was to survive.

During the first lean years, he and his wife made ends meet from her position as an account executive at a local television station. Dr. Watkins spent a lot of time visiting general dentists throughout the area and teaching continuing education classes on periodontics for general dentists through the local dental society so that he would become known. Now, in its fifth year, Dr. Watkins's periodontics practice is solidly established, with a lengthening list of grateful patients and with dentists of many ethnic backgrounds comfortably referring to him.

Two patients sit in Dr. Watkins's operatories today. Alonso Nelson has been referred by Dr. Jack Chong, who services a group of patients from the dental program of the city's transit workers union. Many general dentists would not have referred Mr. Nelson, preferring to keep the work and trusting that their skills were up to it. Dr. Chong is not unusually cautious about periodontal disease, but he has found collaboration with Dr. Watkins very constructive. Instead of worrying about what the specialist will tell his patients about his work, Chong knows that Watkins will communicate with him if anything needs attention and will encourage patients to work with Dr. Chong and take advantage of his skills. Watkins has also given Chong useful advice about a couple of patients and has always taken Chong's advice about his referrals seriously. So rather than doing a procedure for Mr. Nelson that Dr. Chong has performed only a couple dozen times since dental school, he sent the patient to a specialist who does it 20 or 30 times a week.

Mr. Nelson arrives in Dr. Watkins's operatory well informed about the condition of his periodontium and about the procedures that Dr. Watkins will likely discuss with him. He suffers from diabetes mellitus and is on a daily regimen of self-administered insulin injections. In spite of a careful program of daily oral hygiene developed by Dr. Chong and his dental hygienist, the vascular effects of Mr. Nelson's diabetes are beginning to take a toll on his gums.

But the healing process from major periodontal surgery involves more risks for diabetics than for other patients. While many indicators for full-mouth surgery are present, after examining Mr. Nelson's mouth, Dr. Watkins thinks it may be possible to buy him some more time before that major step is taken. Mr. Nelson will need to work closely with Dr. Chong and his dental hygienist, and make regular visits to Dr. Watkins's office as well, so that the periodontal disease doesn't suddenly get out of hand. But putting off the risks of full-mouth surgery even for one more year are, in Dr. Watkins's judgment, worth the effort.

Before communicating this judgment to Mr. Nelson, Dr. Watkins calls Dr. Chong's office. Chong is with a patient at that moment, so Dr. Watkins asks Mr. Nelson if he can wait a few more minutes at Watkins's office until Dr. Chong is free. When Chong is free, Watkins explains his view of the case and asks Chong if he thinks anything has been missed. When he has determined that he, Dr. Chong, and Dr. Chong's hygienist are in agreement, Dr. Watkins gets Mr. Nelson on the telephone with them, and the four of them go through the treatment plan in detail, with Mr. Nelson agreeing with every step and grateful to have the surgery postponed for a time.

Meanwhile, in Dr. Watkins's other operatory, is Kathleen O'Gara, who now works at the same television station as Watkins's wife, having recently moved to the area and so left the practice of the dentist who treated her since she was a teenager, Dr. Herbert Schmidt. Pain in chewing sent her to a local clinic, where she was informed that she had severe periodontal disease and periodontal surgery was recommended. She couldn't believe this, since Dr. Schmidt had never mentioned such a thing. So having heard from someone that Sarah Watkins' husband was a periodontist, she found him in the telephone book and made an appointment.

On examination, Dr. Watkins finds advanced periodontal disease, as the clinic dentist had said. Ms. O'Gara is very angry at this diagnosis and tells Dr. Watkins that she expected the husband of a friend to say something less frightening. (Dr. Watkins has never heard his wife mention Ms. O'Gara, and his wife subsequently confirms that she barely knows her.) Dr. Watkins then asks Ms. O'Gara whether Dr. Schmidt had ever spoken with her about periodontal disease.

"He would look at my teeth and he would always clean them with that little rubber thing on the drill," she answers. "The last couple of visits, he said he found some deposits or something, and he would scrape it off. But it made my gums bleed and I really didn't like it. Once in a while he would have to do a filling. But he said my teeth were very strong; he said that every year, twice a year, since I was 15. That's 17 years of strong teeth. Now I move away and I am told my teeth are in wretched shape. I want to know what is going on."

"I am a specialist, Ms. O'Gara, but I did practice for 5 years as a general dentist before going into this specialty, and I would judge that Dr. Schmidt was quite justified in saying that you have strong enamel and a good bite, which are characteristics of excellent teeth. That is why I asked if Dr. Schmidt ever specifically discussed the health of your gums with you, because strong teeth need healthy gums to do their work. The scraping he did on your last two visits might well have been aimed at treating a periodontal condition, especially if Dr. Schmidt was scraping down below the gum line."

"He is a very good man. I can't imagine that he would have forgotten to tell me anything important about my teeth. He is the only dentist I ever went to who was kind and considerate. The dentists my parents took me to when I was little were like dictators and they had no compassion. I used to cry and scream every time I had to go, until I went to Dr. Schmidt. My girlfriend's mother recommended him when I was in high school, and I went to him and never went anywhere else after that. He certainly would have told me if something was wrong with my gums. Couldn't all of this have happened since my last appointment with him?"

"How recently was that?" asks Dr. Watkins.

"I moved here 8 months ago. I had a check-up about 6 months before that. I was due for another check-up and cleaning when I left Greenville, but I figured I would wait until I found a new dentist here, and then I never got around to it. I was nervous about starting with a new dentist, I guess, since I had so many bad experiences before Dr. Schmidt."

"Periodontal disease does not sneak up on a person," says Dr. Watkins gently. "Could I ask you whether he took X-rays of your teeth when you got your regular check-ups, especially after he began to do that scraping. X-rays can often indicate if a periodontal condition exists."

"I don't like X-rays, doctor, and Dr. Schmidt understood that," says Ms. O'Gara. "He used to take them when I was younger, but when I became aware of the risks, I told him I was opposed to them, and he stopped."

"It looks like you might be experiencing some bleeding around your gums. Has that been going on for a while?" asks Dr. Watkins.

"Yes."

"Did you ever discuss that with Dr. Schmidt?"

"It didn't happen very often until recently, maybe last spring. Before that it was just now and then. I don't remember being concerned about it, but I suppose I might have mentioned it to him. Like I said, his scraping made my gums bleed, so I might have mentioned it then. Are you saying that he should have been paying more attention to my gums?" asks Ms. O'Gara.

"Your periodontal disease has undoubtedly progressed since you last saw Dr. Schmidt if that was 14 months ago," says Dr. Watkins. "But it is most unlikely that there were no symptoms at that point. Perhaps Dr. Schmidt thought that the scraping plus your regular oral hygiene would be sufficient to keep it under control and did not want to alarm you. Perhaps he figured he could keep a close eye on the condition because you were so regular with your check-ups. Did he teach you to floss as part of your regular cleaning of your teeth?"

"No, he never mentioned using dental floss or I would have gotten some. You are saying he would have found something 14 months ago if he had looked, aren't you?" asks Ms. O'Gara.

"Well, I wasn't there, obviously, and I haven't spoken to him or seen his records. But I can certainly say that the disease is far enough advanced in your mouth that it would be extremely unusual for it to progress from being undetectable all the way to this point in so short a time as 14 months."

"Then what are you going to tell me to do?" Ms. O'Gara is clearly upset.

"You obviously have had a very positive relationship with Dr. Schmidt," says Dr. Watkins, "and that is something to build on now with a new dentist. He also seems to have done a fine job of regular cleaning and filling cavities when that was needed. If you wouldn't mind, I would like to contact him to see what he noted about your periodontal condition and whether he had any plan in mind regarding it. I can provide the best care when I can work closely with a patient's regular dentist, and he is the one who has cared for you the most recently. But since he is 400 miles away, I would recommend that you contact a general dentist here in this area, with the hope of establishing a good long-term relationship like one you had with Dr. Schmidt. As for your periodontal disease itself," continues Dr. Watkins, "I understand how disappointed you must feel, learning about it all of a sudden. But there is plenty you can do. It is not so far advanced as to be a serious health threat if you begin to take action now. I would be happy to develop a treatment plan for you, if you would like. It will include some periodontal surgery, and also working closely with my dental hygienist to help you develop a plan of self-care to prevent the condition from worsening now or recurring later. I would also work closely with your general dentist here when you get one."

Ms. O'Gara silently studied Dr. Watkins's face for a few seconds, then stood up from the chair, took her purse from the counter, and headed for the door. "I don't think I can ever trust any dentist again," she said, and was out of the office before Dr. Watkins could say another word.

Ms. O'Gara never returned to Dr. Watkins's office and declined to speak with his receptionist on the telephone. Several weeks later, though they barely knew each other, she went out of her way to tell Sarah Watkins, "I have nothing to say to you." Dr. Watkins later made a few inquiries of other periodontists in the area, but none of them ever heard of Kathleen O'Gara or treated her.

He also called Dr. Schmidt in Greenville shortly after Ms. O'Gara's visit. He told him that Ms. O'Gara had visited his office and was suffering from severe periodontal disease. Dr. Watkins explained that she had left suddenly and without treatment, although its importance had been explained to her. He wanted Dr. Schmidt to be aware of this in case he heard from her or perhaps wanted to take the initiative of calling her about getting treatment. Dr. Schmidt told Dr. Watkins that he remembered Ms. O'Gara very well and that he had been treating her for a periodontal condition when she was his patient. "It was completely under control at that time," he explained. "In a case like this, a little scaling and regular use of the toothbrush is all it takes. I sometimes wonder how you periodontal specialists stay in business."

Dr. Watkins wished Dr. Schmidt well and ended the conversation without trying to answer his question.

COLLABORATION VS. THE MYTH OF THE LONE RANGER

Many strands of American culture, and many aspects of dental training as well, conspire to inculcate a picture of dental practice, and of human life in general, as something that is principally accomplished alone. Many important and undeniable facts about dental practice give the lie to this picture. All dentists are continually dependent on the work of dental and biomedical researchers, and these researchers are in turn dependent on dentists in practice for data and to articulate the needs their research responds to. General dentists are unavoidably dependent on specialists for cases they can't or do not want to handle, and specialists depend on general dentists for referring patients to them in the first place. All dentists depend in a number of ways on the educational and therapeutic initiatives of public health dentists, and public health dentists depend in turn for much of their success on the educational and preventive activities of dentists in office-based practices. Dentists' success in practice also depends in many ways on their working together through formal organizations and informal groups of many sorts. Nevertheless, these facts somehow fade in significance under the influence of our culture, and it is the picture of the dentist as lone ranger, single-handedly confronting the challenges to patients' dental health, that most often dominates both dentistry's and the public's imagination.

Because of this, the most underdeveloped of the eight categories of professional norms, not only for dentistry, but for all our society's professions, is the category of *ideal relationships between co-professionals*. Many readers may even be surprised that the authors consider this a category of professional norms for dental practice, since, as most dentists are aware of, guides for conduct in this area may well seem more like rules of etiquette among dentists than norms of professional conduct. But in fact, some guides for conduct about the relationships of co-professionals are already clearly matters of professional obligation for dentists, and a general ethical commitment to collaboration, the authors hope to show, ought to be considered such as well.

Some of the more familiar categories of norms have clear implications about the relationships of dentists with their co-professionals. For example, the norm of competence obviously requires that dentists not practice beyond their expertise and hence that they refer patients whom they cannot care for adequately to other professionals who can. But both the central value of autonomy and the ideal relationship between dentist and patient require that this referral not undermine the patient's relationship with his or her general dentist, as Chapter 9 stressed frequently. If dentists believed that it made no professional difference how they viewed and treated one another, however, then this and many other of dentists' obligations to their patients would be almost impossible to fulfill.

· Suppose that both the general dentist and the specialist viewed themselves as lone rangers, responding to patients' dental needs without dependence on collaborators. Each would work to strengthen his or her own relationship with the patient, and connect with the other practitioner only grudgingly because the limits of his or her expertise had been reached, rather than trying to bring the patient the greater benefit of two heads and two lives of rich professional experience working together. The authors submit that this is only one of many aspects of dental practice in which the relationships of co-professionals are not matters of professional indifference. Dentists are professionally obligated to practice collaboratively and to develop in themselves the habits of perception and action regarding co-professionals that will facilitate such practice.

Because this component of the professional-ethical practice of dentistry has been so little examined, this chapter will survey a number of areas of dental practice in which, in the authors' judgment, a self-conscious commitment to collaboration with one's co-professionals makes or would make a clear difference. Working out more subtle issues and more difficult cases will require more extensive dialogue on this topic both within the dental community and between it and the community at large.

COLLABORATION BETWEEN GENERALISTS AND SPECIALISTS

The most obvious example of professionally required collaboration is the one stressed in the examples used so far, namely, collaboration between the general dentist and the specialist. But as was just noted, general dentists can send their patients to specialists, and specialists can treat them and return them, without a spirit of collaboration. Where such a spirit exists, where working with another dentist is viewed as a positive component of good patient care, then the general practitioner is not motivated to practice right up to the limits of his or her expertise. Thus fewer errors about the limits of one's technical capabilities are made, and patients receive better care. General dentists are also not afraid that the specialist will fail to support, or will even undermine, the general dentist's relationship with and work for the patient. For when the care of the patient is viewed collaboratively, then one principal task of the specialist, as Chapter 9 stressed, is to support and strengthen the general dentist's relationship with the patient.

Nor will the specialist begrudge "returning" the patient to the general dentist. For in the specialist's view, if care of the patient is genuinely collaborative, the patient has never "left" the generalist's care. At its best, in fact, collaborative care of a patient is team care. The generalist and specialist view themselves as caring for the patient with combined knowledge and combined skills, each respecting the contributions of the other and each working to integrate his or her own contribution with the positive contribution of the other (rather than working to have the patient view his or her own contribution as the one that is just now the most important).

This picture is admittedly somewhat idealized because of the frequently conflictual natural of dental practice in today's society, because of the social and economic history of American dentistry as a profession practiced almost exclusively solo, and because of the demands of daily practice on each dentist's time and energy.

First, dentists work in a changing economic environment that seems to put them increasingly into competition with each other, and sometimes into conflict as well. (See Chapter 14 for discussion of the ethical issues directly connected to these economic pressures.) They also practice in a society where many people seem as prone to sue as to negotiate to further their interests, and their suits frequently draw dentists into conflict with one another as well. But dentists should ask themselves whether they should passively allow economic, social, and legal trends that have nothing to do with the bases of their professional commitments to define how those commitments are understood by themselves and by the larger community. Dentists can say to the larger community: our society has created pressures that draw us into conflict; therefore that is how we shall live and practice. But this is not necessary, and it is certainly not the best way for dentistry to serve its patients, individually or collectively.

If dental care is inherently collaborative, and is increasingly so as dental knowledge and skills grow increasingly sophisticated and specialized, then dentists must affirm this reality about their profession in their actions and in their education of the larger community about dental care. They must point out the misfit between the conflictual pressures upon them and their professional commitment to collaborative care for people's health, and they must try to practice collaboratively, as the circumstances of each case require, in spite of these pressures. This topic will be examined in greater detail in the next section.

Second, history seems to be against the ideal of collaborative dentistry as well. Since dentistry's earliest days as a profession in the United States, social and economic forces in American society have shaped dentistry so that it has been practiced almost exclusively solo. It is this history, much more than the conflictual pressures of the current scene, that makes the myth of the dentist as lone ranger appear true. For almost all dentists, until very recently, practiced alone, and for many years most practiced as the sole professional in their offices.

There is one respect in which every professional does practice alone. For to be a professional is to be independently capable of expert judgments about clients' needs and the means to redress them or fulfill them, and in every professional-client interaction, there is a moment—or many moments—when the professional makes a judgment about the client's need and chooses appropriate interventions. Even when the practitioner is on a team, and even within the most interactive of relationships with a client, these moments of professional judgment and choice must still precede—for every professional involved—what the team, or the professional(s) and the client as a unit, then judge and choose together. This is a moment that belongs to oneself in the exercise of one's own expertise, even if the fruit of this moment will not become effective until it is blended with the fruits of other practitioners' similar exercise of their expertise, together with the judgments and choices of the client, and even if much will be reconsidered and reconstructed in the process. At that moment of judgment and choice for one's client, one practices one's profession only as oneself, no matter how interactive and collaborative the larger setting of one's practice.

But this fact about professional practice must not be confused with the idea that the larger setting of one's practice should not be or is not really collaborative. Nor should social and economic accidents that have made dental offices for the most part places where just one dentist serves patients be taken as defining circumstances for what it means to practice dentistry at its best. Particularly as changes in the surrounding environment seem to try to pull dentists apart, they ought to think carefully about the real nature of dental practice and the real nature of its ethical roots, and they should reaffirm and reemphasize in word and action that it is a collaborative enterprise. For it is a collaborative enterprise whether it is practiced in groups or as one dentist to an office and regardless of the economic structures by which patients and dental care are brought together.

Finally, this picture of dentistry as collaborative—in the present example in the relationships between general dentists and specialists—is idealized because of the demands of daily practice on each dentist's time and energy. It takes more time and more energy to actively support positive collaboration. It takes extra phone calls and memos and the special effort of communication among equal experts with differing areas of expertise and different practice experiences. It takes compromises in planning and subtlety in communicating about dis-agreements without giving up on working things out together. It also increases the level of effort required to communicate properly with the patient and to support as interactive a relationship with the patient, for both dentists, as is possible.

Many dentists, both general practitioners and specialists, may find them-selves asking who is going to pay for this extra time and effort, for it is time and effort that does not fit into the most common picture of dental practice. But that is the picture of the dentist as lone ranger, a very common picture, but one that does not represent the dental profession at its best. No ethical dentist would ask: who is going to pay for the time and effort needed for me to practice competently? The commitment to practice competently comes with the commitment to practice dentistry at all. Our proposal here is that a commitment to collaboration is equally fundamental to the proper practice of dentistry. The myth of the lone ranger is just that, a myth, and dentists ought to practice according to the correct picture and ought to represent their prac-tice and educate the larger community in the image of dentistry as collabora-tive as well. (This does not answer the question about who is going to pay for changes in practice patterns that practicing true to this commitment would require. But it does place the question in its proper context.)

WORKING TOGETHER THROUGH CONFLICT

Chapter 9 examined many kinds of situations in which conflict, rather than collaboration, seems almost inevitable because a dentist is caring for a patient experiencing a bad outcome from another dentist's work. How could an enhanced exercise of this collaborative ideal contribute to these situa-tions? How can it counter the effects of the litigiousness of this society on dentists' efforts to work together?

Part of the answer to this question has already been formulated in Chapter 9's emphasis on support for the patient's relationship with his or her general dentist. Although this dentist is, in many of the situations examined, the one whose work has had a bad outcome, nevertheless even when the other dentist judges that the bad outcome is the result of that dentist's bad work, the most appropriate basis for the next judgment, whether it is an instance of gross or continual faulty treatment, is still open communication with the first dentist. In addition, with only the rarest exceptions, the second dentist's obligation to support the patient's relationship with the first dentist remains in place and calls upon the second dentist to continue to work collaboratively with the first dentist.

But in this litigious society it may take special courage to respond to this obligation and to work collaboratively with and thus affirm one's colleague-ship and professional respect for a dentist whom this patient may now sue, since the second dentist has rightly informed the patient about the bad out-come. Both the desire to retain the patient's respect, and also his or her work, and especially the desire to not be drawn into the possible suit, make it very difficult to positively associate oneself with the source of the bad outcome, especially if the second dentist considers it a probable instance of bad work. These fears may even motivate a dentist to judge the other dentist more harshly than the evidence justifies, to act as if the myths of infallible dentistry, discussed in Chapter 9, were true, as if all bad work was inexcusable, and as if infallible practitioners were common.

How can dentists counter such fears, which isolate them and put them in conflict with one another and which make them feel like lone rangers even if they recognize intellectually the falseness of that myth? A valuable antidote is to challenge the myth of the dentist as lone ranger at its root, that is, to self-consciously emphasize the collaborative character of dental practice from the beginning of one's relationship with another dentist. The dentist who views another dentist as collaborator from the start and who acts accordingly in the degree and character of his or her communication with the other dentist, as they care for the patient together, will have laid powerful groundwork for later resisting the fears and pressures that might isolate them from one another if a bad outcome and even bad work should arise.

A relationship between dentists that begins self-consciously as collaboration and proceeds collaboratively in deed as well as word is far less likely to fall apart into conflict. This is also the context within which, more than any other, the patient can be effectively educated to understand that not all bad outcomes are the result of bad work, that most bad work causes little harm or risk of harm, and that occasional minor bad work is inevitable in the practice of even the most superb practitioners because they are fallible human beings (like the second dentist and even the patient).

Collaborative practice is challenged even more severely when a patient actually sues a dentist. The success of such suits depends on expert witnesses, and the dentist who quite properly described a bad outcome to a patient is often made to feel as if he or she initiated the suit for having done so, as if he or she was thereby being disloyal to the profession rather than fulfilling its ethical requirements, and all the more so if the dentist agrees to testify in the suit. In an environment in which the dentist as lone ranger is the dominant image, the two dentists (and often two groups of dentists, as each side looks for more expert witnesses) in a suit can easily view each other as mere competitors, supporting opposite sides of a dispute about proper dental care and therefore justly able to think of the other as deserting the cause of good dentistry and as disloyal to the dental profession.

The effects of such thinking are well known and are widely considered a great loss to the dental community and to the community at large. Why is this? Is it merely because it makes dentists fearful and uncomfortable? Is it only because it motivates dentists to practice defensive dentistry, with someone paying its unnecessary (from the point of view of good treatment) costs? Or is it also, and more basically, because the practice of good dentistry suffers, and the community who are its beneficiaries thus lose something important as well?

Again, we propose that the latter is the case, that collaborative practice is the ideal relationship that dentists are professionally committed to work for, and is so because of what it contributes to dental care for the profession's patients. The pattern of thinking and acting just described is founded not only on a false view of dental practice as fundamentally solo rather than collaborative. It is also in direct conflict with the norm of integrity and education, which requires dentists to base their clinical judgments on fact and to communicate them accordingly and to support the profession's collective effort to protect the community from misuse of dental expertise.

So dentistry's first question about how dentists ought to deal profession-ally-ethically with litigation should be how the ideal relationship between co-professionals can be maximally achieved in so conflictual a setting, while at the same time respecting dentistry's other professional commitments and tak-ing account of dentists' other commitments in the situation, including their obligations as citizens to support the society's system of justice.

If dentists viewed their practice as collaborative from the first moment that they were caring for the same patient and conducted themselves with the patient and communicated with the patient and with each other accordingly, many of today's suits that arise from patients' acceptance of one or another myth about infallible dentistry would not arise. Many more patients would understand that a bad outcome does not always mean bad work and that most bad work is minor and inevitable and poses no risk of further bad work or serious harm. Moreover, in such a collaborative environment, dentists who have bad outcomes might be far more comfortable raising the issue of redo-ing the work, whether bad work was involved or not, so patients did not auto-matically think they needed legal action to get the outcome they intended.

But regularly in our environment, and even occasionally in the ideal envi-ronment just described, suits will still be filed. Some suits will occur because a patient accepts one of the myths about infallible dentistry, in spite of den-tists' best efforts to educate and explain, or the patient sees an opportunity for profit because so many juries accept the myths. In others, perhaps the dentist cannot acknowledge that bad work is involved when it is, or if only a bad out-come is involved, then perhaps the dentist for some reason will not negotiate to get the patient the outcome that the patient and dentist originally intended.

In this less-than-ideal environment, dentists called upon to act as witnesses must be responsive to many ethical standards at once—both when choosing whether or not to be a cooperative witness, and in their actual testimony if called. As citizens they have an obligation to support the system of justice through the courts, and they also have fiduciary obligations toward their patients. But neither these obligations nor any of their professional obliga-tions already discussed ordinarily requires a dentist to volunteer to testify in any particular case when other dentists could provide the needed information equally well. Thus the ADA's *Principles* rightly states, "Dentists may provide expert testimony when that testimony is essential to a just and fair disposi-tion of a judicial...action" (1-H). When actually called, whether voluntarily or not, dentists' obligations as citizens and their professional obligations to com-petence, to integrity and education, and to the central values of patients' oral and general health all require them to answer all questions about the condi-tion of a patient's mouth truthfully and accurately, to the best of their judg-ment.

The dentist's obligation to practice collaboratively complicates these deci-sions. First of all, as soon as a dentist is asked to render a professional judg-ment about the condition of a patient's mouth or appropriate treatment for such a condition, that patient is now that dentist's patient, regardless of the dentist's previous relationship or lack of one to that patient. This means that because of dentists' obligation to practice collaboratively, the dentist is also now a collaborator with other dentists caring for that patient, including the dentist being sued if he or she is one of these. We propose that the idea that a dentist can testify without being a collaborator in patient care with the dentist involved in the case is simply false. The testifying dentist must consider what the obligation to practice collaboratively, along with other relevant professional norms, requires in each such situation. Under no circumstances, however, will it justify deliberately speaking falsely about his or her own honest judgment of the clinical facts and other features of the case.

In one sense, it is true that this obligation requires dentists to testify only in support of one another, but wording the conclusion in this way definitely oversimplifies the matter. Supporting a dentist who is at risk of great loss because a patient accepts the myths of infallible dentistry, or hopes to profit from a jury's acceptance of them, may mean voluntarily testifying to educate about the difference between bad outcomes and bad work, or between occasional, minor, inevitable bad work that yields no risk of future bad work or harm, and gross or continual bad work that does carry such risks. Achieving this end will require a difficult strategic judgment whether the dentist can effectively educate when a skilled lawyer intends to manipulate the dentist's testimony to serve his or her client's needs. But if no dentist ever testified with such education as an aim, American juries and the larger society would learn that much more slowly that the myths of infallible dentistry are myths indeed.

We submit that dentists who would testify in support of these myths and against the distinctions just mentioned not only do dentistry harm and its patients no service but they actually violate professional norms of competence and of integrity and education, and possibly the central values of patients' oral and general health and patients' autonomy, by miseducating about the causal processes operative in dental care. But in all testimony the first rule must be that the dentist speak truthfully according to his or her best judgment, whether the testimony challenges these myths or not.

Even more complex is the question how a dentist ought to support a dentist being sued because he or she has made an ineffectual business judgment, but who has not failed in competence, because only a bad outcome—but not bad work—is involved, and has not failed in any other aspect of professional-ethical conduct either. Even when the dentist being sued has probably done bad work in the second dentist's judgment, but is unable or unwilling to acknowledge this, it is not clear that either testifying to this judgment or refusing to testify is invariably the best form of support. Depending on the situation, either of them might be. The obligation to practice collaboratively does not determine actions generically in these difficult, conflict-laden situations. What it determines is the frame of mind with which the dentists ought to—and ought to consciously work to—view one another's actions in these situations, and it identifies one of the several crucial professional-ethical standards that ought to guide their judgments and actions when they are in these situations.

Finally, there are the peer review structures established by dental organizations or licensing boards. Many dentists who sit on such committees view themselves as fulfilling an educational role rather than one of "competency police." When peer review groups are engaged in routine oversight, the emphasis on education is fairly easy to see. But these groups ordinarily hope that even their most aggressive interventions will occur early enough that the dentist involved can still recoup the deficits that have brought him or her into difficulty and can continue to practice in a competent and ethical manner. This is certainly true when a review committee responds investigatively to a report of probable gross or continual faulty treatment, and all the more so if the investigation confirms the faulty practice. Dentistry's commitments to the larger community require that such oversight activity be undertaken, but dentists' commitment to collaboration requires that it be viewed first and foremost as educational and constructive for those whose work needs improvement.

The conflictual pressures of our times, however, have prompted some dentists to view peer review as an intrusion on their prerogatives as professionals and experts in dental care. But becoming a professional does not make one capable of practicing wholly independently of other practitioners in any profession. The authors have argued, moreover, that in the dental profession the norm of ideal relationships between co-professionals requires that dentists view themselves as collaborators in the provision of dental care and act accordingly. So there is no prerogative in dentistry to practice as a lone ranger. The relevant question is whether actual peer review structures are functioning in support of collaborative dentistry and in accord with the other norms of professional practice.

Once again, the most constructive step to assist in this process is a commitment on the part of all dentists to view peer review structures from a collaborative point of view from the start, to interpret their actions in accord with that view, and to interact with them and their members accordingly.

IMPAIRED DENTISTS

Very few dentists would view the plight of an impaired colleague with indifference or make their first response a punitive one. Most physical and many psychological afflictions are not within a person's power to control, and even substance addictions, though their victims retain an important measure of responsibility for their condition, may seem almost inexorable in a person under the physical and emotional strains that are common in dental practice. So dentists impaired in their practice by any of these conditions are ordinarily viewed sympathetically and with the hope that they will be able to overcome their condition and continue to practice competently or return to competent practice after treatment, if treatment is necessary.

But these sentiments could easily be the sentiments of persons who share only knowledge, skills, and mode of occupation but who have no particular obligations to one another. They fail to express an element of dental professional obligation that binds every dentist to every other in certain respects, an aspect of the commitment to collaborative practice not evident in the examples discussed so far.

The point was made in Chapter 9, and is clear from dentistry's obligation to assure the community that the profession will prevent dental expertise from being used inappropriately, that every dentist's patient is, in some sense, every other dentist's patient. It is also this fact—that in more than one sense the whole community is every dentist's chief client—that justifies the existence of the peer review committees discussed in the previous section and active support for the public health and educational efforts mentioned earlier.

In the present instance, where the obligation to collaboration is under discussion, this fact has a further implication. If every member of the community is my patient, from the point of view of securing at least a minimum of dental health and protection from misuse of dental expertise, then every dentist is also my collaborator in these respects. In these aspects of dental care, we who are dentists practice together as a team, all of us.

If any dentist is impaired in his or her practice, then it is my collaborator who is impaired. Just as I would not react only with sympathy if a close, more obvious collaborator were impaired, just as I would work not merely to protect our patient from bad work but also to help my collaborator correct the deficit and be restored to full and competent practice, so I should respond to this more distant collaborator.

As has been said often in this chapter, the response will be first in one's mind set. The impaired colleague is not a lone ranger in trouble; he or she is someone to whom I am bound by ethical ties. I may not ethically be merely sympathetic; this collaborator's well-being is my concern, for his or her sake and for the sake of our common patients. Whether more specific action is in order, directed to a certain needy individual or to institutionalized assistance programs or the like, or one chooses to make one's professional sacrifices in some other way, a dentist may not ethically view the impaired collaborator as someone with a problem that is only his or her own.

In addition, the term *impaired* can be read more broadly to include dentists who suffer from conditions that have not yet compromised their competence in practice, but which have a natural progression that makes such compromise very likely. Those who collaborate closely with such persons and who see indications of a condition of this sort could not ethically stand by as the condition ran its course. Their obligations to patients and their obligations to their co-professionals would require them to look for ways to alert the practitioner to the problem and to then help him or her recoup before the impairment actually compromised appropriate practice. Since dentists are properly viewed as collaborators, though more distant, with all other dentists in the society, they have an obligation to attend to the signs and symptoms of such conditions and to alert those who suffer from them and help them take action before patients and practitioner alike suffer significantly.

Here again, concrete details of the situation will determine what course of action a person should take to act in accord with the commitment to collaborative practice regarding such conditions. But the obligation to collaboration, as the clearest directive of the norm of ideal relationships between co-professionals, most certainly applies.

OTHER COLLABORATORS AND OTHER CHALLENGES

Dentists are not the only co-professionals that dentists work with, so collaboration with other dentists is not the only implication of the norm of ideal relationships between co-professionals. But as the range of possible collaborators extends, the tendency to view relationships with these collaborators as merely matters of business judgment or etiquette grows stronger. However, our proposal is that important aspects of these relationships are professionally significant.

The larger community, with whom the dental community has a dialogue to determine the contents of its professional commitments, would certainly be amazed to learn that dentists viewed their relationships with dental hygienists, patients' physicians, mental health professionals to whom they refer patients, and others to whom they entrust a share in their fiduciary responsibilities toward patients, to be merely business relationships or relationships governed only by some sort of rules of etiquette. For patients' well-being and the quality of many patients' relationships with the dentist depend in turn on the character of the dentist's relationship with these collaborators. Dentists may not ethically relate to them simply in whatever ways are convenient, mutually agreeable, or profitable. The character of their relationships to these collaborators is a matter of professional obligation.

The most obvious nondentist co-professionals that dentists work with are dental hygienists. In many dental practices, dental hygienists are assigned principal responsibility for the initial examination of patients, for prophylaxis, and for patient education about self-care and follow-up. Some state licensing laws may establish a legal relationship of independent-practitioner-to-dependent-agent between dentist and dental hygienist. But dentists' and hygienists' legal relationship does not answer the question how they are related professionally.

To determine that, the first questions to ask are whether the hygienist is possessed of professional expertise and whether the hygienist exercises that expertise in independent health care judgments and interventions for patients. While dentists may be legally considered their supervisors in all aspects of their practice, most hygienists in fact make numerous detailed judgments and interventions, particularly in providing prophylaxis and education, that dentists do not supervise in detail precisely because the hygienist is considered fully competent to practice independently in these matters, and the same is true even for many aspects of patients' initial examinations, where most dentists play their closest supervisory role.

From this it is obvious that the first three of the characteristics of a profession are clearly evident in the daily practice of dental hygienists: (1) expertise that consists of both theoretical knowledge and skills for applying it in practice, (2) providing important benefits to others through the exercise of this expertise, and (3) independent exercise of that expertise. The fourth characteristic also characterizes the dental hygiene community as a whole and each of its members individually, namely, that they have special obligations in their role, obligations that correspond to the eight categories of professional obligation that have been discussed throughout this book. Formally demonstrating this characteristic of dental hygiene would take this discussion beyond its intended limits, but there is little doubt that dental hygiene possesses it. In sum, dental hygiene is rightly considered a profession and dental hygienists co-professionals of dentists because they are professionals caring for the same patients together.

In many dental offices, dentist and dental hygienist practice collaboratively as co-professionals, each respecting the other's expertise and positive contributions to patient care and each working to make the judgments and choices they need to make together for patients as much the work of professional equals as possible. If one emphasizes the number of procedures that the dentist is expert in, it might appear that the dentist's expertise is much broader than the hygienist's. If one emphasizes the aspects of a patient's life that the professional must consciously address and integrate in treatment decisions, however, it is the expertise of the hygienist that is the broader. For the expert one-on-one dental educator must, especially in difficult cases, address feelings and life-style issues that touch almost every aspect of human life.

The most reasonable view, the authors propose, is to consider both forms of expertise essential to the complete dental care of patients and to look for modes of collaborative practice to make sure both kinds of expertise are available to help the patient to the maximum degree. (The fact that most dentists could perform prophylaxis as expertly as hygienists do if they did so as often and that most dentists could educate as effectively if they were better trained in this area of dental care does nothing to lessen the importance of hygienists' expertise— no more so than dentists' professional expertise is lessened in importance by the fact that most hygienists could perform, for example, restorative procedures expertly if they had the relevant training and experience.)

The reason this is the most reasonable view is that both forms of expertise are essential to complete dental care. Providing chairside treatment without educating, motivating, and assisting patients in self-care is as truncated a view of caring for patients' oral and general health as providing assistance with self-care, but not access to chairside interventions.

The dental professions, like all professions, are not obligated to attend expertly to every aspect of their patients' well-being. Each profession is committed to working specifically for certain values; in dentistry's case, we have proposed, that means the hierarchy of central values examined in Chapter 5. (Clear articulation of the central values of the dental hygiene profession would be a valuable advance in that profession's understanding of its distinctive expertise and its specific contributions to dental care.) But this does not mean that a holistic ideal of health has no place in dental practice. For achieving the values that the dental professions are committed to for their patients brings dental professionals in touch with most aspects of human life, and finding the best ways to achieve them requires more forms of expertise than any one professional can possess. The ethic of collaboration being considered in this chapter is grounded on the conviction that only by melding together the expertise of many professionals can patients be served in the best way possible.

The relationship of dentist to dental hygienist as professional collaborators, which is not effectively mirrored in their legal relationship, is further hindered in many offices by their business relationship as employer-to-employee. (In addition, the character of their legal relationship may often render any alternative business relationship legally impossible.) Culturally based but challengeable assumptions that women are typically less able to master theory-based expertise, less effective as decision makers, and less capable of strenuous work also hinder mutual respect and collaborative practice by dentists and dental hygienists in many settings. So does another culturally based but challengeable assumption, much less examined than the previous one, that longer education renders a person's expertise more valuable than shorter education rather than rendering it certainly rarer and probably more costly, but with judgments of comparative value requiring much more subtle discriminations. Similarly, collaborative practice by the two pro-fessions is hindered by patterns of political conflict between their profes-sional organizations and by stories of personal wrongs and enmity that, even if true, somehow acquire the additional status of legends.

Dentists, we propose, are obligated under the norm of ideal relationships between co-professionals to seek collaborative relationships with the dental hygienists with whom they work and to work together with them against the challenges to collaborative practice just mentioned. The authors believe that dental hygienists have these same professional obligations for their part. In both cases, as has been stressed, these obligations derive from the nature of good dental care, which cannot be properly achieved without the conjoined expertise of these two professions and, in special cases, several others as well.

Dentists do not need to consult patients' physicians in every case, of course. But when the patient's oral or general health require it, the obligation to contact the patient's physician is not simply an implication of the dentist's obligations under the norm of competence and his or her commitment to the central values of life and general health. The norm of ideal relationships between co-professionals is also relevant because the relationship between a patient's dentist and physician will not benefit the patient maximally if either professional views the other, or either thinks he or she is viewed by the other, as a subordinate.

As in the collaboration between dentistry and dental hygiene, and in the collaboration of general dentist and specialist, each professional's expertise is essential and each one's expertise is partial and inadequate without the other's. Neither can properly ask the other to simply hand over information, or even a recommendation, to then be applied by the receiver. For health care practice cannot be broken up into pieces in that way. A health professional cannot properly render a judgment about diagnosis or intervention for a patient independently of a relationship to that patient. This fact, plus the internal connection between all the parts of the patient's life that was just stressed in the discussion of holistic care, means that the health professionals serving a patient must view each other as peers, with no one subordinate to the others. One of them should have the principal relationship to the patient, to integrate the contributions of all into a meaningful whole for the patient's decision-making, but that is the role of a first among peers, not of a superior over subordinates.

There are many pressures that make the ideal of collaborative practice between a patient's dentist and physician difficult to achieve. Limits of time and energy, noted in discussing the relations of general dentists and special-ists, are obviously relevant here. So also is the questionable cultural assump-tion just noted that longer education yields a more valuable form of expertise. Two other questionable cultural assumptions, that death is the worst evil, and that physicians' expertise is principally in preventing death, also contribute to dentists feeling that they are viewed as subordinates when working with physicians and, unfortunately, to both physicians and patients, often enough, agreeing with that ranking.

The authors believe that physicians have a similar obligation to maintain-ing a collaborative practice with their co-professionals that requires them to work against these challenges, to practice collaboratively with dentists, and to view dentists as professional peers. But other than by occasionally being able to educate physicians about their mutual obligations for practicing collaboratively (for which task hospital-based dentists may have the most frequent opportunity), dentists will generally only be able to take care of their own house in this matter. For their part, then, dentists are obligated to practice collaboratively with physicians when the latter's role in patients' care is important and to work against the pressures that tend to throw either party into a subordinate position. One particular obligation of the last sort that dentists should be sensitive to is to watch out for the defensiveness to which their feeling of being, and especially their actually being treated as, subordinates so readily gives rise and which can mar actual relationships with a collaborating physician and become harmful to the patient as well.

Similar reflections about collaboration with mental health professionals are also in order. Each profession's obligation to practice collaboratively requires efforts on both sides to work together effectively and with mutual respect for each professional's distinctive expertise to benefit the patient from their combination. Often enough, the challenge to collaborative practice regarding mental health professionals will run in the reverse direction from the challenges vis-a-vis physicians. For the professional whose expertise is based in the "hard" biological sciences may consider the professional in psychology, social work, and so on to be "soft" and hence typically inferior in importance, decision-making ability, and ability to help the patient. Cultural biases in favor of the "hard" sciences are challengeable on theoretical grounds, and all the more so when the goal at hand is to help the patient deal with his or her oral health needs when doing so is for some reason especially difficult. In any case, the dentist's obligation, grounded in the patient's need for integration of the forms of expertise required to respond best to his or her needs, is again to practice collaboratively with the mental health professional.

Finally, there are the nonprofessional collaborators with whom, in spite of their nonprofessional status, the dentist shares important fiduciary responsibilities in the care of patients. This group can include dental assistants, office managers and receptionists, and many other kinds of staff, depending on the particular responsibilities they are assigned in a given office or institution. The relevant question is whether the duties assigned to such a person put that person in a fiduciary relationship with the patient. That is, is this person asked to make judgments and engage in actions in relation to the patient that are extensions and expressions of the dentist's professional judgments and interventions or of the dentist's professional relationship of commitment to the patient's well-being?

The distinction here may be a subtle one. Some dentists assign duties to some or all of their staff that make it clear that even if they interact effectively with patients and make them comfortable, the staff person's actions are his or her own and the staff person is carrying out a job that is not part of the dentist's care-giving relationship to the patient. Other dentists assign duties their staff in such a way that the staff understand, and communicate in word, manner, and deed to the patients, that they represent the dentist to the patient and, in carrying out their tasks, are extending his or her expert care for the patient. These latter, because they represent and extend the actions of the professional, have fiduciary responsibilities to the patient. If they fail in a task in this role, they have not only done a job poorly, but have detracted from the relationship between dentist and patient and lessened in some measure the dentist's achievement of the values he or she is committed to serving for the patient. If they succeed, they directly actualize those values in some measure and contribute to the relationship between patient and care giver. In other words, if those with fiduciary responsibility fail in something, the dentist has failed in it; if they succeed, the dentist has succeeded.

We do not believe that dentists' obligation to practice collaboratively requires them to assign such fiduciary roles to any, much less all, of their nonprofessional staff. But it does require that those staff to whom they do assign fiduciary roles be considered to that extent collaborators in the care of the patient, and that all involved view their care of the patient to that extent as the work of a team. The reason for this subtle requirement is the same point noted above, namely, that a health care practitioner's judgments, actions, and relationship to a patient cannot be separated into independently deliverable pieces. They are part of a single, complex activity, and as such, they must function together.

The precise implications of this obligation in the daily life of an office or institution will depend on the actual fiduciary duties assigned. Dentists who act on this obligation will certainly view good professional care as the work of the whole team, rather than solely as the work of the office's professionals, and they will share credit accordingly. They will certainly heed the insights of fiduciary staff about patients, and may share certain forms of decision making with them as well. The point is that good care of patients requires that those who are given the role of collaborators in fact must be enabled to function in that role effectively and respected for fulfilling that role when they do so.

This is related to an obligation that a dentist would have as an employer, as a matter of justice, in any case. It is the obligation to match employees' opportunities and relationships with their responsibilities so they have the opportunity to perform in the manner expected of them and to be affirmed for doing so. But dentists have this obligation, with regard to fiduciary employees, for another reason. For they are required to practice collaboratively, as has been explained above, and therefore are obligated to shape whatever collaborative relationships they create for patient care as positively for patient benefit as possible.

THINKING ABOUT THE CASE

The case provides a number of specific examples of professional collaboration and lack of it. But the first comment on the case concerns the theme of discrimination on the basis of race, ethnicity, and gender. Dentists are obligated to collaborate in any situation in which their combined expertise is needed for the patient's benefit. Their choice of collaborators is obviously to be determined by the kind of professional expertise that the patients' needs indicate. Particularly in large metropolitan areas, general dentists may have a wide range of specialists in each area of specialty care to choose from. In making their choice of specialists, dentists ought to pay attention to the technical and communication skills, manner, and philosophy of dental practice that will benefit the patient most. They ought not pay attention to race, ethnicity, gender, or any other factor irrelevant to the best patient care and to effective collaboration between dentists to that end.

The ADA's *Principles* expresses an obligation of dentists that the larger community now requires of all professionals and persons in many other roles of society. Namely, "dentists shall not refuse to accept patients into their practice or deny dental service to patients because of the patient's race, creed, color, sex, or national origin" (1-A). This obligation is required of dentists in their role as citizens, in their role as business persons, and in their role as health professionals as well.

The literature of dental professional ethics rarely mentions the further point that it would be a strange irony if such discrimination were unethical in regard to patients, but acceptable in regard to professional colleagues. Dentists' obligations toward their co-professionals clearly exclude such discrimination and clearly require that professional relationships be based on professional qualities that will benefit the patient both directly and through the building of strong collaborative relationships among the professionals involved.

In a society with a long history of racial discrimination, official and especially unofficial in later years, it is not surprising that daily life in the dental profession has been touched by such discrimination and has only very recently begun to bear significant witness to its decrease. The case that introduces this chapter is fictional. But the success story attributed to Dr. Watkins is intended as a reminder of something that is not fictional: that members of every racial and ethnic group can make excellent dentists and excellent collaborators in the care of patients.

In this connection, consider this interesting fact about the story of the Lone Ranger, who has served as this chapter's running image of noncollaboration. The Lone Ranger is almost always accompanied by the astute and skillful Native American, Tonto. Tonto contributes subtle stratagems and other effective assistance to nearly every adventure of the Lone Ranger and occasionally saves the Lone Ranger's life as well. Yet, though the Lone Ranger is almost always aided by this skillful collaborator, he is always thought of as "lone." Why so? Because Tonto is invisible. He is a Native American. In so many legends of America, there are whole classes of people who disappear from the story, who are not peers, who do not count. This is one feature of our culture that dentistry must not imitate.

In the case at the beginning of the chapter, the collaboration of Dr. Chong and Dr. Watkins is intended to underline the ways in which mutual respect, trust, and close dialogue can benefit the patient and provide both professionals with a strong sense of support from a respected colleague. Mr. Nelson will receive his periodontic surgery from a skilled specialist rather than a dentist with limited experience in the procedure who would be practicing that much closer to the limits of his expertise. In fact, because of his greater training and experience in the area, Dr. Watkins is able to develop a treatment plan that actually postpones the surgery and its risks for a time.

In addition, by not waiting to refer until his own efforts prove inadequate and the case "blows up on him," Dr. Chong enables Dr. Watkins to enter the case when he is able to do the most good, rather than later when the worst has already happened. This is obviously better for Mr. Nelson. But it is also a vote of confidence and professional respect for Dr. Watkins's expertise from a colleague who is knowledgeable enough that he could be doing more, though not as well.

By contacting Dr. Chong and carefully discussing his findings and proposals with him, Dr. Watkins also obtains another colleague's feedback to strengthen his clinical judgment about the case, again benefiting Mr. Nelson with the value of two heads and two dentists' professional experience. At the same time, Dr. Watkins's consulting Dr. Chong affirms his positive judgment and respect for Dr. Chong's expertise and the latter's good relationship with the patient, thus providing the general dentist with the support of a respected colleague as well.

Further, by their active collaboration, the two dentists educate Mr. Nelson in the ways of professional expertise at its best, not as the work of lone rangers, but as the joining of different skills and lives of professional experience for the patient's benefit. Even if a bad outcome would occur, their collaboration on the treatment plan is more likely to leave Mr. Nelson convinced that both dentists did everything good dentists could do just because he knows that each was there to strengthen the other's contribution and protect him from errors. This not only leaves the two dentists legally more secure, which although it is not a matter of professional-ethical significance, is no mean benefit, but it also correctly educates this patient and others he might talk to, correctly representing how dental expertise is applied most effectively.

Finally, both dentists clearly work closely with their dental hygienists, Dr. Chong so closely that he brings her into the telephone conversation with Dr. Watkins and then Mr. Nelson. Both dentists value the special contributions of the dental hygienist in patient education and in developing self-care plans that fit a patient's particular needs and lifestyle. Each of the benefits to the patient and to the two dentists discussed in the previous paragraphs is now enhanced still further in the collaboration between dentists and dental hygienists.

The collaboration described in the treatment of Mr. Nelson undoubtedly idealizes a bit. The challenges to collaborative practice discussed in the previous sections are not at all apparent in the relationship of Dr. Watkins and Dr. Chong or their relationships with Dr. Chong's hygienist, or any of these practitioners' relationship with Mr. Nelson. But in many real practice settings, general dentists and specialists and dentists and dental hygienists do overcome these challenges and practice collaboratively according to the ideals articulated in this chapter. The challenges to collaboration are real, but so is the possibility of achieving collaboration in daily practice.

The story of Ms. O'Gara is obviously less happy, in spite of a long, generally positive relationship between her and Dr. Schmidt and the efforts of Dr. Watkins to help the story come out right in the present situation. Dr. Watkins is correct to say that he cannot provide Ms. O'Gara with a judgment about Dr. Schmidt's role in relation to her advanced periodontal disease. Without talking with Dr. Schmidt, and even after he does so, he may not be able to piece together what evidence Dr. Schmidt actually had of the progress of the condition 14 months earlier or before that, nor would he be able to form a clear picture of how much Ms. O'Gara understood of what Dr. Schmidt told her about it, if anything, or her level of cooperation with recommended self-care or treatment, if there was any.

But the focus for this chapter is not on whether Dr. Schmidt did or did not perform bad work for Ms. O'Gara, nor on how Dr. Watkins should speak to that issue. Dr. Schmidt is clearly a dentist of considerable competence and skill in relating to patients, even if his diagnosis and treatment of Ms. O'Gara's periodontal disease was lacking. He is portrayed here because he is also an example of something else that is at the center of this chapter's attention. He is a lone ranger. He practices solo, not only in the sense of being the only professional in his office, but in his view of dental practice. For him, the practice of dentistry at its best is the work of one person, the general dentist, meeting all the challenges of patient's oral health by his own wits and professional wisdom alone. He does not have the expertise of a dental hygienist to properly identify and treat the early stages of periodontal disease if his own training or experience are patchy in this area, and therefore he practices at the limits of his competence regarding it. He also looks doubtfully on the need for specialists, trusting his own judgment and skills even at their limits.

The case does not provide enough detail about Dr. Schmidt to form a very careful judgment of his practice, or even his care of Ms. O'Gara. But he can easily be imagined embodying the image of the dentist as lone ranger, as the epitome of solo practice, going it alone instead of viewing dental expertise as collaborative from the start. It is a close judgment call whether the circumstances provide Dr. Watkins with enough of an opening that he should try to educate Dr. Schmidt about a more collaborative view of periodontic care and of dental care in general. Perhaps he could be faulted for ending the telephone conversation when he does, rather than making an effort to help his colleague overcome this obvious deficit in his view of dental practice. But in either case, Dr. Watkins knows something very important about dentistry that Dr. Schmidt does not, that there is a professional obligation of every dentist to collaborate effectively with his or her co-professionals.

Finally, a word is in order about patients. Chapter 8 stressed the importance of efforts by the dentist to elicit and support cooperation by patients in dental care, and the crucial ethical importance of the dentist supporting the dentist-patient relationship has been emphasized often. But up to this point, nothing has been said about the patient's obligations within this relationship. Do patients have an obligation to collaborate?

Patients certainly take on a role when they seek a dentist's assistance. This role is not one that the patient can simply create out of whole cloth in each dealing with a dentist because in establishing norms for the dental profession, the larger community and dental community in dialogue have also, at least implicitly, established parameters on conduct of patients. For one thing, at one extreme, if capable patients are uncooperative enough, a dentist may "fire" such a patient, as Chapter 8 discussed. But at the other end of the question, patients do not have a role-based obligation to undertake significant sacrifices for the dentist's well-being. So whatever commitments a patient can be said to have made in establishing a patient-dentist relationship, they certainly involve "less"—they are both less demanding of sacrifice and are less precise in what they require—than the obligations that health professionals have toward their patients.

If patients do take on a role, then, it is not some sort of categorical mistake to say that an uncooperative patient is acting inappropriately, not simply from the point of view of maximizing benefit to the patient, but in terms of a relationship that the patient has taken up but is now hindering or rendering ineffective by his or her conduct. But people change paths often in life, and the mere fact that a person has started on one course and then changes to another is not automatically a moral fault. What, if anything, justifies the conviction of so many dentists that something morally significant is at stake in patients' conduct and that the capable patient who refuses to collaborate with the dentist without some very good reason is morally at fault?

The reason for this conviction, we propose, is not some social role of being-a-patient that is analogous to the health professional's special role with its sizable set of norms governing the professional's conduct. The moral significance of the patient's being cooperative or not derives rather from a more fundamental, nonconventional set of obligations between human beings that is a part of justice and is most naturally summarized under the word "reciprocity." This is the aspect of justice in human relationships that pertains to a fair or equal distribution of burdens within human relationships.

When a social arrangement requires one group of people to bear all or most of the burdens of a relationship when others bear none or few, and when there is not comparably unbalanced distribution of the benefits, many people would declare that distribution of burdens unfair or unjust. The provision of dental care requires considerable sacrifices on the part of dentists, in particular the pattern of sacrifice for the sake of patients' well-being that is required by professional norms and that is the necessary support for the pattern of respect and trust of health professionals on which effective health care by a professional depends. Admittedly, dentists make these sacrifices by their own choice and have given up simply opting out of these sacrifices by becoming professionals. But from the point of view of the distributive patterns, how one came to have certain burdens is not as important as who has which ones.

Being a patient involves some burdens, too, most especially the burdens of cooperation and resisting fears and desires that would lead to uncooperative behavior. Admittedly, some patients' fears, apprehensions, and desires are so great that they effectively have no option but to be less than cooperative, but the ordinary patient does not have this much trouble bearing the burden of cooperation. However, the burden is ordinarily viewed by dentists as significantly less than the dentist's burdens of sacrifice as a professional. Thus a patient who is unwilling to accept his or her burden of cooperation, but still expects the dentist to bear his or her burden of professional sacrifice, is often judged to act unjustly and so to rightly earn the moral criticism of the dentist. It is not that the patient has a role-obligation to be cooperative, but there is an obligation as a matter of justice and reciprocity.

How can dentists facilitate patients' acceptance of this burden? The first answer to this question is the same as the first answer to every other "how to" question in this chapter. The dentist facilitates collaboration by viewing the enterprise as collaborative from the start and speaking, acting, and transacting accordingly. If the dentist treats the patient as a collaborator, the patient in more likely to act like one; if the dentist treats the patient as a passive recipient of services, with the dentist alone as possessed of relevant understanding, judgment, and so on, then the patient is likely to follow the role assigned him or her in this model. The lesson here is the same lesson proposed many times in the preceding chapters: that the most effective and appropriate relationship between dentist and patient is an interactive one in which the patient and dentist emphasize their standing as moral equals, as collaborative judges of the best courses of action, and as choosers together of the path they will follow together.

Clearly, dentists' patients are not to be considered co-professionals. But the ethic of collaborative practice, most important in guiding dentists' interactions with other professionals, is rightly seen as relevant to their relations to patients as well. For it mirrors in its implications about patients the lesson of the norm of an ideal relationship between dentist and patient, discussed so often in these pages, namely, an obligation to work for as interactive a relationship as possible with every patient.

CHAPTER 11

HIV and AIDS in Patients

Case: The Thoughtful Patient

Joe Shovich is a 46-year-old divorced architect who has been a patient of Dr. Michael Lewis for 10 years. Shovich provides good self-care for his teeth and appears faithfully at Dr. Lewis' office every 6 months for a check-up and cleaning. Shovich has needed little work beyond that, except for the placement, over the years, of five crowns on teeth damaged by caries in Shovich's youth. In those five cases, the remaining enamel could no longer support multiple deteriorating amalgams from years ago. Dr. Lewis has been keeping an eye on the lower left second molar for some time as well, for the same reason.

At 1:30 on Friday afternoon, Joe Shovich called the office. He was in considerable pain and thought he had seriously damaged a tooth in the left lower jaw while chewing a handful of beer nuts at a business luncheon. Could Dr. Lewis squeeze him in somehow this afternoon to take a look at it? The receptionist spoke with Dr. Lewis and, luckily for Joe, Mrs. Burns had canceled her 4:30 appointment. Instead of going home a little early, Dr. Lewis would see him.

Shovich's mouth looked exactly as Dr. Lewis expected it would after he had checked Joe's chart. The enamel holding together two two-surface restorations, placed before Lewis ever met Shovich, had finally given out. Fortunately, there was still enough coronal structure that Lewis could place a crown without having to do anything more radical with the tooth. He explained the situation to Shovich and proposed to proceed right away to prepare the tooth for a crown, take the impressions, and place a temporary crown until the permanent one was fabricated—all of this on the condition that x-rays revealed no other problems with the structures below the gumline.

Shovich was delighted that Dr. Lewis could begin the process right away and quickly agreed to the proposed treatment plan. They discussed possible materials for the crown, with Shovich quickly settling on gold, and radiographs were taken.

Dr. Lewis's assistant was just leaving the operatory to develop the films when Shovich asked Lewis to close the door because he wanted to talk with him about something. "You have been my dentist for 10 years now," Shovich began, "and you've given me good care and have been a very decent person to deal with. So I feel that I owe it to you to tell you something that I learned about myself on Wednesday.

"I'm divorced, you know, and I've had a number of different sexual contacts, all with women, over the last several years. I decided that, just to play it safe, it would be good to get tested for HIV.

"Well, on Wednesday, I learned that the results of that first test were positive. I was told beforehand that if the results of the first test are positive, then a second test is done before any conclusions are drawn. Both are what is called a Western blot test. I don't know if you are familiar with all of this, but there can be false positives from that test. So if the second test is also positive, then they would do a different kind of test to confirm the results.

"So no one is saying yet that I have the AIDS virus in me. I know I don't have any symptoms; in fact, I have been very healthy lately. But I thought it might be important for you, since you are going to be working on my teeth, to know that the first test was positive, in case it affects how you would do things.

"I would also be willing to call you to tell you the results of the second test, or a third one if they do it, if that would be helpful to you. But I want it understood that this information is just between the two of us, unless you want to talk it over with my physician. He already knows about it, of course."

"It is very thoughtful of you to tell me about this," said Dr. Lewis. "My staff and I all practice the Universal Precautions that the Centers for Disease Control and Prevention recommends to protect our patients and ourselves from possible infection. But it is important for my proper care of you that I know this information, and I appreciate your candor about it very much. How are you handling this information yourself?"

"I'm dealing with it the best I can," said Joe. "I just thought I ought to let you know."

What ought Dr. Lewis do, and why?

THE ETHICAL CHALLENGES OF HIV AND AIDS

HIV and AIDS have intruded abruptly and powerfully on dental practice in the last 15 years and have changed dental practice as a result. Terrible, fatal, blood-born epidemics have not been part of dental practice for many generations, if ever in its history, and certainly not since dentistry became highly successful in preserving and restoring patients' oral health. Thus the kinds of questions that HIV and AIDS raise about appropriate professional conduct in dental practice have not been carefully discussed in the past. There is no store of well-thought-out answers to these questions to which dentists can turn. That is why these questions are being raised and discussed so intensely today, uncomfortable though they are.

They are uncomfortable questions because, as has been stressed in previous chapters, most of a dentist's actions, like most of the actions of an experienced practitioner in any field, derive chiefly from habits acquired and supported over a number of years. It is the nature of a habit to be conservative in the literal sense of that word: to conserve, to preserve ways of seeing, valuing, judging, and acting that have proven themselves valuable. When a question arises that challenges such a habitual pattern, or when a set of facts arises that habitual patterns have not taken into account, that question and those facts will naturally seem to put the values and norms of the profession at risk.

For one thing, several generations of dentists, and of health care professionals in general, have been educated and gone into practice without seriously considering the possibility that providing care to their patients might place their lives at risk by a fatal infection. Nor is it likely that even if the possibility of a fatal virus becoming epidemic had been foreseen, it could have been guessed that infection by such a virus would also involve the powerful social stigma that HIV infection and AIDS unfortunately have in our society. So it is hardly surprising that the professional norms of conduct that today's practicing dentists learned in their formative years don't seem to provide clear answers to the questions that dental professionals face today because of HIV and AIDS.

This chapter and the next will examine two sets of these questions with the hope of advancing the reflection of both the dental community and the community at large about them. The present chapter will focus on professional-ethical issues regarding HIV-positive dental patients. The next chapter will focus on issues regarding the HIV-positive practitioner.

THE OBLIGATION TO ACCEPT RISK AND ITS LIMITS

For many centuries, indeed up until 50 or 60 years ago, becoming a health professional meant accepting a significantly higher risk of contracting a life-threatening infectious disease than would be faced by someone in another walk of life. For the last several decades, however, it is medical science's successes in controlling fatal infectious diseases that have received the attention, rather than care givers' risk of infection. Consequently, for many health professionals in practice today, neither in their training nor in their daily practice until recently did they give much thought to the possibility that they have made a commitment that includes the acceptance, for the sake of their patients, of greater-than-ordinary risk of contracting a life-threatening infection.

The arrival of HIV and AIDS has changed this. There is a lot of thought being given by students in the health professions and by practicing members of these professions to the risk that HIV and AIDS pose to their lives. In the same way, the community at large is gradually realizing that medical science's permanent defeat of lethal infectious diseases was a myth, and a dangerous one at that.

But what did not change during the era when this myth was dominant, and what has received renewed clarity since our knowledge of HIV and AIDS began to grow, is that both the community at large and many members of the health professions share the view that those who become health professionals are professionally committed to accepting a greater-than-ordinary risk to their lives if this is necessary for the proper care of their patients.

Demonstrating this conclusion in detail, by examining the patterns of action and expectation and the patterns of what are judged acceptable reasons for acting and refraining in certain relevant ways—which is what counts as evidence of an accepted social norm—is a very complex task. It requires a detailed comparison of a variety of different case scenarios to identify under just what circumstances a health care professional is or is not obligated to treat a patient when HIV or AIDS is a risk factor. But when these patterns of action, expectation, and so on are examined, as several will be below, what they reveal is a basic obligation on the part of health care professionals to accept a greater-than-ordinary risk of infection if it is necessary for the proper care of their patients. Moreover, there is no evidence to suggest that dental professionals have been or should be viewed any differently from the other health professions in this regard.

The ADA's *AIDS Policy Statement* is in concert with this view, rejecting as unprofessional and unethical any refusal to treat an HIV-positive patient, or a patient with active AIDS, solely on the basis of the increased risk that such treatment involves for the dental care provider. But as scenarios are compared in search of the patterns of action and expectation that identify the contents of professionals' obligations, it also becomes clear that the dental professional's obligation to accept risk in order to treat HIV and AIDS patients is only one part of the story. For there are also *limits* to this obligation for dental professionals and for health care professionals generally. These limits are of two kinds. One concerns the extent of the identifiable risks to the health professional's life, along with the care giver's capability to control those risks through caution. If the risks are great enough and are not the product of the practitioner's lack of caution, there is good reason for the larger community, in dialogue with the dental professions, to decline to oblige the professional to provide full, appropriate care if doing so would add unjustifiable risk to the care giver's life, and the larger community may even require that dental professionals limit their care-giving for certain classes of patients.

The other limit concerns the relative benefits to the patient if the needed care is not provided. For if providing a certain form of care does not yield sufficient benefit to the patient when compared with the extent of the risk to the care giver, then again it is reasonable for the larger community and the dental profession, in dialogue, to decline to oblige a dental professional to provide it and possibly to even require that it not be provided.

To understand these limits, it is necessary to try to articulate the reasoning process that goes on in the dental profession, in the community at large, and especially in their dialogue with each other as these professional norms are formulated. Consider for a moment the account of the Greek historian, Thucydides, in the second book of his *History of the Peloponnesian War*, of a plague that struck Athens in about 430 B.C.: "a pestilence of such extent and mortality [as] was nowhere remembered." Neither "human art," he tells us, nor "supplications in the temples" were of any avail against it. Nor were the physicians "of any service, ignorant as they were of the proper way to treat it." But the physicians continued to care for those who were infected. In fact, the physicians "died themselves the most thickly, as they visited the sick most often."

Now, no thoughtful community would want to have its physicians dying "the most thickly" like this. No thoughtful community, lay or professional, would accept professional norms that would place the lives of health care professionals at such great risk that the community would soon have to do without them, nor would a provident community let them face grave risk when they could achieve very little good for their patients by doing so. Instead, the community and its professionals would establish norms of professional practice that would preserve the ranks of health professionals to provide needed services to those who survive the crisis, and they would also measure the risk the health professionals ought to face by the benefits they can effectively bring to their patients. Thus they would take a long-term, whole-community approach to the weighing of risks and benefits as they examine alternative ways of understanding the obligations of health professionals in the face of risk.

Consequently, it is very unlikely that any society's view of the obligations of its health professionals, in regard to facing risk to their own lives, is that this obligation is unlimited. It is also likely, to put the same point another way, that if the AIDS virus that we are familiar with were able to pass far more readily from patient to care giver than it can, then the community and the health professions would quickly begin to regulate the contact between care givers and patients so that the ranks of care givers would not be wiped out and people in need of health care be left without assistance.

The presumption in this thought process, as has been pointed out, is that the health professional has already made a commitment to accept greater-than-ordinary risk for the sake of proper care of the patient, but that other considerations, having to do with the long-term well-being of the whole community, may indicate limiting this obligation and even identifying classes of cases in which the health professional should not be bound by that obligation. Thus while the health professional's relationship to the individual patient remains one of care for the patient's needs, he or she is still professionally committed to attend to the needs of the whole community over the long run as well. Sometimes the latter considerations will take precedence over the former.

When will they take precedence? What are the limits of the dental professional's obligation to accept risk? Neither our health professions nor the community at large, in the various ways in which it contributes to the ongoing dialogue on professional norms, has been particularly precise or articulate about this point. But a few types of cases do seem fairly clear.

It seems certain, for example, that if a health care professional refused to provide life-saving treatment, in the form of CPR, to a patient committed to his or her care when a breathing tube and gloves were available, and the refusal was made out of concern that doing so would slightly increase the risk to his or her own life by reason of a possible lethal infection from that patient, then such a practitioner would be acting unethically and unprofessionally. But this conclusion does not follow so clearly if we change the example so that the benefit to the patient is considerably less, and the risk to the provider is considerably greater. In general, then, health professionals are committed to accepting a greater-than-ordinary risk of infection, even lethal infection, if it is required for the proper care of patients committed to their care. But this is not an unlimited obligation. There are classes of cases in which it is in the long-term interest of the community at large that health professionals *not* accept such risk, cases in which the risk to those who would provide full and proper treatment is too great, or in which doing so produces too little benefit for the patient in comparison with the risk to providers.

This is why the judgment of the Centers for Disease Control and Prevention (CDC), and of other organizations whose judgments have agreed with CDC, about the ordinary degree of risk of HIV transmission to care givers when the CDC's recommended "Universal Precautions" are being observed is so important. This is essential data for the professions and the larger community in weighing the risks to care givers against the short-term and long-term benefits of care to determine in what kinds of situations a health professional's ordinary obligation to accept risk should be overridden. In general, the judgment of the CDC is that the Universal Precautions are sufficient to keep the risk to providers in ordinary treatment situations at a minimal level. The clear implication of this judgment is that, when Universal Precautions are employed, health care professionals are obligated to provide all ordinary treatments that patients need.

How does this reasoning translate to dental care? Dental professionals rarely provide treatment to patients that is directly life-saving, so it might seem to be in the community's interest to exempt dental care providers from the obligation of accepting greater-than-ordinary risk to their lives for the sake of their patients on the basis that the benefit to patients is not worth the risk. But the dental community frequently provides patients with relief from intense oral pain and enables patients to maintain forms of oral functioning that are of great psychological importance, not to mention nutritional importance, to most human beings. In other words, although life is only rarely directly at stake in dental care, dental professionals still serve patients in ways that they value greatly.

Consequently, the quick conclusion that the larger community would not sacrifice the lives of its dental care providers for the sake of the benefits of dental care because lives are not at stake is too simplistic. Rather, as an analogue to the previous case, if a dentist failed to treat a patient's severe oral pain when employing appropriate barrier techniques out of concern that doing so would place the dentist's life at a slightly increased risk of possible lethal infection from that patient, the community at large and most health professionals today would find that dentist guilty of unethical and unprofessional conduct. But if the risk were far greater, or if the benefit to the patient were far less important, then it is likely that the community's long-term interests would be better served if the obligation to accept risk were overridden in such circumstances.

If the CDC's conclusions about the effectiveness of Universal Precautions are taken in to account, then the implication is that dental professionals are obligated to accept the minimally increased risk involved in providing ordinary dental care. This is precisely the conclusion offered in the American Dental Association's (ADA's) *AIDS Policy Statement*: "Current scientific and epidemiologic evidence indicates that there is little risk of transmission of infectious diseases through dental treatment if recommended infection control procedures are routinely followed. Patients with HIV infection may be safely treated in private dental offices when appropriate infection control procedures are employed. Such infection control procedures provide protection both for patients and for dental personnel."

Although it is not explicit about the point, this Policy Statement should not be interpreted as claiming that dental care providers have an unlimited obligation to accept risk to their lives for the sake of their patients. It should be interpreted rather as holding that the level of increased risk is so minimized by the use of Universal Precautions that otherwise important limitations on this obligation are not relevant in ordinary dental treatment of HIV-positive and AIDS patients. In other words, because the risk is so limited, the limitations are therefore not relevant in ordinary dental treatment. So the Statement holds that dental professionals are committed to providing all the ordinary forms of diagnosis and treatment that their patients need. It would be unprofessional and unethical of a dentist to decline to provide full, appropriate care solely because of the increased risk to the provider by reason of the patient's actual or likely HIV status.

Of course, a patient with active AIDS, for example, a patient who is immunosuppressed, may need treatment of a special sort or in a special location, *for the patient's own protection*. There are also dental procedures that would not be performed for such a patient because the benefit to the patient does not outweigh the risk of the procedure *to the patient*. Such patient-centered reasons for not treating a patient or for referring a patient for treatment elsewhere are not central to the issues under consideration here.

Some dentists, along with some professionals in other health fields and some members of the larger community, have expressed serious doubts about the adequacy of the CDC's and other institutions' judgments about providers' risk of HIV infection from patients. If the judgments of the CDC and of the other researchers who have supported them were to be proven inadequate, then obviously the question would have to be reopened whether ordinary dental diagnosis and treatment involves sufficient risk that dentists' obligation to face that risk should be more limited. But the weight of scientific evidence currently rests with the CDC and the other scientific organizations and institutions that support its judgments in these matters. So the burden of proof that there is sufficient scientific evidence to reopen the question regarding limiting dentists' obligations to provide ordinary dental care certainly rests on the challengers at the present time.

CAUTION BEYOND THE UNIVERSAL PRECAUTIONS

Every dental practitioner knows that the CDC's Universal Precautions cannot completely eliminate the possibility of blood-to-blood contact between patient and practitioner. The instruments used in dental diagnosis and treatment are very sharp, and accidents occur in which an instrument penetrates not only the practitioner's glove, but the practitioner's skin as well. When such an accident occurs, the chances of blood-to-blood contact between patient and practitioner are increased as is the risk of infection if the patient is the carrier of a blood-born disease. (It is important to note, however, that this increase in risk has not been sufficient to prompt scientists studying the matter to change their judgment that the chances of patient-to-provider and provider-to-patient spread of infection are minimal.)

It is possible, however, for the dental professional to reduce the chances of an accident during diagnosis or treatment by practicing with greater caution. Perhaps he or she can employ more light, or station the mirror more carefully each time to keep a fuller view of each movement with a sharp instrument, or change his or her posture more frequently so that muscles do not strain and control of the instruments is always at absolute maximum. In four-handed procedures, sharp instruments are not passed, but each is carefully picked up by the practitioner who will use it, and so on. In addition to efforts such as these, which will vary in their usefulness from practice to practice, dental professionals can also simply move more slowly and attend with a higher degree of focused concentration to each movement so no instrument goes where it is not wanted. Additional examples of "caution beyond the Universal Precautions" will surely come to mind for every dental practitioner who reads this.

Few dental professionals who provide care for patients known to be or likely to be HIV-positive, or even for patients just suspected of being HIV-positive, do so without practicing some measure of additional caution beyond the Universal Precautions. In fact, a dental professional who failed to practice additional caution when caring for a patient known to be HIV-positive might even be acting *un*professionally. For the interests of the larger community in protecting and preserving health professionals surely require them to protect themselves when there is no diminishment of care for the patient or when there is some small diminishment of care, but it is outweighed by the increased protection of the dental professional's ability to practice.

Now, it is important to notice that the pattern of reasoning at work in the previous sentence is the same pattern that was operative throughout the previous section. The perspective of the community and the dental professions when they consider the long-term oral health of the whole community requires them to consider both the provision of care to individuals who need it and the preservation of those who are capable of providing that care. This reasoning is necessarily in terms of *classes* of cases and *general* characteristics of *types* of patients, *types* of needed care, and the *types* of professional expertise needed to provide it. Reasoning in this way, it is easy to see why it is a norm of the health professions that health professionals accept a greater-than-ordinary risk of infection; otherwise, the community would have no general assurance that they would be treated when suffering from serious infection. But it is also reasonable that there be *limits* to this obligation because otherwise the community could surely expect its health professionals to soon be ill and dying—like the Athenian physicians—"the most thickly" and hence to be unavailable to provide health care to those who will need it in the future.

With regard to caution beyond the Universal Precautions, it is similarly reasonable that health professionals be permitted to practice with additional caution when they are faced with known additional risk and can practice such caution without severely compromising the care they give. If such caution compromised care too severely, however, the extra caution would not serve the long-term interests of the community. If the increase in risk to the provider in a particular class of cases was very great, on the other hand, then at some point along the spectrum of risk to providers the community might in fact require its health professionals to practice with such added caution that the care patients received was significantly compromised. Indeed, at some point still further along that spectrum, as has been noted, there might be a class of patients whom the community even prohibited health care professionals from treating, apart from comfort measures, because of the extreme risk to their lives if they were to do so, or the community might permit only a certain limited group of health care professionals to face such risk.

To see this pattern of reasoning in operation in another aspect of health care practice that is much more common, but where this pattern of reasoning is often overlooked, consider the following. It is certainly the case that any patient whose behavior does not place him or her in a high-risk group for infection and who has not tested for seropositivity could still be a carrier of the infection. This is why CDC and the professional organizations urge all dental professionals to apply Universal Precautions to all patients, in other words, to make these precautions *universal*. But it would certainly be possible for dental professionals to practice with additional caution beyond the Universal Precautions on all patients and in all procedures that could possibly produce a wound from a sharp instrument.

If this policy were followed, far fewer patients could be seen, and far fewer examinations and procedures would be completed. Far less dental care would be provided, and the care that would be provided would cost far more in time and human effort than it does now. The loss to the community in total dental care provided would likely be very great, so much so that this proposal seems completely impractical.

A DISTINCTIVE PATTERN OF THINKING

Notice that the pattern of reasoning involved in the preceding paragraph is the same pattern referred to above. That is, the focus is on the overall long-term negative effects on the community as a whole that this particular way of practicing would produce. These effects are then weighed against the overall long-term benefits, in the form of reduced risk of infection for dental practitioners as a group because the community will depend on them for dental care in the future. Weighing losses and benefits to all affected parties and comparing alternatives in terms of such losses and benefits is precisely how reasonable people judge the details of social roles and social policies of all sorts, including the relative merits of alternative patterns of professional practice and alternative ways of conceiving of the professional obligations of a given group, such as dentists.

Reflecting on how dentists ought to act in the face of HIV and AIDS is therefore not only difficult because it often takes place during a time of fear and anxiety. It is also difficult because it requires a difficult kind of reasoning that is different from our ordinary ways of thinking about things, reasoning from the point of view of the long-term benefit of the whole community. If a dentist responds to the questions of this chapter solely from the perspective of his or her own well-being, hoping to secure appropriate dental care for self and loved ones, and to protect self and loved ones from HIV infection, this dentist's reflections will not come anywhere close to dealing with issues of professional practice and professional obligation specifically as *professional*. For these are matters of *social* institutions, and they require a *social* kind of thinking, one which examines matters from the point of view of the community at large over the long run.

This is a difficult kind of thinking for at least two reasons. First, most of us are influenced by the emphasis on individualism in American culture and are led by it to think that no matter what the challenge, we can, if we choose, go it alone. It is also a characteristic of many people that when they are afraid, they feel even more strongly that they are alone and that they have no choice but to face their challenges without the rest of humanity. Now, there are many important values in individualism, and most of us also believe that there is unique worth in every human being which must not be ignored or violated. But health is one thing that no one can achieve or secure alone, and major epidemics surely ought to remind us, as few other things do in life, that we are all in life together, mutually dependent on one another's strengths and weaknesses whether we like it or not.

This is one principal reason why we have social institutions in the first place, to help us live together and respond to life's challenges together more effectively over the long run. But to shape and reshape these institutions so they meet our needs, we have to be able to *think socially* in the sense just described.

There is a second reason why this pattern of *social thinking* is difficult, at least for most health professionals. Health professionals, for the most part, serve their patients one at a time and face-to-face. When they think of their professional obligations, they think first and foremost of their obligations to the individual patient, probably imagined most often as an individual patient in the chair before them.

Of course, all dentists should recognize that they have obligations to the patients in the waiting room and in the other operatories and to all their patients of record. Granted, a small percentage of health care professionals actually make the health of the whole public their central concern. But for most health professionals it is taken for granted without much thought that health professionals' first obligations are to the individual patients before them, and that any obligations they do have to other patients who are not presently before them will eventually be discharged to those patients in the same way, namely, face-to-face, one at a time, though at a different time even if it is only a few minutes away.

It may even seem to some health professionals that the kind of social thinking described above and proposed as being necessary for careful consideration of professional obligations in relation to HIV and AIDS is, in fact, very close to being in violation of the spirit of professional obligation in health care because it focuses on the well-being of the whole community over the long run, rather than weighing most heavily the well-being of the individual patient in the chair.

Now social thinking of this sort does require that the well-being of the present patient be weighed against the long-term well-being of the community. But even the individual patient in the chair comes to the dentist not as to someone who just happens to be helpful, but to someone who is *already a professional*. The encounter between them, however personal or not, nevertheless presupposes the existence of the dental profession and its norms and the practitioner's membership in that profession and his or her conformity to those norms. That is, it is an encounter that presupposes *social thinking*, the social thinking that shaped and must continually reshape the dental profession and its professional obligations for the sake of the people of the community, including this patient.

The point here is not that the dentist is supposed to think socially about each patient in the chair. If the dentist acts professionally and ethically toward that patient, in accord with the norms of his or her profession, which are already based on careful social thinking, then the patient will be properly served. But when the questions at issue are about *what* those norms *are* and about *what* they *ought to be* if they are to be more precise and better suited to the circumstances at hand, *then* the thinking must be explicitly *social*. It must be conducted in terms of the well-being of the whole community over the long run.

The proposal being made here is that from the perspective of such social thinking, dental professionals have a general obligation to accept greater-than-ordinary risk of infection if proper care of their patients requires it. But at the same time, this obligation is limited by the degree of risk, its avoidability through reasonable caution, and the extent to which care actually benefits the patient, among other factors.

THE OBLIGATION OF CONFIDENTIALITY

It has long been an accepted component of the professional obligations of health care providers that they respect the confidentiality of what they learn about their patients. These obligations derive in part from obligations of confidentiality that all persons have toward one another by reason of the impact that certain categories of information about us can have on our lives and relationships as well as the value we place on determining for ourselves who will know what things about us. But in addition, health professionals have, specifically as health care professionals, obligations in regard to confidentiality, obligations that derive from the kind of social thinking described in the previous section and that modify the general human obligations about confidentiality in important ways.

For health professionals to employ their expertise for the benefit of patients, they need to know many facts about patients' lives, including facts about their bodies, about their behavior, and about their values, goals, and fears, that most people would not reveal to many other people, if to any, and certainly not to people with whom they had no long-standing personal relationship. Therefore health professionals have and proclaim an especially stringent obligation of confidentiality regarding the facts they learn about patients so that patients can feel secure when providing the information practitioners need to care for them. Only with such a stringent professional standard in place can the community expect that its health professionals will be able to work effectively for their patients over the long run. The accepted standard is that every fact revealed to the health professional by a patient is, in principle, subject to the requirement of confidentiality, so that nothing may be revealed to anyone else without the patient's permission.

But this standard has several built-in limitations that are widely accepted and that are taken for granted in daily practice. First, it is taken for granted that other health professionals involved in a patient's care may be told the facts they need to know about the patient to provide effective care. Second, it is taken for granted that some persons who are not providers of health care, but who administer its provision (by keeping records, managing financial affairs, managing the institutions in which care in provided, and so on), will need to know some of the facts revealed to health professionals by the patient to carry out their job. Finally, it is an accepted limitation of the health professional's obligation of confidentiality—although many patients may not think about it very often—that relevant facts revealed by a patient may be communicated both to other health professionals and to student health professionals, who are not involved in the patient's care, when this is done for educational reasons. (Facts about patients are also revealed, of course, in biomedical research, but current practices regarding informed consent require that patients' explicit permission be sought for research uses of information about patients, so this practice is not a limitation of the basic obligation that information about a patient may not be revealed without permission.)

Unfortunately, the settings in which health care is provided have grown increasingly large and complex over the years, and the institutions involved have grown increasingly interconnected. As a consequence, the effect of the three limitations just mentioned is that many people learn facts about patients that were originally revealed confidentially to a single provider of health care. Moreover, many of those who learn these facts are not health professionals. While they are bound by the ordinary obligations of all human beings about confidentiality, and while the other roles they fill may impose on them additional role-based obligations of confidentiality, these persons frequently have no one-to-one relationship with patients to reinforce their experience that there is a particular person who could be harmed and who would in any case be betrayed if confidentiality were violated. Unfortunately, therefore, what is intended to be a very stringent obligation, with three very carefully controlled limitations, often functions more like a sieve, or even a conduit, of sensitive information about patients to parties far removed from their health care, untouched by the health professionals' specific obligations to protect confidentiality, and often with a very doubtful need to know.

The advent of HIV and AIDS has sharply heightened patients' sensitivity to this pattern of relatively ineffective efforts by health professionals to secure the confidentiality of what patients tell them. One reason, obviously, is that a profound stigma has been attached to HIV infection and AIDS in American society. In addition, our health care system is one in which many people are at constant risk of losing insured access to health care goods and services, and insurers will use information about HIV status to cancel or modify patients' health insurance. Thus those who are or who even fear they might some day be HIV-positive are extremely concerned that information about a patient's HIV status not pass through the sieve, much worse find its way to a conduit that takes it to an insurance company or to persons socially connected with a patient who would stigmatize him or her.

Admittedly, many people in American society currently consider HIV infection to be something that will only strike people in other groups—"them"—and never one of "us." This pattern of thinking is both evidence of, and a consequence of, the widespread stigmatization of HIV-infected persons. But to anyone who can take the point of view of the infected person or can consider that the infected person could be a loved one, or who more generally applies *social thinking* to the matter, the relative ineffectiveness of current protections for confidentiality within the health care system must be a cause of deep concern. Moreover, even if being HIV-positive or having AIDS did not involve social stigma, it is still the case that the patient ordinarily ought to be the one in control of the information that he or she has a terrible, fatal disease.

But at the same time, health care providers, including dentists, certainly need to know if a patient has active AIDS to properly weigh for that patient the benefits and risks of needed dental treatment, and knowledge that a patient is HIV-positive will also affect what a dentist looks for during diagnosis. As some hospitals have done, perhaps dental offices and other dental care institutions need to establish a two-tiered system of record keeping and information transmission. In such a system, special regulations govern what is to be done, and not done, with certain categories of particularly sensitive personal information revealed to a health care professional. Typically, psychiatric information is covered, and now patients' HIV status. These fall into a category of information that is to be kept fully confidential by the care giver receiving it, unless the information is essential to another care giver for the sake of proper care of the patient or unless the patient grants specific permission that it be communicated to others.

Information about a patient's HIV status or AIDS, however, must not only be received and properly communicated for the patient to receive the best possible care, in addition to unavoidable administrative uses and possible use in teaching situations. More importantly, it is also information about an *infectious* disease that is fatal and that can infect dental care workers if there is contact between the patient's blood or certain other body fluids and open wounds or mucous membranes of the care giver. So now the question must also be asked whether the risk of fatal infection to dental professionals, and through it the risk to the health of the larger community, is sufficiently great in general or in particular types of cases that it can outweigh the benefits of protecting confidentiality to the individual patient and to other members of the community who will be patients in the future.

One possible answer, based on the judgments of the CDC and other health organizations referred to above, is that the care givers who might receive information that a particular patient is HIV-positive are or ought to be already adequately protecting themselves from HIV infection through the use of Universal Precautions. Consequently, this argument would conclude, the breaking of confidentiality to inform another care giver, whether a specialist or a member of one's own staff, of a patient's HIV status can yield no significant benefit to anyone. The patient would be betrayed and would also be put at risk of harm if control over the information were somehow lost in the process, and the care giver would not benefit significantly since that care giver, if professionally responsible, would already be adhering to the Universal Precautions. Therefore according to this argument, neither in the individual case nor if the pattern were generalized is it justifiable to break confidentiality to protect another dental care provider. (In circumstances in which one knows that the other professional is not using the Universal Precautions, the proper intervention is not to break confidentiality but rather to educate the colleague about the need to employ the Universal Precautions.)

On the other side, it can be argued that there is a level of caution beyond the Universal Precautions, as has already been noted. Moreover, dental professionals are ordinarily permitted, from the vantage point of social thinking, to act with this extra caution in caring for HIV-infected patients unless there are significant losses involved in doing so. Therefore if this extra caution would significantly reduce the risk of infection for care givers by reducing the number of accidental penetrations of gloves, for example, as it seems is reasonable to assume (although solid empirical evidence of this point would strengthen this argument), then the question is whether the benefit so provided outweighs the potential harms. That is, does the decrease in risk to providers and hence the risk of loss of providers to the community, outweigh the potential harm to both present and future patients, including those who might be less candid with health care providers if such breaking of confidences were the accepted practice.

It is important to note that if it becomes an accepted limitation on health professionals' obligations regarding confidentiality that they may inform others caring for the same patient that a patient is HIV-positive or has AIDS, not for the patient's sake but to better protect these professionals from infection by their use of additional caution, then such warnings would *not* then be betrayals of patients' confidentiality. For if such warnings became an accepted pattern within the framework of health professionals' professional obligations, there would be no legitimate expectations of confidentiality of this sort to be betrayed. So the issue is only whether there is enough decrease in risk for the other care givers, as compared with the increase in risk of benefits lost or harm done to patients.

The two-tiered system of managing patient information that was referred to above would lessen the risk of a patient's HIV status becoming known against the patient's wishes. In addition, the settings in which dental care is most often provided ordinarily involve fewer people and less complex institutional structures than large hospitals where patient information seems to travel so fast. Therefore aberrations from the ideal professional practice of strict confidentiality probably occur somewhat less often in dental offices than in large hospitals. But these facts are not sufficient to settle the matter.

Both of the arguments outlined here are reasonable and have some measure of factual and common sense support, and neither has been conclusively subscribed to by either the dental professions or the community at large, much less by both in dialogue. It seems most accurate to say, then, that at the present time the dental profession and the larger community have not yet resolved the question whether a dentist would violate professional obligations regarding confidentiality to inform another professional caring for the same patient of the patient's HIV status not for the patient's benefit, but to protect the second care giver from infection.

Still, although no clear answer to this question has been given as yet, there is a rather clear implication from an answer to another question that has been given. For the position is widely accepted that the Universal Precautions are sufficiently effective to keep the risk of patient-to-provider transmission of HIV extremely small and within acceptable limits from the point of view of the larger community preserving its health care professionals from harm. Consequently, the burden of proof would be on those who would claim that a patient's confidentiality may be reasonably violated to reduce that risk still further. If the level of risk is acceptably handled by the Universal Precautions, and if all dental professionals are already obligated to employ the Universal Precautions conscientiously, then the further reduction of another care giver's already adequately controlled risk of infection is not sufficient to justify a breaking of confidentiality simply for that purpose.

Yet this implication of current practice also admits of an important exception under special circumstances. Suppose that there were special classes of patients for whom the health professions and the society at large accepted mandatory HIV testing prior to treatment so that additional caution besides the Universal Precautions can be employed or so that such patients can be excluded from treatment. The reason for this would be that the severity of risk to providers in such cases was so great and insufficiently reduced by the Universal Precautions alone that it outweighed in importance to the community the risk of violations of confidentiality. If such exceptions to the accepted pattern existed now or were to develop, then in those classes of cases a warning of another care giver about a patient's HIV status might be justifiable for the same reasons. For the time being, however, it seems necessary to consider situations in which such a warning would be professionally justified to be truly exceptional in the special degree of risk to the health professionals involved.

A related question concerns confidentiality and risk to third-parties, especially the sexual partner(s) of an HIV-positive patient. Suppose a dentist raises the issue of risk to sexual partners with a patient who has revealed the results of positive HIV testing in the course of an examination or treatment. Suppose further that the patient informs the dentist that he or she has no intention of making changes in his or her patterns of sexual behavior, nor of informing partners about the infection, nor of taking any steps to protect partners from it. Does the dentist have any professional obligation to take further action, beyond educating the patient as fully as possible, to protect this sort of third party?

The question whether health professionals are obligated to violate confidentiality to protect third parties is not new, but previous discussions of it have not identified clear answers that can be imported here. Many states have long had laws requiring physicians and laboratories who determine that a patient has a sexually transmitted disease to inform the state department of public health, and in some states, that department will attempt to identify and inform such persons' sexual partners of their risk. In some such states, HIV seropositivity is a reportable condition. So it might seem that the larger community (or certain geographical parts of it) consider this kind of violation of confidentiality to be justified since it provides information, through public health departments, to sexual partners who might be infected.

Dental professionals are not principal sources of such reports. More importantly, even physicians and laboratories, who are the principal source of such reports, are not themselves required to try to identify patients' sexual partners and contact them. This is done by public health officers. Even when an infected patient's sexual partner is also a patient of a physician who learns of the former's seropositivity, it is not clear that the physician has a professional obligation to inform the sexual partner, nor is it clear whether the physician *may* do so without violating professional obligations. The obligations of dentists are even less clear.

On this issue, as with the previous one, the health professions and the larger community have not reached a clear conclusion regarding possible limits on the health professional's obligation to protect the confidentiality of information about the patient. But the burden of proof in all ordinary cases again lies with anyone who claims that the value of a dental professional preserving a patient's confidentiality is outweighed by the reduction of risk of infection for parties who are, from the point of view of social thinking, capable of adequately protecting themselves by conscientiously applying information readily available to them.

THINKING ABOUT THE CASE

It may seem much too easy for us to simply declare that Dr. Lewis ought to set aside his fear of HIV infection and treat Mr. Shovich. It may seem much too easy for us to declare that Dr. Lewis may only share the information of

Mr. Shovich's probably being HIV-positive with his staff if doing so is necessary for the proper care of Mr. Shovich. But that is the direction in which the current understanding of the professional obligations of dental professionals points for Dr. Lewis and for the dental hygiene professionals on his staff as well.

Admittedly, the more frightening something is, the more difficult it is to respond to it as someone who has undertaken special obligations in regard to it, and HIV and AIDS are understandably very frightening. But fear and the anxiety it produces do not erase the obligation that comes with undertaking a professional role.

As has been argued above, the individual practitioner does not determine the content of the obligations he or she undertakes when becoming a dentist. That content is the fruit of a subtle but genuine conversation between the expert group and the larger community. Questions about what is required of members of the dental profession must be referred to that dialogue, and if it is reasonably clear in its directions to individual practitioners, then that is how they are obligated to act in their professional role.

The case has been made in this chapter that dentists are obligated to accept a greater-than-ordinary risk of infection if it is necessary to provide needed care for their patients. The sole proviso is that the level of risk to care givers should not exceed a certain limit, which is determined in turn by what will secure the greatest long-term well-being of the community in balance with the well-being of present patients. It was also argued that current understandings of the level of risk to dentists in providing ordinary dental care to HIV-positive patients, provided the Universal Precautions are being followed, does not exceed this limit. Barring special considerations not evident in this case, then, Dr. Lewis is professionally obligated to treat Mr. Shovich.

It was also argued that, although the matter is more ambiguous, the burden of proof is on anyone who claims that patients' confidentiality may be violated in the matter of their HIV-positive status to provide protection to other care givers beyond the Universal Precautions that they ought to already be conscientiously employing. The current judgment of the community at large, it was argued, regarding the level of risk of transmitting HIV infection is that in an office in which the Universal Precautions are carefully followed by all staff, as Dr. Lewis claims they are, the risk is not serious enough to justify violating a patient's confidentiality on this matter. So Dr. Lewis may not ethically inform his staff of Mr. Shovich's HIV status for this purpose.

May Dr. Lewis ask Mr. Shovich for permission to inform his staff, at least those who will actually be caring for Mr. Shovich? Provided that he abides by Mr. Shovich's choice in that matter, Dr. Lewis may certainly ask for permission, but only on the condition that he fully informs Mr. Shovich of the reasons for the request. That is, Dr. Lewis must tell Mr. Shovich that there is no reason to believe that the staff will care for Mr. Shovich any better with this information than without, at least at the present time when Mr. Shovich is asymptomatic and not at any higher risk of infection than any other patient.

He must also explain what the reason for telling the staff is, presumably so that they can practice caution beyond the Universal Precautions, and why they would be doing that and what are its likely effects on Mr. Shovich's care. For example, it is very doubtful that caution beyond the Universal Precautions will improve Mr. Shovich's care, and there is a real chance that it will be a detriment to it. Moreover, the reason for telling the staff is either for their greater ease or to actually increase the level of protection for them, even though the level of risk provided by the Universal Precautions is extremely low and is already low enough for those who are dental professionals to be obligated to provide care. That is, Dr. Lewis may be hard pressed to find good reasons that would persuade Mr. Shovich to take the risks that accompany breaching the wall of confidentiality that protects his communication of his HIV status to Dr. Lewis.

Finally, it is important to reiterate that a person can obviously have multiple obligations in a given situation and that some of these may direct the person to undertake different and mutually exclusive actions. A dentist may judge that obligations to family or other commitments conflict with his or her obligations as a dental professional to provide care, even at the risk of infection, to an HIV-positive patient. The fact of such a conflict does not mean that the professional obligations automatically "win" and determine what the dentist ought to do, all things considered, nor that they automatically "lose" either. As was indicated in Chapter 6, reflecting on such conflicts requires attention to the underlying *reasons* for the two sets of obligations, the benefits and harms that each serves, and so on. So if very special circumstances face a dentist with conflicting obligations to treat and not to treat an HIV-positive patient, or to inform and not to inform a third party about a patient's HIV-positive status, there is no simple formula available for resolving this conflict.

But as was also said in Chapter 6, if the circumstances in which the person conscientiously acts contrary to his or her professional obligations are arising regularly, then the person needs to examine carefully whether he or she is in the right profession. A dentist who judged that he or she was justified in routinely refusing to treat HIV-positive patients or in routinely violating patients' confidentiality about their HIV-positive status should carefully examine these judgments and the circumstances that prompt them to see if he or she is no longer practicing in accord with the professional norms of dentistry, as they are currently understood in our society. To present oneself to the community as a dentist but to decline to practice according to the accepted norms of that profession requires at the very minimum that the person should warn the public before they come for care that they will not be getting what they think they're getting.

On the other hand, especially after information about the HIV virus became more plentiful and came to be supported by more conclusive scientific evidence, most members of the dental community have recognized their obligation to accept greater-than-ordinary risk of infection in order to provide needed care for their patients. Most also recognize their special obligation of confidentiality regarding information about patients' HIV status because of the powerful social stigma associated with it. They and their staffs are understandably afraid of HIV infection, but they have mastered their fears to provide care according to the professional norms they have accepted. This takes a high level of courage and commitment, quite a bit more of both than most members of the larger community realize are involved. For persevering in the provision of care in the face of this epidemic, the community owes a great debt of gratitude to its dental professionals and to its health professionals generally.

CHAPTER 12

The HIV-Positive Care Giver

Case: Best Friends

Bill Prohaska was from Milwaukee. Jack Corrigan was from Portland, Maine. Both were sons of dentists, and both had found more interesting things to do in high school than hit the books. Jack had focused on playing his guitar and on the people who appreciated his playing and the marijuana they smoked together. Bill had played football and baseball for 4 years, had made the minimum grade requirement to stay on the teams by the skin of his teeth, and had filled the rest of his time with a busy social life and a goodly amount of beer.

It was no coincidence that neither young man was interested in college when high school was over. It was quite a coincidence that two young men with such similar backgrounds should find themselves working side by side, and thinking about what they had done so far with their lives, side by side, on a U.S. Navy cruiser in the South China Sea somewhere off Da Nang, Vietnam, in the summer of 1969. A friendship blossomed that supported both men until their Navy hitches were over and helped each to put together a plan for what would follow.

Both men realized that they wanted to give dentistry a try, and they decided to plan their undergraduate applications so they would have a chance of studying at the same school. They were both admitted to Notre Dame, roomed together for 4 years, graduated *cum laude* as the reward for their hard work, and made their applications to dental school, hoping again to be studying somewhere near each other.

Jack was married the summer after college, with Bill as his best man, of course, and Bill was engaged that same summer. Jack went to the dental school of University of Illinois, in Chicago, and Bill was accepted at Loyola's dental school a few miles down the road. Their spouses became good friends, and both men showed as much ability and worked as hard in dental school as they had as undergraduates. The only difference between them was that Jack's car was struck by a hit-and-run driver in the summer after his first year. His leg was pinned in the twisted metal and had to be freed by Fire Department blow torches. He lost a lot of blood before he reached the University of Illinois Hospital Emergency Room. Apart from his leg, however, his injuries were not serious, and his two months in the hospital did not set him back significantly in his studies. But the accident left him with an obvious limp that he would have for the rest of his life.

In May, 1978, Dr. John Corrigan and Dr. William Prohaska held a joint graduation party in Chicago for both their families. Both of their fathers had entertained hopes that their sons would join them in practice, but the two had long dreamed of practicing together. They stayed in Chicago, and in 1984 were able to buy the large practice of a retiring dentist in a Chicago suburb. They were fine men and good dentists, and their joint practice thrived. Their friendship was strong enough that they could disagree and work through it, and they and their families were still able to have fun together when their white coats had been hung up for the day.

But last week, Jack called Bill into his office with a serious look on his face. Jack had decided to be tested for the HIV virus. The two men had discussed their obligation to treat HIV-positive patients a number of times, and had established the Universal Precautions as the routine for themselves and their staff. But to the best of their knowledge, none of their patients so far had been HIV-positive. Jack wasn't quite sure why he had asked his physician to include the test for HIV in the blood work for a routine physical. Perhaps he intended it to be a baseline for comparison if they ever started seeing HIV-positive patients, he said. But he really couldn't remember why his request had seemed right to him at that moment. His physician, he later learned, thought he was doing it because of contact with HIV-positive patients in his dental practice, but decided not to ask about the reason unless Jack brought it up in case it was something more personal.

The results of the test were positive, Jack told Bill, and some further inquiries made it most likely that Jack was not infected by a dental patient but from the transfusions he had received after his accident in 1975. In any case, he was an HIV-positive dentist now, and the question was what they should do about it. Should he quit practice, Jack asked his colleague, or should he keep practicing? If he continued in the practice, were they obligated to inform his patients of his HIV status? What was the right thing to do, Jack asked his best friend and partner, now that he was an HIV-positive dentist?

THE HIV-POSITIVE DENTIST AND THE RISK TO PATIENTS

There are three questions that need to be asked about the professional obligations of dentists regarding the HIV-positive dentist. The first of these asks whether an HIV-positive practitioner has an obligation to refrain from treating uninfected patients to eliminate all risk of practitioner-to-patient transmission of the virus, or whether HIV-positive dentists at least have an obligation to refrain from certain classes of treatments that are judged particularly high in risk of such transmission. The second asks if infected dental professionals have a professional obligation to inform their patients of their positive HIV status. The third asks if dental professionals have a professional obligation to be tested for HIV. This and the next two sections will address these questions in order.

Prior to 1991, there was not a single instance of verifiable transmission of the HIV virus from a dental practitioner, or any other health care provider, to a patient. Then, in January, 1991, the Centers for Disease Control and Prevention reported first three, then later possibly five probable instances of HIV transmission from a dentist to a patient, all involving the same dentist, Dr. David Acer. These reports received a great deal of media coverage, but very little attention was paid to the apparent likelihood that Dr. Acer was inconsistent in following the Universal Precautions. The media focused intensely on the tragic deterioration of one of Dr. Acer's patients, Kimberly Bergalis, who had contracted AIDS and who, before she died, urged the public and eventually the Congress in Washington to subject all health professionals to mandatory testing, to provide severe penalties for infected practitioners who infect patients, and to require all infected practitioners to inform their patients of their HIV status.

The emotional level of discussions during this time was extremely high, and efforts to address the issues involved from the perspective of *social thinking*, described in the previous chapter, went mostly unheard. Luckily for the health professions, no legislative body enacted on the Bergalis proposals, although various interim reports from the CDC and from a number of the professional organizations did, for one reason or another, at least implicitly support the Bergalis claim that infected health care providers constitute a significant risk of infection to their patients.

There were a number of mistakes in these reactions to the report about Dr. Acer. One of them was well expressed in an article by Glantz, Mariner, and Annas:

> The transmission of HIV from David Acer to Kimberly Bergalis focused public concern on *who* transmitted HIV, not on *how* HIV was transmitted. What was feared was the *person—a dentist, and* by extension all physicians and other health care practitioners—not *what* a dentist did or did not do. Personalizing HIV infection diverted attention from the particular techniques and behaviors that can spread infection to particular groups of people.
>
> Defining persons as the problem makes removing the persons the obvious solution. This reaction perpetuates the destructive stereotype that there are categories of people who are dangerous, previously limited to gay men and intravenous drug users, rather than behaviors that are dangerous, such as unprotected sex with multiple partners, needle sharing, and poor infection control techniques.

A second mistake in these reactions was to ignore the fact that the Acer report is not evidence of a significant risk of transmission from dentist to patient, even from an HIV-positive dentist. Five probable instances of transmission by the same dentist, out of many millions of contacts with patients by infected care givers, including dental professionals, physicians, nurses, and others, over the last decade and more, does not constitute significant risk to patients, particularly when it is also probable that Dr. Acer did not consistently employ the Universal Precautions. Glantz, Mariner, and Annas summarize the evidence:

> The risk of transmission of HIV from a physician or nurse to a patient is unknown since it has never happened. The risk of transmission by a dentist is also unknown, even though one dentist transmitted the virus to his patients. This is because the Acer case is so strange and unique, especially given the fact that there have been no reported cases of HBV [Hepatitis-B virus] transmission from a dentist to a patient since 1987, and HBV transmission by the same route is at least 100 times more likely.

What happened in this reaction to the Acer report and to the plight of Kimberly Bergalis is that the genuine seriousness of the harm, because of the emotions to which it gives rise when it occurs or when it is imagined, is being mistaken for *likelihood* of its occurrence. But there is no connection between the two. Even the CDC, perhaps trying to stay in step with the national mood in its interim reports, made this mistake. It offered "estimates" that the risk of practitioner-to-patient transmission range from 1/260,00 to 1/2.6 million for dental procedures. But these "estimates" did not rely on any statistical evidence of such transmission, but instead on a series of "what ifs," for example, what if a practitioner punctured a glove, and what if the sharp then penetrated the practitioner's skin, or what if there was already an open wound there, and what if the practitioner's own blood then found its way back into the patient's body?

The Office of Technology Assessment (OTA) of the U.S. Congress subsequently analyzed each of the CDC's "what ifs" and concluded that there is no dependable data regarding whether or how often they occur. Consequently, the OTA concluded that CDC's proposed calculations are unreliable and likely to be overestimates. Former Surgeon General C. Everett Koop made the same point when he stated that the risk is so remote that it will probably never be measured.

When we actually focus on the *likelihood* of practitioner-to-patient transmission, given the evidence of practitioner-to-patient contacts and transmission to date, the conclusion has to be that the risk of such transmission is *extremely* slight. That is, there is every reason to believe that the Universal Precautions, conscientiously employed in dental offices, will continue to be the proper way to prevent transmission of the HIV virus from infected dentists to their patients. Consequently, infected dentists who conscientiously employ the Universal Precautions (and perhaps additional caution beyond the Universal Precautions if they judge this appropriate and no significant loss to patients occurs) would not be violating their professional obligations by providing care to their patients.

Of course, if there were no negative effects of removing infected dentists from practice, then it might be less unreasonable to claim that their practicing should be considered professionally unethical on the grounds that there is still some slight, speculative risk that could be avoided in this way. But every dentist certainly knows, from his or her own point of view, that enormous negative consequences would arise from such a shift in professional norms. Any effort at social thinking about such a policy would be inadequate if it failed to weigh the losses and suffering of individual dentists and their families, and also of their regular patients, who would be affected by such a shift. These negative consequences must be weighed against the marginal benefit of eliminating a slight, speculative risk of transmitting the infection from infected practitioners to patients.

In addition to these more dramatic, because more personal, effects of such a shift in professional norms, there would be important negative public health consequences as well. First, infected dentists provide clinical services for their patients. The sudden loss of many or most of these services would be a real loss for the dental health care system. Second, fear of seroconversion on the part of dentists and prospective dentists would likely be strongly heightened by such a shift in professional norms. So there would be good reason to expect an additional loss of professional services due to changes in careers and career plans by noninfected dentists, by dental students, and by persons contemplating a career in dentistry.

3 Third, any policy requiring dental professionals to know their HIV status will place strains on the resources for HIV testing, in addition to the fact that these resources are far more efficiently employed for persons who engage in high-risk behaviors than for health care professionals who do not, particularly where the risk of provider-to-patient transmission is minutely small. Such a policy would also markedly increase strains on current systems of information control to protect the confidentiality of those who are tested. 4 Fourth, since the risk of transmission from patient to practitioner is estimated to be many times greater than the risk of transmission from practitioner to patient, such a shift in professional norms would almost certainly prompt a corresponding increase in pressure that all patients also be tested for HIV. The costs involved in this, the consequent disincentive for practitioners and patients alike to not avail themselves of the health care system, and the impact of the significant numbers of false positives (which are estimated to run at 1 out of every 40,000 to 50,000 tests under ideal testing conditions) are all additional negative factors that would need to be weighed, together with those previously mentioned, against the slight benefit of eliminating a minute, speculative risk of practitioner-to-patient transmission.

In sum, given the significant body of data currently available to us, there seems to be very strong evidence for saying that the risk of practitioner-to-patient transmission of the HIV virus, when the practitioner is conscientiously employing the Universal Precautions, is extremely low. There are also very serious negative consequences that the health care system would have to bear if, to prevent such transmission altogether, professional norms were changed so that dental practice by infected practitioners was considered unethical. Not only from the point of view of the suffering and loss to individual dental professionals, their families, and patients, but just as surely from the point of view of the long-term well-being of the whole community, such a shift in the understanding of dental professional obligations is not warranted.

At the same time, it must be stressed that the principal protection of the larger community from transmission through practitioners, like the principal means of protecting the practitioners themselves for their own sake and for the sake of the community in the future, is the conscientious employment of the Universal Precautions. While a change in our current understanding of dentists' obligations is not warranted, for the reasons indicated, every dental professional is surely obligated by the strongest of professional obligations to practice the Universal Precautions conscientiously, not only to protect each patient from possible harm, but to protect the long-term health of the community as well.

As in many other matters, it is by the professionalism of the dental community, practiced in this instance through the Universal Precautions, that both the individual and the collective well-being of the community is most effectively secured. (Throughout this discussion, it is taken for granted that every dentist who, for reasons of health, whether HIV infection, AIDS, or any other health condition, or for any other reason, is unable to practice competently or is unable to perform certain kinds of dental care competently, is professionally obligated to refrain from doing what he or she cannot competently do. Nothing about HIV and AIDS changes this fundamental obligation of every dental professional.)

SHOULD PATIENTS BE INFORMED OF THE DENTIST'S HIV STATUS?

A second question about infected dental practitioners asks whether they have an obligation to inform patients of their positive HIV status. The argument offered in support of such an obligation depends on two claims. First, it is argued, the patient needs to know all the risks attendant on the reception of dental services, along with all the likely benefits, in order to make an informed choice of dental services. Second, the patient has a right to make such an informed choice before the dental professional provides any such services. (The implications of this argument for patients who are not capable of fully participating in treatment decisions would follow the lines developed in Chapter 7. Only fully capable adult patients will be considered in this discussion.) If the infected dentist fails to inform a patient of the fact that he or she is HIV-positive, it is argued, then the patient is made incapable of informed choice regarding dental treatment and the patient's right to make such a choice is violated.

The basis of the patient's right to make an informed choice prior to dental treatment has been articulated in several different ways. Some ethical theorists hold that it is a fundamental moral right of every human being to control whatever is done to his or her body by another human agent. But, as was noted in Chapter 4, so specific a right is more likely to be derivative from some more general and more fundamental right regarding personal choice or autonomy. In addition, as the same chapter argued, from the point of view of the professional obligations of dentists, there is an ideal relationship between practitioner and patient that the dentist ought to be striving to achieve with every capable patient, and the patient's participation in treatment decisions by way of a fully informed choice is certainly a component of this ideal. Even though the fullness of this ideal may not be achievable with every capable patient, the dentist is professionally obligated to strive for it. Therefore whether it is correct to speak of this matter in terms of the patient's rights or not, the dentist is certainly obligated to provide the patient with sufficient information that a fully informed choice of dental care can be made. That much is clear.

But is it true that patients need to be explicitly informed of *every conceivable risk* to make a fully informed choice of dental care? The answer to this question is clearly "No" for two different reasons. First, there are many "conceivable" series of events that would have untoward outcomes for dental patient that there is no need to communicate about with the patient because there is no dependable evidence that indicates any likelihood of their occurring. There are, in other words, myriad "what if" scenarios that no thoughtful professional would consider mentioning and no thoughtful patient would want to discuss.

What if, for example, the structural members of the building were to shift, or there was an earthquake, so that the dentist was jostled while examining the patient with a probe, and the probe cut into the patient's tissue. The risk of this and an immense number of other untoward possible scenarios is not simply zero, but it is minute and speculative, and because of this, there is no need for the patient to consider it in order to be fully informed about the risks of the proposed dental care. Consequently, neither the patient's rights nor the dentist's obligations are violated when some of the "conceivable risks" in this sense are not discussed.

There is no agreement that the risk of practitioner-to-patient HIV infection, when the Universal Precautions are being conscientiously employed, can legitimately be called "minute and speculative" in the same sense in which this phrase was used in the previous paragraph. That is, it is not agreed upon whether discussing such a risk would or would not be analogous to discussing the weakening of building beams. Nevertheless, given the sizable body of current data about practitioner-to-patient contacts and transmissions, the similarity is worth considering. More likely, however, because of the great seriousness of HIV infection and AIDS, such comparisons will seem inappropriate and out of place. In making this judgment, however, it is important to remember that the *seriousness* of a harm is distinct from, and should not be confused with, the *likelihood* of its occurrence. These considerations make a strong, if not conclusive, case for saying that the dentist's HIV status is not a piece of information that a patient has a right to or needs in any important way to make a properly informed or even an interactive treatment decision.

A second line of reasoning about the obligation of an infected dental professional to inform patients of his or her positive HIV status, when the Universal Precautions are being conscientiously employed, compares the risk of transmission in this situation with other instances of accepted risk. Suppose, in other words, that we understand "every conceivable risk" to mean every risk with serious untoward outcome and with any significant likelihood of occurring. The likelihood of building beams weakening, or of an earthquake, it might be argued, is so minute that discussion of these possibilities is not required. But, it might be argued, the risk of practitioner-to-patient infection is greater.

The response to this argument is that as far as our data can inform us— and it is not a small body of data, but concerns many millions of practitioner-to-patient contacts over the whole health care system over more than 10 years—the risk of practitioner-to-patient transmission *is* minute, is *extremely small*. For example, even the CDC's what-if-based estimates mentioned above would place the risk of transmitting HIV infection during a dental procedure at from less than half to less than $1/20$ the risk of a patient treated with penicillin having a profound adverse reaction (anaphylaxis) resulting in death. Note that in this comparison, the subject is at risk of an even more serious negative outcome, immediate death, and that it is considerably more likely to occur (from 2 to 20 times more likely). Yet we do not ordinarily consider physicians who have properly inquired whether the patient is known to be allergic to penicillin—that is, who have taken the step analogous to the Universal Precautions in this situation—to be unprofessional if they do not then inform the patient, regardless of his or her answer, of the small risk of anaphylactic shock.

In other words, our current understanding of health professionals' obligations to inform patients about the risks of professional care so they can make properly-informed choices regarding it do not include information about the risk, even of very serious negative events, *if the degree of risk is extremely low*. Once again the point to be made most strongly is that the patient's and the community's chief protection against the spread of the HIV virus in patient-to-practitioner interactions is the conscientious employment of the Universal

Precautions. If the first set of considerations yielded a strong if inconclusive argument, we submit that, taken together with the second set of considerations, these constitute a conclusive argument that the risk of practitioner-to-patient transmission is currently too slight for an HIV-positive dentist to be professionally required to inform patients of his or her HIV status.

The objection might be raised at this point that a policy in which infected dental professionals are not obligated to inform patients of their HIV status is demeaning to the dignity of patients, that it is a paternalistic refusal to provide them with information for their own good. But given the reaction of many people to Kimberly Bergalis' case when it was being played out in the media, there is some reason to ask whether people in general are well enough skilled in interpreting the relevant epidemiologic data or whether they would likely draw incorrect conclusions from information about their dentists' status. This line of reasoning was developed thoughtfully in a document of the ADA Council on Ethics, Bylaws, and Judicial Affairs regarding the ethical acceptability of a dentist's advertising the negative results of HIV tests. Most readers of these advertisements, the Council argued, would be unlikely to interpret the data they provide about HIV status in an appropriate and reasonable way.

Moreover, apart from the question whether patients would be able to properly and reasonably weigh data about individual dentists' seropositivity and the previous question of whether the risk of harm is great enough to require disclosure, there is another very important reason why the withholding of information about dental professionals' HIV status is not simply a paternalistic refusal of information for the patients' own good. This reason concerns the effect on the infected dental professional of revealing such information to patients. For, first of all, there is every reason to expect that many, even most, patients would likely seek dental care elsewhere, thus effectively destroying the established practices of these professionals, even though there would be no significant risk to their patients in their continuing to practice. This would have approximately the same negative effect on the community's actually used supply of dentists as reducing their numbers by requiring infected dentists to cease practice.

Second, patients are not bound by the same obligations of confidentiality regarding HIV status that apply to dental professionals. There is every reason to believe that information about a dentist's HIV status would spread rapidly and would do immense harm to the practitioner and his or her family, particularly in our current situation in which there is still a severe social stigma associated with positive HIV status and in which other important social and financial consequences, for example, loss of health insurance, can follow such revelations.

Thus, even if there were good reasons to think that patients generally would be able to properly interpret information about a particular dental professional's HIV status, and even if there is some reasonable and appropriate contribution about significant risk that such information might make to a patient's informed choice about dental care, the possible benefits of providing patients with such information would still have to be weighed against the very severe negative consequences for the dental professionals who are required to make such revelations and the significant negative effects on our society's dental health care system, analogous to those discussed in the previous section.

In sum, given our current understanding of the professional obligations of dental professionals and health professionals generally, HIV-positive dentists do not seem to have a professional obligation to inform their patients of this fact. Nor are there any solid reasons currently available to suggest that this understanding of dentists' professional obligations should be changed. What is appropriate, rather, is a much more effective education of the whole community about HIV and AIDS, about how to prevent infection, and about the minimal but unavoidable risks of many sorts that attend all forms of care by health professionals, and almost every other aspect of human life.

TESTING DENTISTS FOR HIV

The question of testing dental professionals for HIV needs to be briefly addressed. Although this issue has been discussed at some length in the literature, its treatment here can be brief. For there are only two good reasons that could be offered for requiring dentists to be regularly tested for HIV as part of their ethical commitments as professionals. One reason would be if, on the basis of such information, dentists should limit their practice either altogether or in some specific ways if they are HIV-positive. The other reason would be if dentists had an obligation to inform their patients of their HIV status. But the discussions preceding this have concluded that dental professionals do not have either of these obligations at this time and that, given the extensive data available about HIV and patient-to-practitioner interactions and HIV transmission, there is no good reason to think that these professional obligations should be changed.

Consequently, although individual dental practitioners may have good personal reasons for seeking HIV testing, there is no good reason from the perspective of social thinking, in other words, from the perspective of the long-term well-being of the community at large, for such testing to be required, either by a change in our understanding of dental professionals' professional obligations or in some other way.

THE COMMUNITY'S RESPONSIBILITY TO SEROPOSITIVE PRACTITIONERS

A community that designs its institutions so that its health care providers undertake an obligation to face greater-than-ordinary risk of life-threatening infection clearly owes any health care providers who are infected more than a polite thank you or even a statue in the park. The community owes practitioners infected in the course of treating their patients the best health care that the system provides, assistance to their families during their illness, and, if death is the result, secure financial protection of their families thereafter. While the people of the United States have given some serious thought in the last 15 years to the obligations of health professions to accept risk of HIV-infection to treat their patients' needs, there is little evidence that this society has paid much attention to the other half of this mutual commitment.

The principal reason for this lack of attention is a set of assumptions that lies behind the economics of the U.S. health care system. The operative assumption for much of the U.S. health care system is that the people in general do not have any responsibility for anyone's ill health, and therefore the people in general have no obligations to provide treatment or any other assistance for those who are ill or for their families. The idea has not been seriously entertained, much less acted upon, that the patterns of distribution of health and illness in a society are very much influenced by its distribution of resources and education and by the environmental effects of its people's activities. So the general idea that the whole community might have obligations for someone's health care because it is at least partially responsible for their ill health has little currency, and this makes it that much harder for the community to believe that it might have special obligations to particular classes of individuals (e.g., health care providers) because of the particular form of service they provide to the society.

If there is any circumstance in human life that ought to teach a society the lesson that we humans are in this business of life together, that going it alone is not an option, it is ill health and the need for health care, especially the experience of a life-threatening epidemic. But the individualism of American culture runs deep, and even in the face of the challenge of HIV/AIDS, there are still many in this land who believe that each of us is best off if we just work our lives out on our own. We do not support this view.

The more general theme of the ethical distribution of health care resources in a whole society, and the implications of the characteristics of this society in relation to that theme, will be explored in Chapter 13.

It is true that in the case that begins this chapter, Jack Corrigan was more likely infected with the AIDS virus through transfusions he received years before rather than by a patient. It is also true that if a dentist or other health care provider became infected with the HIV virus by reason of his or her own lack of caution, especially if the person was not conscientiously following the Universal Precautions, then the community's obligations to that person would be lessened in proportion. But these qualifications aside, the point to be stressed here is that the same process of social thinking that determines that the norms of the health professions should include an obligation to accept greater-than-ordinary risk of infection for the sake of patients' well-being should also identify the larger community's obligations toward those who face such risks if they become infected. It is profoundly unjust to hold that dentists and other health care providers are simply on their own if they are infected by the HIV virus in the course of providing needed care for their patients.

A DENTIST'S STAFF AND SEROCONVERSION

The issues of justice raised about the whole society in the previous section pose important questions in a different way within the setting of the individual dentist's office. The dentist's staff are also the dentist's employees, and so it might seem that the obligations relevant to providing health care and other assistance for infected staff members fall exclusively upon the dentist/employer. If the society at large provided universal health coverage for all of its citizens, of course, or if it had a system of coverage and other assistance specifically for health care providers who become ill in the course of caring for their patients, then the question of the dentist/employer's obligations in this connection would not even arise. But neither of these systems is yet in place, and any such system that might soon come into being could well contain large gaps in the kinds of coverage and assistance that it provides, especially for the family members of HIV-infected care givers. So the question about the obligations of the dentist/employer remains significant.

One relevant point is that the dental hygienists who are in a dentist's employ are themselves health professionals. Their acceptance of the risk of HIV infection, and of other forms of infection, is not grounded in their contract with the dentist, but in their commitment to the larger community as health professionals. In their case, for the reasons explained in the previous section, the principal responsibilities fall on the society as a whole, just as in the case of dentists. If as a way to attract and retain dental hygienists of high quality, a dentist contracts to provide additional benefits over and above what the society at large owes the hygienist in return of accepting greater-than-ordinary risk, this is a contractual commitment between the two parties, not something the dentist would owe independently of their contract.

With regard to other staff members, however, who are not ordinarily considered to be bound by the norms of a professional role and so not ordinarily presumed to be obligated to accept greater-than-ordinary risk, such assumption of risk as they do undertake is undertaken as part of their contractual relationship with the dentist. The first ethical issue then concerns how effectively the dentist communicates to his or her staff the nature and degree of the risk of HIV infection they will face in caring for patients in that office. Obviously, there must be careful training in conscientious use of the Universal Precautions (for *everyone's* protection) and in the use of caution beyond the Universal Precautions where it is justifiable and of benefit. But beyond this, in the course of contracting, the dentist must also be certain that prospective staff members understand whatever risks they are undertaking before they commit to serving in that office.

The issues of confidentiality must also be discussed. In our view, this issue involves the policy that was argued for in the previous chapter, namely that confidentiality about a patient's positive HIV status is not to be broken with staff unless doing so is necessary for the best treatment of the patient. Furthermore, the dentist would be well advised to discuss clearly, and in advance of any need for the information, exactly the extent of his or her contractual obligations in the event that a staff member seroconverted as a consequence of patient care in that office.

It is difficult to offer a precise guideline about the extent of health care coverage and other assistance that a dentist ought to make available, particularly because the dentist's obligations in this regard will partly depend on his or her overall resources and the degree of risk of infection in that particular practice, among other things. But it is surely wrong for the dentist to simply say "let the buyer beware" as he or she presents a potential employee with a contract. Since the staff member may be facing risk of serious harm, even possibly a lethal disease, and doing so not because of a professional commitment to the larger community but because he or she contracts with the dentist to do so, the dentist has a proportionate obligation not only to properly inform the prospective employee of the risk, but to offer the employee a just program of benefits and other assistance in the event of the employee's falling ill, as the dentist's part of the bargain.

In addition, the dentist may conclude that he or she has important obligations to hygienists and other staff members, not contractually or by reason of their professional roles, but as human to human, and co-worker to co-worker. The spirit of cooperation and the importance of relationships of mutual respect among health co-workers that was emphasized in Chapter 10 would lead to and support a sense of mutual obligation, and as the party who ordinarily has the greater measure of resources, the dentist may view himself or herself as especially obligated in this way.

THINKING ABOUT THE CASE

The patterns of social thinking set out in this chapter lead directly to the conclusion that Dr. Corrigan has no professional obligation to withdraw from dental practice or to limit his treatment of patients in any way, provided only that he and the staff continue to conscientiously practice the Universal Precautions. Nor does he have any professional obligation to inform his patients of his positive HIV status. Nor does Dr. Prohaska or anyone else in the office have a professional obligation to be tested for the HIV-virus.

So long as he shows no symptoms, Dr. Corrigan could, with a clear professional-ethical conscience, practice as if nothing new had happened to him. He might wish, in point of fact, to practice with additional caution beyond the Universal Precautions, not because he is obligated to protect his patients by doing so, but in the interests of protecting himself more effectively from other forms of infection, to which, in due course, he will likely be susceptible. If he does so, and if the use of additional caution affects the quality of his treatments in any significant way, he would need to seek patients' permission to do so. Here there would be an ethical challenge, since he may quite reasonably not want patients to know of his HIV-positive status, but would need to give patients not just a plausible explanation of his use of additional caution, but in fact an honest one. This fact would likely restrain him in the use of additional forms of caution that adversely affect the quality of practice, but it would be important not to become insensitive to these adverse effects as his desire to protect himself more effectively grows greater or more urgent.

He might also wish to practice with additional caution out of a generous desire to protect patients additionally from the already minute risk of provider-to-patient transmission of the infection. His motivation in this matter may be quite admirable. But again, if the effect of the use of additional caution is to lower the quality of treatment significantly, he may not ethically do so without the patient's permission. For the patient may rightly expect that only treatment of the usually acceptable quality will be provided unless additional explanation is offered and consent is given. The fact that the patient benefits is not a sufficient reason for engaging in additional caution because the patient benefits, in this instance, by a lessening of a level of risk already judged too slight to require the patient's consent in the first place. So a crucial question in all use of caution beyond the Universal Precautions and other ordinary forms of caution in dental practice is whether its use has significant negative effects on the quality of treatment.

If and when Dr. Corrigan's infection becomes symptomatic, either with AIDS-Related Complex (ARC) or with the beginnings of AIDS itself, then an additional set of questions must be posed by Dr. Corrigan. For, as was noted above, no dentist may attempt to practice in a manner for which he or she is incompetent. So Dr. Corrigan will need to ask himself whether the effects of his disease are such as to significantly inhibit his ability to practice. It is likely that certain elements of dental practice would be affected before others, depending on the progress of the disease in a particular patient. He will have to question himself carefully and honestly to respond properly to the professional norm of competence in these unfortunate circumstances.

It is at this point especially that Dr. Prohaska's professional obligations to their patients would begin to require specific action on his part. For so long as Dr. Corrigan's ability to practice competently is not impaired, Dr. Prohaska has no special professional duties regarding his colleague's disease. But since it is known that some effects of ARC and AIDS on its victims can adversely affect their abilities, Dr. Prohaska is obligated to watch carefully for such effects, particularly since Dr. Corrigan, out of understandable love of his profession, his desire to continue to be of service to his patients, and many other motives and feelings, may prove less sensitive to deficits in his ability to practice than an independent observer.

It is worth asking, additionally, whether Dr. Corrigan has any special obligation to inform the office staff of his infection for their protection any sooner than when it begins to impinge adversely on his ability to practice (for at that point, his professional obligation would be to ask all of his co-workers to help him maintain his level of competence and be on the alert for deficits in it to assure that their patients are competently cared for). It has been argued above that there is not enough risk to care givers to violate the confidentiality of patients who are HIV-positive, and the level of risk of provider-to-provider transmission is probably less than that of provider-to-patient transmission, which is both minute and considerably less than the risk of patient-to-provider transmission. Consequently, the level of risk does not seem to justify a requirement, under the norm of professional obligations to co-professionals, that Dr. Corrigan inform his staff of his HIV-positive status.

Yet the subtle relationships of trust and loyalty on which effective cooperation in the health care team depends may require, for their maintenance, or at least as an implication of what they say about the several parties' connections with each other, that Dr. Corrigan inform his staff anyway. It is not so much that he would be professionally obligated to do so as that his relationships with team members and co-workers would suffer sufficiently that he ought not do otherwise, at least if the ideal of cooperation discussed in Chapter 10 is operative in this office. On the other hand, he might conclude that until informing the staff is necessary to protect patients from less competent practice, the staff's knowledge of his situation would interfere with their collaboration, out of feelings for him that would distract from their attention to their patients. There is an important judgment call here that cannot be made without much more information about the two doctors and their staff than the case has provided.

There is much else that would likely take place in the relationship between two such close friends and colleagues as Bill Prohaska and Jack Corrigan, now facing so great a tragedy. We leave it to the readers' imagination to reflect on how they would respond if practicing with a close friend and colleague under similar circumstances. These aspects of the friends' responses to one another are not matters of professional obligation, of course, and in some respects not matters of obligation at all, but flow from their deeper humanity, as acts of friendship and love. Were any of us infected with HIV in the practice of dentistry, we might hope it would be under work circumstances like these.

CHAPTER 13

Social Justice and Access to Dental Care

Case: But It Will Show!

Dr. Sandra Mosiek purchased the practice of Dr. Giulio Berardinelli in 1981 after working as his associate for nearly 5 years. In 1981 it was a thriving practice. There were not a lot of dentists in Montclair, and even with two dentists in the office, nonemergency patients often had to wait 3 or 4 weeks for an appointment. Sandra actually considered hiring an associate to help her during the first year after Dr. Berardinelli retired. But she worked long hours herself instead, and was able to pay off more of her debts for the effort.

Unfortunately, more than half of Dr. Berardinelli's patients when Dr. Mosiek bought the practice were in their late fifties or older. They had become his patients years earlier, when he first came to Montclair, and stayed with him. Now they were retiring to warmer climates if they could, moving closer to children in their later years, or just dying. Most of their children had already left Montclair as well, a small city whose once robust industrial base was now largely gone.

By 1988, a new patient could get a convenient appointment within the week, and Dr. Mosiek had begun to worry about where this trend would end. Several insurance companies had approached her with the prospect of accepting capitation plans. She could use the business, but she was suspicious of what they had to offer. Even if it provided secure annual revenue and guaranteed patients, she worried that she would feel financial pressure to provide less than the best treatments for the capitation patients. On the other hand, some dentist needed to care for these patients.

She was also distressed at the dental insurance that many of her retired patients and some of those still employed had through their labor union. The insurance company would pay for only the cheapest acceptable treatment, regardless of the individual patient's circumstances. Few of these patients could afford to pay for their dental care without the help of the insurance. The depressed economy of Montclair left many of them, even those still employed, very much in a bind.

Clara Thomson, for example, was a retired beautician in her late sixties. Her husband, Herb, 71, was a retired machinist for the only large manufacturing company that had made a commitment to stay in Montclair in return for important concessions from the union. The couple lived on Herb's modest union pension and their social security, plus what Clara earned by giving beauty demonstrations and selling La Beaute beauty products to groups of women in Montclair and the smaller towns around it. Herb and Clara were widely admired in the area because they had made the sacrifices necessary to raise and care for their mentally retarded son in their home, in addition to raising three other children, and had been very active in the Special Olympics program when they and their son were younger. William, their son, was now 47 chronologically, but he functioned at about the mental level of a 3-year-old. Clara and Herb worried greatly, of course, about what would happen to William if anything happened to them or if their income fell any lower.

Clara had lost a filling from her upper left first premolar, and had come to Sandra Mosiek to get it replaced. But Dr. Mosiek could see at a glance that this would not be simple. There was another old restoration in the tooth that was fractured and ready to fall out itself. The most appropriate treatment for Mrs. Thomson would be a crown, preferably porcelain-fused-to-metal since Mrs. Thomson's work as a beauty products consultant and salesperson required that she look her best. The tooth would certainly show whenever she smiled, and, being the kind of person she was, she did that often.

But the Thomson's dental insurance would cover only the cost of a three-surface amalgam restoration. Dr. Mosiek was certain of that, and a quick telephone call confirmed it. It was the difference between a $75 charge and a $500 charge. The more attractive crown was obviously very important to Clara's work, not to mention her self-image and her sense of her dignity, but the Thomson's did not have $500, or anything close, to pay for it.

"Why are they so insensitive to an old woman's circumstances?" Mrs. Thomson asked Dr. Mosiek.

"You are not an old woman," said Dr. Mosiek warmly but firmly. "You are vital and alive and attractive. Everyone admires you, and you just keep going and going, and your smile brightens everyone's day."

"Yes, my smile," Clara said with feeling. "What good is this other thing to me, this three-surface thing you said the insurance wants you to do?"

"It would be functional. You would be able to chew comfortably. And it would be strong; it won't give you any trouble."

Tears welled up in Clara Thomson's eyes. "I know all that," she said. "But it will show!"

SOCIAL JUSTICE

One central thesis of this book has been that dental care is not only a matter of relationships between individual dentists and individual patients. Those relationships occur in the context of a complex social institution, the dental profession, whose norms are the product of an on-going dialogue between dentists as a group and the larger community. Whether a dentist's particular actions toward a particular patient are ethical or not cannot be resolved without considering the dentist as a professional, and therefore examining the dental profession and its dialogue with the larger community and the norms of dental practice that are this dialogue's result. Dentistry, even when it is most one-to-one, is also and by its very nature a broadly *social* enterprise as well.

The point of this chapter is that there is another broad social structure, or set of social structures, that is directly involved in dental practice, even in the most direct one-to-one encounters of dentist and patient. This is the set of social structures that distributes a society's resources and governs their exchange so some are used or exchanged by some people, others by others. Moreover, like the institution of profession and the particular profession of dentistry with its particular norms, the set of structures that governs the distribution and exchange of a society's resources can be ethically sound as it exists in a given society, or not. Since our own society's structures for the distribution of resources have such great impact on what kinds of dental care dentists provide to their patients, they deserve to be examined here and the question explored whether they are ethically sound in their impact on dental care or whether they ought to be rejected in favor of other, more ethical structures for distributing dental care resources.

When a society's structures for distributing resources are ethically sound, a common adjective used to describe such a society is *just*. When a society's structures are ethically deficient, one proper term is *unjust*. Aristotle labeled as *distributive justice* the effort to determine which kinds of distributive structures are ethically sound and which are not, and the label has stuck. But to emphasize the fact that this aspect of dental practice connects each dentist and each dental patient with the whole society's structures, another expression will also be used here: *social justice*.

What are the characteristics that make a society's distributive structures just? This is not an easy question to answer. Aristotle's description of justice at the most general level provides a starting point. He observed that justice of every sort, in every aspect of life where talk of justice is appropriate, has to do in general with treating like cases alike and different cases differently in proportion to their relevant similarities and differences. This tells us something important about ethical distributions, but we won't be able to apply it to any practical area of life until we can answer the further question: In the area of human life under consideration, which similarities and differences between people should be considered ethically *relevant*?

With regard to the recipients of dental care, then, we need to ask which kinds of similarities and differences should determine differences in how much and what kinds of dental care resources each patient ought to receive. The next four sections will examine this issue, first in general terms and then in connection with the current structures for distributing dental care resources in the United States. The final section will examine the connections between these issues of social justice and the specifically professional obligations of dentists in commenting on this chapter's introductory case.

BASIC NEEDS AND THE JUST DISTRIBUTION OF DENTAL CARE

A number of different criteria for distributing a society's resources among its people have been proposed. But a detailed discussion of even a representative sampling of these criteria would be too large an undertaking for this chapter. Instead, a brief account of some of the most important criteria will have to do. As each of the criteria is discussed, the reader should be asking: Is this the criterion (or one of several) that should determine what and how much dental care ought to be available to each dental patient in an ethical, just society, and why or why not?

The values not only of American culture but of cultures and peoples in many parts of the world today make it fairly easy to reject one historically important criterion for distributing resources, namely *social class and birth-*

based social status. There is a broad consensus that these are not relevant characteristics for determining the distribution of dental care, or any other form of health care, and that a society that distributed dental care on the basis of social class or birth-based social status would be unethical and unjust. It would be a useful exercise for the reader to pause here to ask *why* this is (or is not) a correct conclusion.

A more complicated criterion supported by many thinkers in recent centuries is *equality*. The claim is that there are *no* relevant differences between people when it comes to the distribution of dental care resources or other kinds of resources to which this criterion is applied. Therefore, these thinkers argue, a society's distributive structures should be arranged so that these resources, in this case, its dental care resources, are distributed *equally*.

But *equally* in regard to what? That is a question that must be answered before this view of just distributions will be clear enough to be put into practice. For example, does "equality" here mean that every person in the society gets exactly the same resources as the next person? So everyone would get the same number of porcelain-fused-to-metal restorations as the next person, for example? This makes no sense. People's needs for particular forms of dental care vary, and most people would agree that the dental care a person ought to receive should be determined by his or her need for that care. So the interpretation of equality that means "equal stuff for all" does not seem very useful here.

Another interpretation of equality focuses on people's access to needed resources, on their ability to actually obtain a certain form of health care or some other resource when they need it. On this view, equality in distribution would exist when people had to bear equal burdens or hardships or could act with equal ease to receive a certain form of dental care. But there is still an ambiguity with this interpretation. One still needs to ask whether this equality of access is equal access to the *same* or *similar kinds* of care, or to *comparable* care, or what? As this criterion is usually understood, it refers to equal access to *needed* care. So the notion of need appears again as an important determinant of social justice. For present purposes, then, let *equal access* be understood here to refer to access to *needed* dental care.

The term *need* has many uses in ordinary conversation. But within health care, distinctions between what is needed or essential care and what is nonessential and therefore optional care are widely taken to be quite clear. In fact, in the contemporary literature of health care ethics and health care policy, the expression "basic health care" has come into common usage as the collective term for health care that is essential and so responds to (basic) needs, in contrast with other kinds of health care that are judged nonessential and that respond, not to (basic) needs, but to the wants and desires that people have over and above their (basic) needs.

But this explanation is still incomplete. We must ask: Essential for what, basic to what, needed for what? Most theorists answer this question in terms of what is considered normal or appropriate human functioning. Thus, as an example, the discussion of oral health as part of the hierarchy of central values of dental practice specified *oral health* as "appropriate and pain-free oral functioning." The reasons why certain kinds of functioning, for example, pain-free functioning, are taken as norms or standards of how humans ought to function, and therefore as standards of appropriate health care interventions and of (basic) *need*, are very complex and well beyond the scope of this book to examine. But the reader would do well to think carefully about these matters, since the goal of such reflection is, in fact, to determine what it is that dentists are aiming at for their patients.

For present purposes, however, the authors shall simply propose that because the dental community and the community at large view certain kinds of human functioning as standards of what ought to be the case for humans, it follows that dental care resources ought to be distributed with those standards chiefly in mind. That is, the proper criterion for ethically distributing a society's dental care resources is the *need* of patients for such care. Every society that has enough resources to do so, therefore, ought to arrange its distributive structures so that whoever has dental care needs in the society can obtain the needed dental care resources to fill them, and any society that has sufficient resources to do this, but fails to do it, is in that measure an unjust society. But we have not yet addressed the question: What kinds of dental care are *essential*? What kinds of dental care are responses to *basic needs*? This question will be discussed later in this chapter.

First, however, several competing views about the proper criterion for distributing a society's resources, including dental care resources, deserve a hearing. For the view that equal access to needed care is the proper criterion is not the only one with thoughtful reasons to support it, and the reader should carefully consider the reasons on all sides before accepting one position over the others.

CONTRIBUTION AND EFFORT AS POSSIBLE CRITERIA

Some theorists hold that a society's resources, including its dental and other health care resources, ought to be distributed according to the value of each person's *contribution* to the society. The underlying idea here is that the resources that a society has are mostly *produced* resources, rather than resources that are already highly useful in their natural form. Therefore because these resources wouldn't exist without the contributions of the humans who produce them, each producer has a legitimate claim on that proportion of a society's resources that he or she has produced. Thus the measure of what each person in a society receives through the operations of the society's distributive structures ought to be the value of his or her contributions. In other words, the ethically relevant differences between people in the distribution of a society's resources are the differences in people's *contributions*.

Only in a world where there was no specialization and no division of labor would people actually want to simply hold onto what they actually produce. Dentists need to eat, and farmers can't provide all of their own dental care. Thus an exchange system develops, but its operation unavoidably involves a "cost" and unavoidably consumes a portion of the available resources in order to run at all. It follows that the value a person receives from their exchanges will always be some faction less than what they put in. This is why the criterion for distributive justice in terms of contributions is actually that each person ought to receive *in proportion to* the value of his or her contribution.

Because children do not contribute much when they are growing up, using this criterion of contribution also assumes an exchange system between generations. Children tally up a debt by receiving without contributing for a time, and then repay that debt when they are able to contribute significantly. (A similar system covers persons who are temporarily unproductive due to accident or illness and whose savings are not great enough to cover their needs during this time.) It is easy to forget, however, how indebted to the society a young adult is when he or she first begins to contribute something of value to it, and how many years of prorating one's return (downward) it might take to gradually pay off that debt. It is also important to note that, if one uses natural resources or resources produced by others' contributions in one's own productive efforts, then these resources also need to be paid for out of the value of one's contribution before what is left belongs unconditionally to the producer.

Objectors to this view identify three problems with it. The first asks what standard is to be used for *measuring* the relative *value* of each person's contribution, so that differences in what people receive will be proportional to differences in the value of what they produce. Some objectors even hold that there is *no standard* of value that is universally accepted or that has some sort of objective status even if it is not universally accepted, nor even a standard that is widely shared within our own society. Therefore, they argue, the comparative judgments of value on which the practical application of this view of justice depends are impossible to make or defend. So it is a useless theory.

When the focus is on dental care, this is a weaker objection than it might be if other kinds of resources were under consideration. For dental care focuses on values such as relief from pain, comfort in functioning, nutrition, appearance, control over one's body, and so on that are very widely considered important for human life, not just for human lives in this particular society but generally. The experience of giving and receiving dental care seems to make it clear that there are some values of universal, or at least of very general significance.

A second objection concerns one troubling implication of the contribution view of social justice. Namely, that those members of the human family who are unable to contribute at all, not only in the present like children or those temporarily unproductive but forever because their disabilities are permanent, ought not to receive *any* resources from their society.

Many people cannot accept this conclusion and would consider providing some resources to those unable to contribute (e.g., resources necessary to meet such people's basic needs) to be a matter of justice for any society with enough resources to do so. But this position cannot be incorporated into the contribution view without changing it radically. Consequently, for many theorists, if contribution has a role in relation to distributive justice, it is only as a criterion for justly distributing whatever resources a society "has left" after its structures assure that everyone in the society has been able to meet their basic needs.

Should patients receive dental care in proportion to the value of their contributions to the society? Or should they receive at least some dental care ("basic" dental care?) in proportion to their need for it, with nonessential, nonbasic care distributed in proportion to their contributions?

A third objection to the contribution view asks a more radical question: Do people really *deserve* to receive in proportion to the value to the society of what they produce? This objection argues that people's ability to contribute something of value depends greatly on their inherited genetic and biological capabilities, over which no one has any control and for which no one can take any credit or any return. A person's contributions also depend greatly on accidents of upbringing, education, opportunity, and luck, and, if we are honest, we must acknowledge that a great deal of what we take credit for in our daily work and other activities involves skills and ideas that we received from others, rather than being able to take credit for them as if they were our own inventions. One British philosopher, L.T. Hobhouse, argued that if we all deducted from our claims on society the part of the value of our contributions that, in all honesty, we can't personally take credit for, we would have to admit that the differences between those who seem to contribute the most and those who seem to contribute the least are in fact very slight. If we take contribution as the proper criterion of distributive justice, but are really honest about what each of us can take personal credit for, he argued, we would see that we should actually distribute society's resources equally, because the differences between us, after everything is properly deducted and prorated, are actually negligible.

But many people would say to Hobhouse. "What about how hard I have worked. Certainly, I have had control over that." In addition, what really bothers a lot of people most is someone who is not working hard at all, but who is receiving the same resources as someone who works hard (which most of us presume we are doing). The focus of this response to Hobhouse is on *effort* rather than contribution. It suggests yet another view of the proper criterion for social justice, namely, that the relevant differences between people, when it comes to distributing a society's resources, are differences in *effort*. How *hard* a person works rather than the value of his or her actual contribution should be the criterion.

Some have argued in response that how hard a person is able to work is partly controlled by genetic and psychological factors over which the person has little or no control. So only insofar as a person is able to put out effort by his or her own initiative or choice may that person's effort be used as the measure of what he or she should receive in the society. In addition, note that if distribution were simply in terms of effort, then great effort would deserve great return, even if it was not productive of anything of value. This makes the use of this proposed criterion of social justice at least paradoxical.

Should a society distribute its dental care resources in proportion to how hard a patient works, with harder working patients receiving more dental care and less hard working patients receiving less dental care, independently of other considerations including their need for dental care? Once again, it seems incorrect to ignore need as a criterion of social justice, where need is understood in terms of maintaining and restoring appropriate human functioning.

The authors' view, proposed in the previous section, is that a just society first arranges its distributive structures to meet all the basic needs of all its members, and only then employs criteria other than need in the distribution of whatever resources are "left over" after that. The reasons for supporting this view are straightforward. The authors hold that, whatever other goals, values, principles, purposes, or ideals a human being might choose to live by, none of these can be effectively pursued unless his or her basic needs are filled. The alternative is to say that a person's being able to live at all by their own goals and values and so on is more important than other people's having this same, most fundamental human capacity; and there is no justification for that. Consequently, meeting people's basic needs must take moral priority in the arrangement of a society's distributive structures. If a society is able to meet all its people's basic needs, this is the first requirement of a just society. The section on Basic Dental Care will discuss what forms of dental care should be considered essential responses to basic needs.

THE FREE MARKET VIEW OF JUSTICE

There is one more view of distributive justice that needs to be discussed, one which rejects the authors' view and every other proposal examined above. This view seems to have a wide following within contemporary American society. But it is not clear that all of those who claim to support it have thought carefully through the assumptions it makes about human beings or the conclusions it entails for human social life. Unfortunately, like the other approaches, it can only be briefly examined here. This view holds that a just society is simply one in which all social arrangements and all distribution of resources are the product of voluntary exchanges of the society's citizens in a free marketplace.

To understand this approach to social justice, consider this example. You and another dentist take a vacation in Las Vegas, and each of you sets aside $200 for enjoying Las Vegas' games of chance. Suppose that the two of you enter the same establishment at the same time, each with $200, and assume, for this example, that the games are not rigged so a player is simply playing against the odds (which favor the house, of course, but everyone knows that).

At the end of the day, you emerge without a single dollar of your original $200. But the other dentist finishes the day with $10,000! Has anything immoral happened in this story, even though there is now a huge discrepancy in the two dentists' final financial position? The correct answer seems to be "no." For the games were fair, and every play that either player made was freely chosen. In other words, in this type of case, the ethical distribution is *whatever* distribution results from adequately informed choosers freely choosing to exchange their goods however they choose to exchange them.

If the dentists had been coerced into playing the games, or if they were lied to or defrauded in some other way, or if anyone had failed to keep commitments to the dentists that he or she had made, then the story would include something immoral, and the final distribution would not be a just one. Some kind of restitution would then be needed for the party who was coerced, defrauded, or suffered someone else's breach of contract, and it might also be right to punish the guilty party in addition to requiring them to make restitution. But so long as no one acted in these immoral ways in the example, it seems that *whatever* distribution results from the participants' freely chosen exchanges is an ethical distribution, regardless of whether it conforms to the criterion of need, or contribution, or effort, or any other.

Supporters of the free market view of distributive justice claim that what makes the distribution ethical in this example is exactly what makes any distribution in any aspect of human social life ethical: the exercise of uncoerced free choice by the participants. Thus in this view, a just distribution is whatever distribution results from the participants' freely chosen exchanges, without reference to its conformity to criteria like need, contribution, or effort. The supreme moral value for all social matters on this view of justice is *respect for people's freely chosen actions* (provided the person does not freely choose an action that violates someone else's freedom).

Applied to the distribution of dental care resources, this view holds that dental care resources are justly and ethically distributed when they have been distributed to whoever the providers of dental care choose to provide them to, on the basis of ability to pay the prices dentists ask for their services, on the basis of need, or on some other basis or some combination of bases. So long as both parties *freely choose* the exchange, then the resulting distribution of resources is ethical and just.

In a society whose distributive structures provided every individual with resources for needed dental care (through universal insurance, vouchers, or some other mechanism), distributing dental care thereafter solely on the basis of freely chosen exchanges between dentists and patients would not conflict with the goal of meeting everyone's dental care needs. But in our actual society, people's resources vary greatly, and for many people, the resources available for dental and other forms of health care are limited, and in some cases are almost nonexistent. Consequently, distributing dental care on the basis of free market justice in our society means that many people are unable to receive the dental care they need. Many people's dental needs go unmet, and many others receive only minimally acceptable forms of treatment rather than forms of care most fully suited to their needs and circumstances.

On the other hand, people's actual starting points in life are not equal in resources or opportunities (unlike the Las Vegas example). So the only way a society's distribution system could provide every individual with resources for needed dental care would be by taking resources from those who start with more resources or who get more opportunities than other people, and then giving those resources, in the form of dental care, to those without. But unless the losers in this redistribution freely choose the redistribution, doing this would violate their freedom and would therefore be unjust, according to the free market view of justice. A society that did such redistributing over the objection of even one of its people would be, according to the free market account of justice, an unjust society.

So long as free market justice prevails as the distributive criterion for dental care in the United States, the only likely way that the oral health of everyone in the society would be voluntarily, and therefore justly, preserved and maintained would be if dentists themselves would provide vast amounts of free and underpaid care, far more than they do now. But, as has been noted, dentists' professional obligations to accept some measure of sacrifice for their patients' well-being are limited. The current understanding of these limits seems to be such that dentists are not professionally obligated to sacrifice a decent standard of living for themselves and their families in order to respond to the needs of patients currently left outside the system. Nor is it likely that a change in this understanding of professional obligations, nor even a massive charitable effort on the part of dentists above and beyond their professional obligations, could effectively meet all these needs so long as the larger distribution system allocates dental care according to free market justice.

The reason for these discrepancies is that there is another ethically crucial difference between the Las Vegas example and the distribution of a society's dental care (besides inequalities in resources and opportunities). The players in the Las Vegas example did not *need* to gamble; it was an optional entertainment. (Admittedly, some people do need to gamble, but this is not considered a normal human need of the sort that basic health care, including basic dental care, is. In fact, if the desire to gamble becomes a need, this is itself considered unhealthy, dysfunctional, something that ought to be responded to with care and treatment if possible.) Therefore permitting opportunity for gambling to depend on whatever exchanges happen to take place in the marketplace may be acceptable. But basic human needs, the authors have argued, are much more important than this. They concern essentials; their absence renders humans unable to participate effectively in other areas of human life, even in free market exchanges about other matters.

Therefore a society's responses to its members' basic needs ought not rest solely on whatever exchanges people happen to make, on free market justice. As we argued in previous sections, an alternative standard of social justice, namely, to meet the basic needs of every member of society, ought to guide the distribution of dental, indeed all health care, resources. Just what practical mechanisms and particular structures should be used to meet people's basic dental care needs, whether by universal insurance, or vouchers, or whatever, and how the structures that meet them should be shaped so as not to interfere with dentists maintaining their professional commitments to their patients and to other norms of their profession are important strategic questions. But they are questions beyond the scope of this book. The principal point of this section is that leaving the distribution of dental care to free market justice alone means leaving many of our society's people with their dental care needs unmet, a situation that we have already argued is unsatisfactory from the point of view of social justice.

BASIC DENTAL CARE

The expression *basic dental care*, namely those aspects of dental care that are included within *basic health care*, has been used so far without further clarification. Now it is time to try to differentiate those aspects of dental care that are essential (because they respond to basic needs and are linked very closely to the maintenance or restoration of normal human functioning) from those aspects of dental care that are nonessential or optional.

The easiest categories of dental care to identify as essential or basic are treatments that end or limit serious oral pain and that restore functions whose loss prevents or severely limits normal nutrition and speech. Note that many different kinds of dental procedures will play a role in achieving these goals, depending on the clinical details of the patient's condition. Determining which forms of dental care are essential or basic and which are optional in the relevant sense is not a matter of putting certain procedures on one list and others on another list. It requires instead that we ask of every procedure under what conditions it preserves or restores essential components of a patient's capacity for normal human functioning.

The categories of treatment just mentioned, relief of severe pain and restoration of functions necessary to nutrition and speech, are most obviously essential when the conditions to be corrected are emergent, for example, the pain is currently debilitating or function is currently severely impaired. But intervening sooner, when the pain or impairment of function is less, is ordinarily included within the category of essential or nonoptional treatment whenever these less burdensome conditions are likely to lead to conditions that will certainly require emergency treatment, as is most often the case. Therefore essential or basic dental care includes not only emergency treatment of these conditions, but treatment of similar conditions less far advanced. This is so not only to limit the patient's suffering but also to subject the undesirable conditions to expert control at an earlier point in their development so as to forestall yet worse complications and, ordinarily, to use dental resources as efficiently as possible as well.

It is important to note that many diagnostic procedures, such as oral diagnosis and radiography, are necessary predecessors of the treatments just discussed, and so are also included, whenever the treatments are, in the category of essential dental care. The same is true of the kinds of patient education, after care, and so on that properly accompany such treatments and without which they could not be effectively performed.

The themes of forestalling worse conditions and using resources efficiently for patients' dental health raise one of the most subtle questions about what should count as basic dental care. Namely, whether routine checkups and prophylaxis, the use of sealants on pits and fissures for younger patients, and general patient education for self-care, should be considered essential or optional care. Certainly the emphasis within the dental community has been to view such preventive care as essential to good dental health. This is a major tenet of most contemporary dentists' philosophy of dental practice. But its inclusion within the specifically professional commitment of dentists does not necessarily mean such care should count as essential, as part of basic health care, from the point of view of distributive justice for the whole society.

But it certainly would seem profoundly foolish and a gross waste of dental care resources to pay no or only optional attention to preventing the need for the more costly and risky forms of dental care and to treat painful and function-impairing conditions only when they actually arise. The U.S. health care system has been remarkably slow to recognize the inefficiency of such an approach, and dentistry is widely admired in the larger community for the providence of its emphasis on these aspects of dental care. But these arguments by themselves only establish a close and very efficient link between these forms of dental care and what is clearly essential for human functioning. If there were no other link, the case for their inclusion in the category of basic dental care might still be unsure.

But there is another link. It concerns the point made in Chapters 4 and 5 that pain and impairments of oral functioning, even mild and occasional pain or impairment, lessen a person's sense of being in control of his or her body. It involves not only a lessening of many people's sense of effective autonomy, but also disrupts a person's sense of the unity of the self, since one part of the self is out of control and working at odds against the rest. To some people, these may seem rather soft and unscientific reasons for emphasizing the elements of preventive dental care, but from the point of view of many who suffer from oral pain and dysfunction, the fear and disruption of normal functioning attendant on them are far more dysfunctional than the modest pain or oral impairment themselves. This is also why support of and restoration of the patient's autonomy is ranked as highly as it is on the hierarchy of central values of professional dental practice, immediately after oral and general health.

If health care resources were so scarce that the several categories of care listed so far could not all be provided to those who need them, patients would certainly choose to forego this last category of care before they went without treatment of severely painful and severely impairing conditions or without treatment of the lesser conditions that lead to them. In that sense, the elements of preventive dentistry and education are arguably less valuable to human functioning than the other two categories. But that does not mean that preventive dental care and education lacks a sufficiently close connection with normal human functioning that it should not be included in the category of essential or basic health care. For this combination of reasons, the authors include it in this category.

An even more subtle question concerns whether those aspects of dental care focused principally on esthetic concerns should be placed within the category of essential or basic health care. Some kinds of dental interventions aimed at improving appearance are clearly nonessential, even granting their psychological importance to the patients who seek them. But it would be a mistake to overgeneralize from these. What counts as a normal appearance (or normal enough) is quite wide. Consequently, even though dentists are professionally committed to being concerned about the esthetic value of their work, many aspects of dental treatment that address appearance will not count as basic dental care in the sense in use here. Nevertheless, there will be circumstances, and not only in the practice of oral and maxillofacial surgeons, in which a patient's need for dental treatment to rectify or preserve appearance will be essential to his or her normal human functioning. When this is the case, such treatment should count as an instance of basic dental care.

If our claim is correct, that a just society arranges its distributive structures to respond to the basic needs of all its people, then it follows from the reasons given above that the categories of dental care discussed in this section as instances of basic dental care should be available to all members of such a society. It also follows that the availability of these forms of dental care should not depend principally on the generosity of or on major sacrifices by the society's dentists, or on the chance workings of the free market, but rather on establishing the meeting of people's basic needs, including basic dental care needs, as the criterion by which distributive structures are judged in that society.

THINKING ABOUT THE CASE

The distribution of dental care in the United States has long been according to the criterion of free market justice, with a few small efforts at meeting the basic needs of certain groups added into the mix in recent years. Whereas we have argued that this system falls short of what a just society would do, it is important to ask about the obligations of dentists within this less-than-ideal situation. What ought Dr. Mosiek do about Clara Thomson's situation in this chapter's introductory case, for example?

Some of the most difficult moral questions that human beings face concern how they ought to act when the social institution(s) that form the context of their actions are less than fully moral themselves. This is the situation for dentists in the United States today, in our view. The first question to ask about Dr. Mosiek's situation is whether she is obligated to make up, out of her own resources, for the ethical deficiencies of the U.S. health care distribution system?

We argued in Chapter 6 that dentists are professionally committed to accepting some measure of sacrifice for the sake of their patients' well-being. These sacrifices include some measure of charity care and other sacrifices to assist patients whom the U.S. distribution system would otherwise leave without adequate dental care. But the discussion in Chapter 6 also stressed that there are *limits* to this obligation.

Little long-term good would be done if a dentist's efforts to care for those the system has forgotten brought the dentist's practice to financial ruin. In addition, we proposed, the current state of the dialogue between dentists and the larger community seems to indicate that these sacrifices need not be so great that a dentist is obligated to risk the fairly good standard of living that dentists typically enjoy in this society. Sacrifices within these limits, then, are all that dentists seem professionally obligated to undertake in response to the deficiencies of the U.S. health care distribution system. Any sacrifices beyond this would be above and beyond their professional duty

On this basis, Dr. Mosiek is obligated to accept some financial sacrifices for the sake of her patients who would otherwise receive no dental care or less-than-adequate dental care because of their limited financial means. But there are many ways in which Dr. Mosiek can make this sacrifice.

One possibility would be for her to spread the sacrifice over her whole clientele by charging lower prices to all patients across the board. But this would be a less desirable way of using her sacrifice for patients left out by the distribution system, since many of a dentist's patients will be able to handle ordinary prices. Not only may Dr. Mosiek ethically set her prices, given the present U.S. distribution system, according to how they are characteristically set in a free market exchange system, namely, she may aim to maximize her income, within the competitive marketplace, up to the level that the market will bear. But, in fact, it would seem far better for her to reserve her sacrifices for those patients who cannot obtain adequate care through the ordinary pricing structure.

Of course, the injustice of the surrounding social institution does not excuse, much less justify, individual injustice over and above it. Dr. Mosiek may not "price gouge," charging more for her services than they are worth by taking advantage of patients' ignorance of the relative value of services and the current market price structure. Such conduct is a violation of justice in the relationship between seller and purchaser. But even before that, it would already have violated her professional obligations concerning informed consent, respect for patient autonomy, and the effort to achieve the most interactive relationship possible with the patient.

Dr. Mosiek could make her sacrifices in the form of free care for some patients and payment plans for others, as was described in Chapter 6. Or she could make them by accepting patients on Medicaid or public aid, where payment is usually well below ordinary charges and is often long delayed as well. Or she could make them by establishing a relationship with a nursing home, a facility for the developmentally disabled, or an orphanage or other child care facility, where the reimbursement level will probably be below standard and where a significant amount of the sacrifice will be in the form of the extra effort needed to provide care, and caring attention, to patients with special needs and deficits.

Or Dr. Mosiek might make her sacrifices by participating in a capitation program, where she knows that some of the patients in the program will need far more treatment than the annual capitation payment can pay for, even allowing for those patients on whose care she comes out ahead. If she were unwilling, or unable because she had already made so many sacrifices in other ways, to assume the cost of the additional treatment, then participating in a capitation plan would place her in a terrible ethical bind. It is precisely this bind, along with the pressure it places on a dentist to consider providing inadequate treatment for patients, that makes so many dentists hesitate to join capitation programs. But if Dr. Mosiek used participation in such a program as her way of making the limited but real sacrifices she is professionally committed to, then she would have resolved the pressure to act unethically in advance by committing herself to always provide appropriate treatment to these patients.

Should Dr. Mosiek do any of these things for Mrs. Thomson? Part of the answer to this question depends on what other forms of sacrifice for her patients Dr. Mosiek has already committed to, something that the case as presented does not discuss. But another part of the answer concerns Mrs. Thomson's need. Is her need for a crown rather than a functional three surface amalgam an instance of basic need or not? This is not an easy question.

Ordinarily, preserving the prettiness of someone's smile is not essential to their capacity for normal human functioning. There may be exceptions for individuals in specific walks of life whose psychological well-being is deeply dependent on their continued success in those pursuits. But even then, exceptions that would cover a first premolar, as compared with a central incisor, would not be very numerous. So Dr. Mosiek might seem fully justified in concluding that this particular need or desire of Mrs. Thomson does not count as a basic need and that assisting Mrs. Thomson in obtaining the crown would not qualify as help for those whose adequate dental care has not been properly provided for by society, since the focus of this requirement is patients' *basic* dental care needs.

But the deficiencies of the U.S. distribution system enter the picture in another way in this case. Mr. and Mrs. Thomson need her income from her beauty consulting and sales to meet their own and their developmentally disabled son's basic needs. If the placement of an amalgam restoration in this tooth would likely hamper their ability to provide for the basic needs of themselves and their son, then the tooth is essential to their normal human functioning indirectly, even though it is not essential directly.

There is a close judgment call here. But given the financial circumstances of the Thomson's as the case describes them, Dr. Mosiek might well be justified in treating the need for a crown as a basic need, not because it is a basic dental need, but because it is essential to her meeting basic needs of other sorts. If so, then efforts on Dr. Mosiek's part to either provide the crown at cost or with an extended payment plan, for example, or to fund it in some other way, would qualify as an instance of the sacrifice for her patients that Dr. Mosiek is professionally obligated to undertake. Even so, however, provided she was meeting her obligation to sacrifice in other ways, Dr. Mosiek could also justifiably decline to assist Mrs. Thomson in meeting this need, even if it is indirectly basic, because there are also limits to the extent of sacrifice that a dentist is professionally committed to accepting.

Finally, we need to ask if Dr. Mosiek or any other dentist is professionally required to be opposed to health care distribution systems that adopt the free market justice criterion. We have argued that the U.S. health care distribution system is unjust because, being dominated by the free market criterion, it fails to meet the basic needs of many of its participants. It might seem therefore that we would condemn as unprofessional any dentist who supported this system and/or the free market justice approach to ethical distribution it employs. But this is not so, for a very specific reason.

It does not seem to be part of the professional commitments of dentists, or of any other health professionals, that they are obligated to be consistent in their moral views. There is an inconsistency, we have held, between the free market justice criterion, which holds that there are no objective values other than, or at any rate as significant as, respecting the free choices of exchangers in the marketplace and the commitments of dentists and other health professionals to the value of health (understood, in this account, in terms of normal human functioning). A health professional must not only practice in accord with this value, but must also—as the norm of integrity and education requires—support and testify to its significance in other aspects of his or her life as well. Doing this conscientiously while also supporting, or at least tolerating free market justice as the criterion of a society's health care distribution system requires a great tolerance for inconsistency of thought, or else a great deal of careful thought aimed at somehow comprehending both commitments into some, presumably larger, internally coherent philosophy of personal, professional, and social life. But, specifically from the point of view of professional obligation as it is understood in this society at this time, eliminating such inconsistencies from one's thinking is not professionally required.

CHAPTER 14

Dentistry as a Business

Case: Happy Smiles

Bob Milford graduated from dental school in 1976 and was able to start a practice in Montclair, thanks to a start-up loan from a local bank and his ability to prove to the bank that the number of dentists per capita in Montclair was very low at that time. His practice grew steadily and his life grew comfortable. But he could see Montclair's industrial base beginning to weaken in the early 1980s, and he didn't see much hope for rejuvenating Montclair's economy for some time to come.

So in 1984 he used the profits of 8 years of successful practice and another bank loan to buy a good-sized practice from a retiring dentist in Ridgeview, a comfortable suburb of the state's largest city about 130 miles from Montclair. At the same time, he put the declining Montclair practice into the hands of the associate he had hired 3 years earlier, retaining ownership of the practice and paying the associate a salary for managing it, plus 35% of the profits and an annual bonus for keeping costs in line. The profits from the Montclair practice would help cover him during the transition in Ridgeview.

Milford also arranged the timing of the move so he could leave Montclair 6 months before the owner of the Ridgeview practice actually retired. He took a wonderful European vacation with his wife and three children during that period, and spent the rest of it attending continuing education programs and workshops all over the country to develop his skills in esthetic dentistry, in pain control and anxiety reduction techniques, and in dental marketing. He saw a down time coming for dentistry, and he had a plan that would enable him not just to weather it, but to come out ahead.

When he returned to take up the Ridgeview practice, he first changed its name to "Happy Smiles, Inc." He hired a marketing consultant and not only contacted all the patients of the previous dentist, but sent a carefully worded mailing to every resident in Ridgeview and six surrounding communities. An attractive cover sheet announced the establishment of a new dental practice that would bring advanced dental technology to the patients of Ridgeview and that would make "happy smiles" the focus of the practice, rather than "the pain, discomfort, and anxiety that many patients experience in the dental office." The enclosed letter described a special introductory offer for an initial check-up for new patients, and for the next check-up for the previous dentist's patients, at a published price that Dr. Milford set well below area dentists' standard charge for a check-up.

The letter also asked its readers if they knew of "all that can now be done, thanks especially to new dental treatments and materials involving the most advanced technology, to improve the appearance of teeth, in addition to dental health considerations that have always been dentists' first priority." This was the new age, when people could get the appearance they wanted, the prospective patients were told. They should look carefully at their teeth and what their appearance communicated to others about themselves. If they wanted to change their image to be more attractive and better received, "improving the appearance of your teeth might be a very direct way to take action toward this end."

A list of possible dental defects in appearance was offered, and a matching list of possible treatments to correct these defects, along with a sentence indicating that these were only possible treatment options and that the dentist's actual recommendations would depend on the results of a careful diagnostic evaluation, together with the patient's goals for the treatment. Dr. Milford's continuing education work in this area was also noted, and a free "dental appearance consultation," including the option of intra-oral video imaging, was offered to both current and new patients in the practice at no charge whatsoever.

Dr. Milford's marketing consultant had some knowledge of the practices of Milford's chief competitors, especially Joseph Kamamata, who had practiced in Ridgeview for 8 years, and Ed O'Brien and Silvia Della Galla, who had a joint practice in the next suburb to the north. On the consultant's advise, Milford offered Dr. Kamamata's office manager a large raise and better medical benefits and offered O'Brien and Della Galla's best hygienist the same incentives plus a contractual commitment to support her completion of her Bachelor's degree at the local university. Both women gave their current employers the chance to meet Milford's offers, but when he proved to be the highest bidder, they joined Milford's new office.

The fruit of all these efforts was not only a well-run office and top quality dental hygiene care to complement Milford's solid technical skills, but above all an immediate jump in new patients and a steady flow of the previous dentist's patients into Milford's practice. Quite of few of the new patients came specifically because of the emphasis on esthetic dentistry. Milford's marketing consultant had matched the advertising well to the upscale lifestyle of the Ridgeview area. But these new patients quickly saw that it would be better to have their regular dental care provided in the same office as their esthetic care, and left their former dentists for Milford for that reason.

After only 2 years in Ridgeview, Milford saw that he needed another dentist in the office. Milford advertised at several dental schools, proposing to pay the new associate, who would focus almost exclusively on basic diagnostic and restorative work, a fixed percentage of gross receipts in three categories: dentistry the associate personally performed, dentistry the associate prescribed that was performed by the hygienist, and cosmetic dentistry performed by Milford that resulted from the associate's educating patients about its value.

Some dental students thought this payment structure included unethical financial incentives to treat excessively. Others had heard horror stories of vague, competitive, or demeaning relationships with employer dentists and welcomed such a clear-cut arrangement. In any case, by now it was 1987, and there were plenty of dental students burdened with $100,000 debts from undergraduate and dental school loans and with no prospects for independent practice. So Milford had plenty of high-quality applicants.

Meanwhile, Drs. Kamamata, O'Brien, and Della Galla were furious with Milford. With considerable support from other dentists who had lost patients to his practice, Drs. Kamamata, O'Brien, and Della Galla submitted a petition to the Ethics Committee of the local dental society, arguing that Dr. Milford's mailings were unethical because they made claims about esthetic dentistry that, if not simply false, were certainly materially misleading. Dr. Milford was a member of the local dental society, but had not participated in organized dentistry very much, preferring to be active in local business organizations and in several health-related charitable organizations, where he was already well respected. He considered the three dentists' petition to the Ethics Committee to be nothing but an act of revenge for his hiring away their employees.

"All they had to do," he said to a friend, "was pay them better themselves. It's just good business, and they weren't willing to do it. If they don't like the effects of my marketing, they should hire a consultant themselves. I don't object to a good fair fight in the marketplace. It's this backhanded business of complaining to the Ethics Committee that I object to. I actually think there are plenty of patients out there for all of us, if we'd only get better at reaching them. Only half the population use dentists regularly for nonemergency care. So why am I some kind of ogre for trying to get them into a dentist's chair?

"We should all be marketing aggressively and telling the people what we have to offer. That's not just good business; it's what good dentistry ought to be about, educating people so we can help them. If we don't get them in the door, we can't give them the education they need, and if we don't educate them, we can't help them. I say that good marketing isn't unethical at all. I say it's good dental education and it's what good dentistry ought to be about!"

NEW CHALLENGES FOR DENTISTRY

Across the United States dentistry looks different today from what was most common in the 1950s, 1960s, and 1970s, at least in urban practices. Dentistry has always been part of the free enterprise system in the United States, with most dental care being provided by individual dentists running their own small businesses. But the culture of the dental community and the understanding, both among dentists and within the larger community, of the content of dentists' professional obligations were such that few of the most prominent characteristics of the free enterprise marketplace were in evidence in dental practice. There was no active marketing of dental services, no competitive advertising, and rarely any serious competition by price. But now all three of these, and many other characteristics of the free enterprise market place, are in plain view in dentistry. What has happened to dentistry in the United States since the 1970s? And, more importantly, what is the relationship of these events to dentistry's claim to be a profession and its members' claim to be ethical professionals?

What has happened to dentistry is no mystery, although it has involved the coming together of a number of fairly independent sets of events, so its causes are multiple and complex. First of all, because dental school admissions were radically increased in the 1960s and early 1970s, the number of dentists grew much more rapidly than the population that dentists serve. It might have been assumed that more than half of the population would begin to use dentists on a nonemergency basis if there were more dentists available, but that did not happen, and still hasn't. Consequently, with many new dental school graduates and no comparable increase in the user population, the United States found itself with more dentists than it could keep busy at previous levels.

At the same time, the dental community had succeeded in persuading the larger community to take preventive dental care seriously to a previously unprecedented degree, not only in the dental office and by better educated self-care, but also through fluoridation of the water supplies in many parts of the country. The result was a large decrease in the frequency of dental caries and so a large decrease in dentists' opportunities to do restorative work for the half of the population who sought regular care. Increases in the provision of in-office preventive care made up for some of this decrease, but not nearly enough to offset it completely. Dentistry found itself facing an increase in the number of providers and a decrease in the need for dental treatment at the same time.

Added to this mix was the aging of the U.S. population, with elderly patients less interested in long-term forms of dental treatment and frequently having fewer financial resources for dental care than other groups, and the entrance of insurance companies into the dental care picture, with their efforts since the 1980s to control health care costs as tightly as possible. Already in difficult straits because of the first two factors, U.S. dentistry now had also to face a fiscal situation in which there were significantly fewer dollars for dental care than there had been before.

Finally, there was a significant change in the situation of dental students beginning in the early 1980s. First, the federal tuition grants of previous years had ended, putting the full burden of tuition on the students themselves, who were already more indebted than in previous generations because of decreases in aid for undergraduate education. Then followed sharp increases in the cost of dental education, for many reasons, but with a prominent factor being a sudden decline in enrollments, presumably because dental school graduates' prospects were now dimmer. Consequently, dental students' tuition bills rose sharply and the amount of their indebtedness rose rapidly with them.

The graduating dentist of a previous generation could ordinarily move directly into a practice with the help of a bank loan and a population waiting for his (and occasionally her) services. Of course, the loan had to be paid off, but it was available to the young dentist to get started. Since the 1980s, however, very few graduates get started with a bank loan because most are already too deeply in debt from the cost of their education to be considered for such a loan. Nor are there open fields for the young dentist to practice in, given the oversupply of dentists that the country has seen for some time now. So even a graduate with very small debts would be hard pressed to persuade a bank to support a new practice under these circumstances.

Dental students have therefore become understandably anxious about their prospects. They know that they will most likely begin their dental career in someone else's practice. They hope they will be lucky enough to serve as the associate of someone who is seeking a younger professional peer, rather than as the mere employee of someone willing to take advantage of their financial need. A world in which dentists are not actively competing with one another is a dream world for them, or something out of the past, because dental students are unavoidably competing from the moment they enter dental school just for the opportunity to practice dentistry in a setting they can feel proud of.

Note that none of these factors that have contributed to such important changes in dentistry has been the product of anyone's ill will toward dentistry nor of anyone's insensitivity to the norms of professional dental practice. The dental profession, like any social institution, is situated among and strongly affected by many other complex social institutions, and many U.S. institutions have played a hand in the changes just discussed, although economic policy decisions and other economic factors seem to have played a particularly important role. It is therefore hard to assign blame for these changes, if there would be any value in doing that anyway. Far better for the dental community to ask how it ought to respond to these changes in order to continue to practice dentistry in as professional and ethical a manner as possible.

Answering this question is more difficult than it might otherwise be because of another set of changes that have taken place, not just for dentistry, but for the whole of U.S. society. These are the changes in the education level of the population and the shift from a production economy to a service economy that were mentioned at the end of Chapter 8. Because of these changes there has been a shift in the kind of relationship between dentist and patient—and between professionals of other sorts and their clients as well—that members of this society consider ideal.

Although the Guild Model might have identified the ideal of this relationship for practitioners in a previous generation, there is no question that it is no longer the accepted ideal. The norms of the dental profession must now stress the value of patients' autonomy and the ideal of an interactive relationship. But this shift in professional norms for dentists connects in complex ways with the other changes that have been noted. It is possible to see a pattern in the two sets of changes that seems to eliminate trust from dental practice altogether, pitting dentist against dentist in the competitive marketplace and patient against dentist as the patient seeks a greater degree of independence within their relationship. This is not how the ideal of an interactive relationship views the dentist-patient transaction, of course, but as the old ways change, this might seem to be the dominant theme.

It is very important, therefore, to reflect on how dentistry can be done ethically and professionally in the changed economic and social circumstances that face dentists today. Every practicing dentist asks such questions daily, and the discussion here can only attempt to survey the most important issues. But there is probably no more prominent set of ethical concerns for today's dentists than these, so they deserve careful attention.

ETHICAL ADVERTISING

The most dramatic shift in dentistry, in the minds of many dentists, has been the elimination of the ADA's prohibition of competitive advertising in 1979 and the consequent proliferation of competitive advertising since then. But none of the five causes of change described in the previous section required or was even directly related to the end of the prohibition of competitive advertising. The proliferation of advertising since 1979 is certainly a sign of a much more competitive relationship between dentists. But the reasons for the competition are the factors just described, not the advertising that expresses it.

Advertising actually has the potential to educate the public about dental services; it is therefore clearly a mistake to view dental advertising as an unmixed evil. Nor may the excesses of some individuals be taken as proof that dentists can never advertise in a manner that is ethical and professionally appropriate. Many, even most, who have advertised since the prohibition was removed from the ADA's *Principles of Ethics and Code of Professional Conduct* in 1979 have done so ethically. But the criteria for determining when competitive dental advertising is ethical and professionally appropriate now that it is not simply prohibited have not yet been fully developed. The ongoing dialogue between the dental community and the community at large has only had a few years so far to consider this matter. One important depository of the fruits of this dialogue is in the Appellate Disciplinary Decisions of the ADA's Council on Ethics, Bylaws, and Judicial Affairs.

In 1979, when the actions of the Federal Trade Commission (FTC) and the courts made it clear to the ADA that it would lose any effort to retain the long-standing prohibition of advertising in its *Principles of Ethics and Code of Professional Conduct*, the ADA prudently entered into a consent order to this effect in order to avoid a costly legal battle it could not win. But the actions of the FTC at that time were at least as likely motivated by political considerations as by a careful reading of the mind of the larger community. So one could argue that the elimination of the prohibition was not necessarily an expression of the community's wishes. On the other hand, the larger community has never had extensive representation on the ADA councils and committees, or on the councils or committees of other dental organizations, that have drafted dentistry's only explicit codes of ethical conduct. So we have the same evidence of the larger community's acceptance of these groups' articulation of dentists' professional obligations as we do of the FTC's actions in 1979, namely, the community at large has not protested vociferously. As is usually the case when dealing with the more subtle contents of professional norms, one is forced to look for more subtle forms of evidence of the community's mind as well.

It is at least relevant, then, that there has been no ground swell of objections to dental advertising on the part of the larger community, much less a strong movement to try to reinstate the prohibition. It seems best, then, to turn to what we do know about the obligations of dentists and ask what these norms imply regarding advertising, rather than mourning the removal of the prohibition.

The categories of norms that will be used here will be the eight categories of professional norms first identified in Chapter 3 and applied to numerous other topics throughout this book. But as shall become clear, the three most important categories with regard to advertising are the obligation to respect patients' autonomy, the norm of an ideal relationship, and the norm of integrity and education. This section will focus on the themes of autonomy and the ideal relationship; the norm of integrity and education will be considered later in this chapter.

Four models of the dentist-patient relationship were considered in Chapter 4, and reasons were offered for judging the Interactive Model to most accurately represent what the dental community and the community at large currently accepts as the ideal relationship. Three of these models—Guild, Commercial, and Interactive—draw important contrasting conclusions regarding dental advertising.

One central theme of the Guild Model is that the lay patient is wholly incapable of making judgments, not only about his or her appropriate therapy, but even about his or her need for therapy in the first place. This is why the Guild Model has no place in it for patient decision-making. Even regarding the original choice of a dentist into whose hands the lay patient then places his or her well-being, the Guild Model must hold that this choice by the patient is blind. For the patient has no understanding of the data that would be needed for the rational consideration of alternatives for such a choice.

Consequently, there is simply no justification for dentists, or any other health professionals, to advertise according to the Guild Model. Since lay patients cannot understand or properly evaluate any advertised data that would be relevant to their choice of a dentist, physician, or other health care provider, advertising is at best utterly useless.

But in fact, if it is done, advertising is worse than useless because it suggests to the lay patient that he or she *can* form properly reasoned judgments about the choice of a health professional. Suggesting this to otherwise unknowing lay persons might then lead them to believe they are capable of properly making other judgments about dental care, for example, about what sort of care is needed or about the quality of the care that is provided. Consequently, advertising runs a serious risk of interfering with the formation of a proper dentist-patient relationship. If the patient comes to believe that he or she is capable of judgments that only the dentist can make, then the patient may become less receptive to the essentially passive role that is the only appropriate role for patients in the Guild Model.

The fact that the Guild Model has no place in it for patient autonomy, together with its inability to recognize the fact that over the last several decades the majority of patients have become increasingly better educated and more knowledgeable about their health, has seemed to some people to support the proposal that we should adopt a Commercial Model of the dentist-patient relationship. The Commercial Model is obviously the approach supported by the Federal Trade Commission.

According to the Commercial Model, the relationship between dentist and patient is simply that of producer and consumer negotiating about possible exchanges in the marketplace. The two parties are viewed as being, from the first, self-interested competitors, each trying to obtain from the other the greatest amount of what he or she desires while giving up as little as possible in exchange. The Commercial model's supporters claim that by the working of the "invisible hand" of the competitive market-place, relationships formed on this model yield the greatest quantity and quality of dental care for the least cost in both natural resources and human effort. The "invisible hand" therefore makes this the most efficient model of social relationships, its supporters argue, as well as one in which the value of every party's autonomy is most respected.

The Commercial Model implies that advertising by dentists and other health professionals is a good thing because, its supporters believe, advertising increases competition. Increased competition is believed to improve efficiency through the workings of the "invisible hand." Moreover, the Commercial Model does not need to worry whether advertising will mislead the lay patient or will adversely affect the relationship between dentist and patient. Their relationship is presumed to be an adversarial relationship from the start and has no positive characteristics other than those the parties themselves create. So there is, so to speak, nothing to harm. Furthermore, because the patient is presumed to be an active participant from the start, the implication of this model that the Guild Model rejected, namely, that the patient's role is to be an active decision maker, is viewed as a positive feature of this approach.

In addition, dentist and patient are here viewed as equal bargainers, for they have no obligations to one another prior to their contracting, except an obligation prohibiting coercion and an obligation to some measure of truthfulness and to keeping one's contracts once they are made. Consequently, providing these minimal obligations are met, the two parties cannot act unethically toward one another. Even the obligation to truthfulness is an obligation only to *truth*, not to the *whole* truth. That is, though the bargainers may not lie, they have no obligation to speak clearly or precisely or to say everything they know. They are not responsible for the other party's understanding. If their statements are not "false or misleading in any material respect," to use the phrase promulgated in the ADA's consent agreement with the FTC, then either party may say anything he or she judges will be useful to enhance the other's desire to engage in an exchange in a manner profitable to the speaker.

Consequently, the Commercial Model not only permits a broad range of advertising language and techniques but views all efforts at advertising that do not violate the minimum obligations as contributions to efficiency. Therefore as the mandate of the FTC also requires, the Commercial Model would oppose any efforts at regulation of such advertising, whether by statute or by professional code, that would test it by any other standard than whether it is "false or misleading in any material respect," in other words, untruthful in the relevant sense.

In the ordinary case, the consumer of dental care views his or her situation as, in part, a lack of the information and skills necessary to meet important needs. Consequently, the dentist is at a significant advantage in the relationship. But, says the defender of the Commercial Model, life is like that: some of us are in situations of advantage at some times and at a disadvantage at others. But no one owes anyone else equality in such matters unless they have voluntarily contracted beforehand to provide it. Therefore the dentist may take whatever advantage of the information and skills at his or her disposal that the consumer will agree to. Dental care is no different from the rest of life, and so the relationship between dentist and patient has no business being different either.

The Interactive Model of the dentist-patient relationship holds both of the previous approaches to be incorrect. The Guild Model fails to support the important value of patient *autonomy* and so is too ready to assume that patients cannot understand what they often can. Even more important, it forgets that dentists' expertise in rendering technical judgments about diagnosis, prognosis, and therapy does not include any special expertise in human values, specifically the values of the patient. Therefore the Interactive Model holds, dentists must have as a central goal of their practice the enhancement of patients' autonomy, often diminished by the psychological and physiological effects of their ailments. This means that they must assist patients to make their own value judgments about what shall be done for and to them, based as much as possible on the patients' own values, goals, purposes, and so on.

At the same time, patients ordinarily *do* lack the technical understanding that is necessary to make sound dental care judgments, and they lack the technical skills that are necessary to carry these judgments out. So they cannot function as equal bargainers with their dentist to judge quantity and quality of alternative dental care options. In fact, motivated to seek dental care by important needs they cannot meet themselves, and often fearful and in pain, patients rarely interact with dentists as equal bargainers as rational market consumers are supposed to. Thus whereas the Commercial Model's emphasis on equality is correct, what is important is the *moral equality* of the patient and the dentist, not their equality as bargainers in the marketplace.

What then does the Interactive Model imply about the characteristics of ethical advertising? Certainly the Guild Model's arguments against advertising are much weakened by the Interactive Model's emphasis on patient decision-making and the on patient's ability to understand, much of the time, with the assistance of the dentist, much of what is relevant to sound dental care decisions. So a blanket prohibition of advertising is certainly unjustified in an interactive relationship. Nor does advertising mislead when it suggests that patients be active decision makers; instead it says something correct and important.

But the Commercial Model's minimal constraint that advertising merely be not false or materially misleading is inadequate when we know that, prior to actual contact with the dental professional, many patients are not yet well informed for the decisions that they have to make, especially the initial decision about who is an appropriate care giver. Consequently, the proposals of many state dental societies that, for example, claims of competency be regulated to guarantee their accuracy and comparative data be required, rather than just vague comments about cost or quality, when comparative claims are made, seem quite justified within the perspective of the Interactive Model.

Before the Interactive Model's implications for ethical advertising can be developed further, however, the audience of this advertising must be considered. For example, a *hardened consumer* will habitually doubt the validity of advertised comparisons in terms of cost or quality and will habitually discount associations of a particular dentist's work with elements of the "good life." At the other extreme, a *wholly receptive consumer* will simply accept such comparisons and associations. A more *reflective consumer* falls in between. He or she will attend to the evidence offered in support of comparisons and weigh its merits and will hold associations with the "good life" up to critical reflection before forming any judgment about the advertised dentist's services.

A dentist hoping to advertise his or her services in a manner consistent with the Interactive Model must therefore consider which of these three groups, or of the many additional variations that lie in between them, are likely to be recipients of his or her advertising. For advertising "puffery" that would not be taken seriously at all by the hardened consumer and that would be evaluated and then ignored by the reflective consumer might be accepted as evidence of quality care by the wholly receptive consumer. Since such a dentist's goal is to assist every prospective patient who receives the advertising in making a careful choice of care giver, the dentist must determine what the likelihood is that the advertising will fail to assist, or even positively hinder, wholly receptive consumers within the projected audience.

Marketers of other goods and services who do not have a professional commitment to preserving and supporting certain values for their clients may be able to justify misleading some recipients of their advertising by reason of the good done for others or for the producers themselves. The ethical questions raised by such a practice are complex and beyond the scope of this book. But dentists may not do this. For they are committed to serving the values of general and oral health and patient autonomy for *every* patient they contact with either information or service.

As was noted when the norm of the Chief Client was discussed in Chapter 3, a dentist's professional obligations are not only owed to patients of record and those who seek out the dentist for emergency care. Whoever receives a dentist's advertising is owed, by the dentist, as interactive a relationship as possible, given the circumstances, and as much respect and support for his or her autonomous decision-making as possible. Since there are likely to be parties in a dentist's advertising audience who will be wholly receptive consumers, the dentist is professionally obligated to advertise only in ways that will assist rather than hinder, or not mislead, much less harm, the decision-making of the wholly receptive consumer.

In summary, we have argued that the changes that have taken place in dentistry since the 1970s were not caused by the removal of the prohibition against advertising. Nor is advertising necessarily a violation of the commitments of dentistry as a profession or of the individual dental professional, providing it is advertising of the right sort. Indeed, when the ideal of an interactive relationship and the obligation of the dentist to respect patients'—and prospective patients'—autonomy are carefully attended to (for example, by considering the implications of the Interactive Model, as above), then the educational effects of properly conceived advertising seem to recommend it as a professionally appropriate activity. What is ethically questionable are certain kinds of advertising.

False or misleading advertising clearly violates the dentist's obligations to respect patients' autonomy and to work for as interactive a relationship with the patient as is possible and is seen as unethical even from the far more accepting perspective of the Commercial Model. But that is not the only kind of advertising that is ethically questionable. Also deserving of professional ethical criticism is advertising that fails to assist, or runs the risk of hindering, the decision-making of the wholly receptive consumer. For it is this consumer whose ability to benefit from dental advertising must be taken as the standard of ethical dental advertising.

There is an additional category of professional-ethical criticism of dental advertising that does not come to light in an examination focused on the norm of the ideal relationship and respect for patients' autonomy. This concerns advertising that, even if it meets the standard just developed, sends the larger community the wrong message about dentistry and that prompts doubts or raises questions in people's minds about values that principally determine dentists' actions regarding patients and prospective patients. Such advertising violates the norm of integrity and education that obligates dentists, within limits, to act consistently with the values they are professionally committed to even when they are away from the operatory and the office. This norm was examined in some detail in Chapter 8. Now it is important to consider its implications for dental advertising.

THE COMPETITIVE SPIRIT AND PROFESSIONAL INTEGRITY

Many dentists who were formed in their views of the dental profession when the prohibition of advertising was in place believed in that prohibition then, and they are critical now for reasons quite different from those discussed in the previous section of some dentists' extensive use of advertising and other marketing techniques. They are concerned that the very activity of advertising and marketing by dentists sends a false and damaging message to the public about dentists and their professional commitments.

At the core of this message, it is argued, is a view of dentistry in which there is something that is more important to the dentist than the well-being of his or her patient. First, to any audience reasonably cynical about the contents of advertising and marketing language—whether the hardened consumer of the last section, or only the reflective consumer—the fact that dentists employ any kind of language or imagery that resembles standard advertising "puffery" suggests that they are not interested in communicating with their clients literally and carefully in terms linked to scientific fact. This suggests that they are willing to place a "sale" ahead of meeting the patient's needs. For it suggests that treatment decisions will be directed by the effectiveness of the advertising rather than by the patient's clinical condition as expertly examined and judged and considered by the patient.

Second, since such advertising and marketing efforts are inherently competitive "against" other dentists, it suggests that there is a measure of successful dental practice that is more important than meeting patients' dental needs and bringing about the other central values of dental practice. Namely, success at "beating" other dentists in the market place, even though those other dentists may be serving their patients' dental needs very well.

The complaint offered against dental advertising and marketing is that such activity communicates a message to the public, regardless of whether the content of the ad or letter is true or false, misleading or not. Such activity, it is argued, communicates to the public that the objective of dental practice is to sell and to "win," and that serving the patient's well-being is only important insofar as it is instrumental to meeting this double, marketplace objective. Such a message surely misrepresents dentistry, which is committed to giving priority to the patient's well-being, both in the sense of working specifically to preserve or restore the central values and in the sense that the dentist makes significant sacrifices of other interests for the sake of the patient's well-being. Such a message also runs the risk of undermining the dentist's ability to achieve its committed goals by undermining the patient's trust that the dentist is so committed.

Sometimes, when such criticism of advertising and marketing is offered, it seems that what is most at stake for dentistry is its prestige and its privilege of exclusive practice. But even if such activities did yield long-term adverse effects for dentistry's privileges and prestige, these effects would not be the most serious concerns here. What should rather be stressed in examining dental advertising and marketing is the dentist's obligations under the norm of integrity and education. Because dentistry stands for, and each dentist commits to practice for the sake of, certain values and certain norms of conduct, the obligations of dentistry as a profession. If it is true that dental advertising and marketing, or certain kinds of them, affect the larger community's view of dentistry in the ways discussed in the preceding paragraphs, then these activities may be in direct violation of the dentist's obligations to profess and live by the central values and other norms of professional dental practice.

The factual question here is a subtle one, however: What effect does dental advertising and marketing have on the community's overall view of what dentistry is about? This is not something easily determined. The answer certainly cannot simply be that the effects of advertising in this regard must be adverse because dentistry has clearly changed so much since the prohibition of advertising was dropped. For, as has been noted, there are many other factors responsible for these changes in dentistry, and the end of the advertising prohibition was arguably only coincidentally connected with these factors in time.

In addition, one of the groups proposed as most likely to draw the conclusion that dentistry has shifted its priorities away from the patient's well-being, namely reflective consumers, is also the group most likely to appreciate the efforts of careful dentists to use advertising to educate rather than to merely sell and out-compete competitors. It is this group that is most likely, in other words, to understand what is going on in ethical advertising and to receive the proper message, namely an educational message aimed at enhancing the community's understanding of the connection between dental care and oral and general health, and a motivational message to prompt people to act on their understanding.

Nevertheless, the claim being raised against dental advertising and marketing by those who criticize it for these reasons is a serious one, even if the factual support on which it will ultimately depend has not yet been gathered in any sophisticated way. In addition to trying to determine the actual effects of dental advertising and marketing on the public's view of dentistry, however, a concerted effort by dentists and the lay community, working together, to formulate clear guidelines for dental advertising and marketing would likely be equally helpful. But these must be guidelines that address the additional issues raised in this section, and not only the question of "false or misleading" advertising that is the usual focus of policy making for dental professional advertising.

Such guidelines, if developed jointly by dentistry and the lay community, may be the most effective way to assist dentists in fulfilling their professional commitments regarding integrity and education in this matter. Unfortunately at the present time an effort to develop such guidelines would have to be constructed very carefully, if it can be accomplished at all, because the power and interest of the FTC in these matters are currently directed at preventing the formulation of new rules or guidelines about advertising and because of the legal force of the consent order entered into by the ADA in 1979 prohibiting regulation of advertising beyond application of the standard of "false or misleading."

It is important to note, in addition, that it is not only by advertising and marketing that dentists run the risk of misrepresenting dentistry's priorities to the larger community. Dentists profess their values and communicate to the public about dentistry and its priorities by many other kinds of words and deeds as well. So the concern raised earlier in this section about the potential for misrepresenting dentistry to the public exists not only for advertising and marketing, but for all forms of speech and communication. Consider, for example, a dentist whose manner at chairside can be perceived as salesmanship rather than an effort at interactive, collaborative decision-making, or whose approach to time management or the management of an office sets other values ahead of the patient's general and oral health. Words, actions, and policies can misrepresent dentistry's commitments just as surely as aggressive advertising or marketing.

Consequently, every dentist needs to regularly examine how he or she pursues the entrepreneurial goals of dental practice and ask what that pursuit communicates to the larger community about the practice of dentistry and its priorities. Each needs to make sure that his or her own words and conduct and the policies and practices of his or her office do not misrepresent dentistry's commitment to the central values and other norms of dental practice.

DIFFERENT MODELS AND PHILOSOPHIES OF DENTAL PRACTICE

One of the central values of dental practice discussed in Chapter 5 is a dentist's "Preferred Patterns of Practice." Effective dental practice requires that many of the component activities of dental practice become habitual, and dentists vary in the patterns of practice that they can effectively habituate. Consequently, within the range of what is acceptable in dental practice, different dentists will quite properly adopt different patterns of practice, and practicing within one's preferred pattern of practice is properly a high value, though not the highest, in dentists' practice decisions.

Different philosophies of dental practice, as one of the most important of such patterns, lead almost automatically to different models of dental practice from a business point of view. A dentist who is unbending from a philosophical commitment to provide only the best imaginable treatment in each clinical situation will almost of necessity have a low volume, high fee business setting for dental practice. A dentist who is philosophically committed to providing extensive care to the underserved in contemporary U.S. society will probably have a large number of Medicaid patients. Another dentist may choose to participate in a capitation program for similar philosophical reasons, and this practice will look more like the Medicaid practice and less like the low volume, high fee practice.

Another dentist may choose what might be called an "average" practice, where most patients have dental insurance and the means to pay a little more besides and they are interested in receiving the kinds of dental services that "everyone takes for granted." Another may choose to run a high volume, lower fee practice, and so on.

Of course, many dentists choose one or other of these business settings for dental practice for economic rather than philosophical reasons. Whether that is the case or not, the economics of each kind of business setting brings its own kinds of ethical challenges. The dentist with a Medicaid or capitation practice, for example, must be careful that the financial pressure from limited income in such a practice does not lead to treatment choices or ways of dealing with patients that violate the minimal standards of care. The low volume, high fee dentist must be careful that the dentist's commitment to a particular philosophy of practice does not lessen his or her respect for and support of patients' autonomy, for example, that it does not lead to a Guild-like pattern of relationship with capable patients.

The dentist with a high volume, low fee practice also has to attend especially to patients' autonomy and the ideal of an interactive relationship. For it is easy for high volume practices to underemphasize patient collaboration in decision-making to practice as quickly as possible, and where fees are low, there is also some pressure to push additional dental services on the patient rather than propose them to the patient appropriately in response to the patient's needs.

One particular ethical challenge that every dentist must address concerns the blending of the topics of the two previous sections and this one. Namely, advertising and other communication to patients, including one-on-one communications with patients at chairside, specifically about the business aspects of one's and other dentists' practices.

Every dentist knows of the ethical—and legal—obligation to correctly inform patients at chairside of the cost of proposed treatments, and it is just good business, as well as professionally obligatory, to inform them about payment plans, the extent and limits of insurance coverage, and the like. But consider advertising language that suggests that this particular practice's charges are lower than others' or that its services are more completely covered by insurance than others' and the like, when actual comparisons have not been done or would not support the suggestion. Or consider similar comments at chairside. For example, a dentist might give the impression that his or her efforts will provide a higher level of insurance coverage for a patient than the insurance company would otherwise provide or than another dentist could arrange, even though the coverage depends on the insurance contract and what the dentist actually contributes is effective communication with the insurance company, proper handling of the paper work and so forth, which the patient justly expects in any case.

Some patients will not believe such suggestions, but others, those described in the section on ethical advertising as "wholly receptive consumers," may accept such suggestions uncritically and therefore be misled by them. For this reason, the same ethical standard proposed there regarding advertising in general also needs to be applied to advertising and other communications with patients regarding price and other business matters of a dental practice. The standard is that the dentist is ethically bound to speak in ways that will not mislead or fail to support the effective exercise of autonomous decision-making on the part of a wholly receptive consumer.

Moreover, for the reasons explained in the previous section, even the hardened and reflective consumers may be misled in another way by such suggestions. For if their content is not believed by the patient, then it is clear to the patient that they must be motivated by the desire to sell more dental care and to compete more effectively with other dentists. These reasons are at fundamental odds with dentistry's commitment to give priority to the patient's general and oral health, and the other central values and norms of practice, in practice decisions. Consequently, such actions miseducate the public and misprofess what dentistry is about, and they violate the dentist's obligations to integrity and education.

Just as different dentists justifiably—that is, in a manner consistent with their professional-ethical commitments—practice dentistry according to different philosophies of practice, so each of the different models of dentistry as a business can be practiced in a professionally appropriate manner. The task for each dentist is to identify and respond appropriately to the particular ethical challenges that the economics of his or her type of business setting produces. It is not the case that one or other of these kinds of business setting is inherently unethical for dental care. The appropriate question is rather how well the ethical challenges of that setting are being addressed, and this question must be asked about every kind of business setting in which dentistry is practiced.

THINKING ABOUT THE CASE

The are many respects in which Dr. Milford's Ridgeview practice differs markedly from the way dentistry was practiced 20 or 30 years ago, and there are many ways in which Bob Milford seems to be a different sort of person from the typical dentist of those years. But differences are not automatically deficits, particularly when everyone acknowledges that the surrounding environment has changed radically for dentistry since 1980 or so. So each of the differences between Dr. Milford's practice and more traditional styles of practice needs to be examined before any overall judgment of his Ridgeview practice can be rendered. We can begin with Dr. Milford's advertising and marketing activities.

The mere fact that a dentist is actively marketing his or her practice to prospective patients is not, we have argued, something that is unprofessional or unethical. This includes, for example, changing the name of the practice, sending mailings to potential patients to inform them of the approach the practice takes to dental care ("happy smiles") and the services offered, and providing a low first-visit charge for a check-up to get patients into the office. The ethical question that needs to be asked, however, is what these marketing activities communicate to prospective patients, especially what content the "wholly receptive consumer" will take from them. That is what needs to be evaluated most carefully.

Organized dentistry prohibited trade names like "Happy Smiles" until the 1979 consent agreement with the FTC. The objection to them was that they made dentistry appear to be a commercial enterprise like any other marketplace activity, rather than an ethical and professional activity aimed first of all at preserving and enhancing patients' well-being. That objection is not a foolish one, as the arguments in the previous sections have demonstrated. But it is not at all clear that trade names like this are taken all that seriously by the public, even the most receptive of them. Consequently, unless the wording is particularly miseducating or misleading—for example, calling a dental practice "Dentistry Chiefly For Profit" or "Dental Health Guaranteed"—a trade name alone is unlikely to violate a dentist's professional obligations.

In combination with various other marketing activities, however, the use of a trade name may cross the line and become, in that context, significantly miseducational and therefore professionally unethical. This possibility of the cumulative effect of marketing efforts that are individually acceptable will be discussed in a moment.

What about Dr. Milford's letter? Here the "happy smiles" motto is explained as indicating an emphasis on dental care that significantly limits "the pain, discomfort, and anxiety that many patients experience in the dental office." Many patients do experience pain, discomfort, and anxiety in the dental office, so this part of the claim is legitimate. But this may still be an unsupportable and misleading claim if the actual wording used by Dr. Milford implies that his office can do this better than other dentists do. However, since Milford has taken continuing education in pain control, among other things, the claim that his office is adept at this is not inappropriate.

To many dentists, Dr. Milford's letter to prospective patients may be most objectionable in its marketing of esthetic dentistry. The increased emphasis on techniques for improving patients' appearance, over and above dental health considerations, has coincided with the downturn in the amount of restorative work available for general dentists to do. In the minds of some dentists, those who now actively propose esthetic options for their patients are violating their professional commitments because they are serving a goal other than health, and they are doing it for financial reasons, not for the sake of patients' well-being. The professional-ethical issues here are subtle and deserve some careful attention.

The first point to be made is that esthetic dental work that significantly impairs a patient's oral or general health involves a violation of the hierarchy of central values of dental practice. Esthetic values are among the central values of dental practice and so are properly pursued by dentists, but at the same time, they rank below oral and general health on the hierarchy. Patient autonomy is also a central value, so that responding in an interactive treatment decision to a patient's request for appearance-enhancing treatment is, other things being equal, a justifiable employment of a dentist's professional expertise. But patient autonomy also ranks below oral and general health on the hierarchy of central values. Therefore the patient's oral and general health may not be significantly impaired in the present or put at significant risk of impairment in the future solely for the sake of a desired enhancement of the patient's appearance. (As was noted earlier, problems with a patient's appearance can sometimes be of such psychological importance to the patient that addressing them is actually part of caring for the person's general health, but such situations are rare exceptions in ordinary dental care.)

The second point is that any dentist who acts against a patient's autonomy and fails to work for the most interactive relationship possible with a patient, for the sake of selling more dental services, is acting unprofessionally, whether esthetic dental techniques are involved or not. For some people, questions about their appearance are not psychologically loaded, so the proposal that a patient might benefit from appearance-enhancing dental work does not impair the patient's ability to make an autonomous decision on the matter. But for many people, the proposal that their appearance is flawed in some way, which is an almost unavoidable implication of the suggestion that it can be improved, is psychologically potent and inhibits autonomous decision-making. It is therefore almost always a violation of the proper dentist-patient relationship for the dentist to directly propose specific appearance-enhancing treatment or to directly identify a specific flaw and the subsequent improvement available to the patient, especially in the operatory, without the patient having taken the initiative to inquire about it first.

This does not mean, however, that the dentist cannot inform prospective patients of the existence of appearance-enhancing dental procedures in general, or that the dentist may never pose the general question to patients whether they have had concerns about their appearance. But to protect patients' autonomy and the interactive character of the dentist-patient relationship, such communications need to take place in a setting in which the patient is in control, and they must not imply any specific deficit of appearance for the patient. Thus for example, the dentist's intake form may ask patients if they have concerns about the appearance of their teeth without creating an inappropriate psychological environment. The patient is still in control.

Similarly, a dentist at chairside may ask if a patient would like to see a close-up of his or her smile through video imaging. But if the dentist initiates the discussion of what the patient sees by proposing that some aspect of the patient's appearance is deficient, proposing it explicitly or even proposing it implicitly by suggesting what could be changed before the patient raises the question, then it is ordinarily a violation of the psychological conditions in which patients' autonomy and an interactive relationship between patient and dentist function most effectively.

Consequently, the professional-ethical questions about Dr. Milford's marketing of esthetic services are whether it violates the priority of patient's oral and general health over esthetic values (the first issue above) or it violates his patients' autonomy and the ideal of interactive decision-making with them (the second). The case about Dr. Milford does not tell us what takes place in Dr. Milford's operatories. It is possible that he is a high-pressure salesman of esthetic services. But it is just as possible, absent evidence, that he is fully respectful of the priority of oral and general health and fully respectful of his patients' autonomy and that he works hard at having treatment decisions on esthetic matters and all others be as interactive as possible. The fact that he calls his practice "Happy Smiles, Inc." and advertises esthetic and other dental services by mail is not evidence of how he treats patients at chairside at all.

With regard to Dr. Milford's actual mailing, again the case does not provide full details. It is possible that other statements in the mailing would be professionally compromising. But the information provided indicates an explicit statement of the priority of dental health over esthetic considerations, a statement that treatment decisions will depend on the clinical facts of each patient's situation, and an indication that treatment decisions will be made by the dentist and patient together. From the data provided, then, Dr. Milford's advertising of esthetic dental services appears to conform to the hierarchy of central values and to the ideal of an interactive relationship that is respectful of patient's autonomy. The claim that his letter is either false or materially misleading or otherwise unethical appears to be mistaken. If there is any ethical problem here, it has to do with the cumulative effect of all of Dr. Milford's marketing efforts together on the public's view of dentistry.

Is it possible that a dentist whose marketing efforts, taken individually, were each ethically appropriate and defensible could nevertheless violate his or her professional commitments when all of them were considered together? The discussion in the previous sections suggests that this possibility cannot be ruled out. The point of the norm of integrity and education is that dentists have a professional obligation to speak and act consistently with the values and norms they profess, over and above conforming their individual actions in practice to these professional norms. So we must ask whether Dr. Milford's overall marketing effort misrepresents the dental profession and miseducates the public about what dentistry stands for, even if his marketing activities are professionally acceptable when examined one by one.

The argument that Dr. Milford's critics would raise is that recipients of the letter will conclude—from its being sent at all and from its use of persuasive language, like the "Happy Smiles" trade name, and other familiar marketing techniques—that dentistry is a commercial, profit-driven enterprise like any other in the marketplace, rather than a profession founded on a commitment to the patient's well-being, even to the point of actual sacrifices for the sake of it. Dr. Milford's reply to this argument is clearly that his mailing is a form of education and motivation of the public to come to a dentist, education and motivation that dentists are, in fact, professionally obligated to undertake under the same norm of integrity and education that his critics appeal to. Who is correct here?

To date, no one has done any careful research into the educational impact of professional advertising on the public's view of professions, much less research specifically on the impact of dental advertising, say since 1979, on the public's view of dentistry. From that point of view, the matter remains an open question, one that the dental community would do well to investigate. But it is important to remember that the principal way in which the public's views of the dental profession are shaped is from direct contact with dentists. This is far more formative of their views about dentistry than their experience with dental advertising, which the public still encounters in relatively small amounts. Provided that each individual instance of dental advertising meets the standards of being true and not materially misleading, which is required even by the minimal ethic of the marketplace, and provided it also conforms to the norms of respect for patient autonomy, the ideal of an interactive relationship, and the priority of general and oral health and the other central values, then the cumulative impact of dental advertising at its present level of use is far less important than the cumulative educational and motivational impact of dentists' communications at chairside. If Dr. Milford conforms to this standard, he is not professionally in the wrong.

Here the contrast with Dr. Prentice, in the introductory case for Chapter 2, is instructive. Once again, as was noted there, we do not have enough detail in the case to make a once-and-for-all judgment of Dr. Prentice's manner of running his practice. But Jack Williamson's reports and impressions, if accurate, strongly suggest that Prentice does not place either the general and oral health or the autonomy of his patients ahead of financial success in his clinics. His marketing, outside the clinic and especially inside in the operatories, is specifically aimed at producing additional business, and does so first by failing to carefully distinguish in treatment decisions between patients' needs and other work that can be done without harm, and then by not informing the patients of this difference when treatments are proposed.

Consider the two dentists' arrangements for their dentist employees. Dr. Milford's arrangements for his associate in Montclair and those proposed for the associate soon to be hired in Ridgeview do place some financial pressure on them to practice in a fiscally sound and productive manner. But it is doubtful that these arrangements would produce any greater financial pressure for these dentists than a solo practitioner already feels today in trying to keep his or her practice financially afloat during these more difficult times. Dr. Prentice, on the other hand, has established per-patient quotas and other quotas regarding work ordered and work done, together with a severe penalty—loss of job—for failing to meet them. These arrangements automatically create powerful pressures on Prentice's employee dentists to persuade patients to have more work done than they would ordinarily be judged to need in a practice run in another way. This is, in fact, the frank reason for Prentice's quotas.

There are, in other words, subtle but professionally significant differences between these two dentists. Dr. Milford's conduct and marketing activities appear, from the limited data available, to be professionally sound, taken one by one. If he is at risk of acting unprofessionally in this regard, it is by the cumulative effect of his entrepreneurial activity and the possibility that it miseducates the public about the dental profession. While this is a genuine concern, his response in his defense is plausible, and the greater educational impact of chairside communication on the public also supports his view of the matter, provided his chairside conduct and communication would prove ethically sound when carefully examined.

Dr. Prentice, on the other hand, seems to have no concern whatsoever for the potential of his practice arrangements and marketing efforts to miseducate the public about dentistry. Indeed, his comments to Jack Williamson suggest that he believes the Commercial Model of dentistry, discussed and rejected in Chapter 2, is accurate. In fact, Dr. Prentice actually seems to think that if his style of practice communicates a commercial view of dentistry to the public, that is as it should be. While the style of practice that Dr. Prentice requires in his clinic may manage to fulfill the market's minimal ethical requirement of informed consent without coercion or fraud, it is hard to say, on the evidence the case gives us, that the priority of patient's general and oral health over other values and support of his patients' autonomy and of interactive relationships are the chief determinants of practice decisions there. But even if these norms of professional dental practice were being met in Dr. Prentice's clinics, he is still misrepresenting the dental profession and miseducating the public about what dentistry stands for as a profession. He is violating the norm of integrity and education.

Why then the antagonism against Dr. Milford among his peers in the Ridgeview area. Part of that ill feeling is understandable because Dr. Milford has hired away valuable employees from two dentists and is drawing patients away from other dentists through his marketing efforts and his emphasis on and skills in esthetic dentistry. But if he is not conducting himself in an unethical manner in these matters, if he is simply a more effective entrepreneur, but is careful that his employment of the tools of the marketplace does not yield professionally unethical conduct, why is he considered to be at fault?

Before the advent of the social and economic changes in dentistry that have been discussed here, most dentists probably shared a fairly similar temperament and style. The dental profession of necessity attracts prospective members from a fairly narrow range of personality types and the particular understandings of the norms of dental practice that were in place in that era, and the relative ease with which good, hard work could earn a dentist an established practice and a fairly comfortable life probably limited that range even further. This is not to say that all dentists of that era liked each other or recognized themselves in one another. But it is reasonable to think that there were significant affinities that would not be as evident now when the environment of dental practice has changed so much.

To enter dentistry in this new era, a person needs to be willing to face great risk, since the possibility of not practicing in a congenial setting or even of not practicing at all is routinely available, and the person also must be able to be comfortable with huge debts and financial insecurity. It would not be surprising, therefore, if there were significant differences in personality type and style between persons who have become dentists during the present era and those who became dentists in the previous environment.

In addition, even among dentists who entered practice in the previous environment, there may well have been differences of style and temperament which had no occasion to manifest themselves until the environment for dental practice became unavoidably competitive. Those who were adept at managing competition, but who felt no call for it in the previous environment, might now be motivated to call up those skills and apply them with energy, and so distinguish themselves fairly quickly from their peers who felt less affinity for functioning in an highly competitive environment.

It is likely that both of these processes have been at work in recent years. But whatever the psycho-social process that has brought it about, it is clear that dentistry now includes men and women of very different temperaments and styles, particularly when it comes to participating actively in the competition that the present environment makes inevitable.

Many dentists, of whatever age and training, prefer to practice in a manner that is largely passive to the competitive pressures around them. Others actively engage the challenge, even though they can see that doing so is a professionally-ethically delicate enterprise for the reasons that this chapter has tried to detail. A few more, like Dr. Prentice, practice at the very edge of professional acceptability, and probably beyond it in some respects, perhaps because their vision of the dental profession has been affected by the changes in the environment and they have mistakenly concluded that dentistry is now simply a commercial enterprise. A few, indeed very few, but unfortunately if they are found out an often well-publicized few, have given over the claim to being professionals—according to a Normative Picture of profession—altogether. They have turned their clinics into frankly commercial enterprises for profit, with dental care merely a commodity and "let the buyer beware" as their motto.

It is extremely important that neither the public nor members of the dental community mistake this last group for any of the other groups, and especially that those in the second group, as Dr. Milford has been portrayed to be, not be confused with the last group or even the second to last, the Dr. Prentice's of the world.

It is our firm conviction that many features of the marketplace can be adapted for use in fully professional, fully ethical dentistry. This is a subtle ethical task and one that requires constant ethical vigilance. But it is not impossible, and a practitioner who attempts it deserves not the criticism of his or her fellow dentists but their support and ethical wisdom. The differences between the dentists in the first two groups are not chiefly differences in professional commitment. These dentists do not live and practice by different norms, nor with different degrees of moral seriousness, sensitivity, or commitment. The differences between these dentists are rather mostly differences of temperament and style. In facing the challenges of this new age, the dentists in both of these groups would benefit far more if they learned to respect their differences, to emphasize their fundamental similarities as dedicated professionals, and to communicate with each other so that the members of both groups can persevere in the ethical practice of dentistry as social and economic conditions continue to change.

CHAPTER 15

The Dental Profession and the Community

Case: Professional Organization or Commercial Enterprise

You have recently become editor of the prestigious (and fictitious) *American Journal of Prosthodontics*, the official publication of the American College of Fixed and Removable Prosthodontics (ACFRP) and a leading journal within the American dental community. You were appointed editor of *AJP* because of years of hard work, careful teaching, and significant research. You now face an important decision about advertising in the journal. Your managing editor and your chief associate editor, who have been with the journal for years, are seated before you. They are deeply divided about an expensive, full color, four-page ad that the Peterswill Corporation wishes to place in *AJP* for its new product, "Capwright."

Peterswill has been a leading producer of dentifrices and other oral hygiene products for years. Its advertising has been a mainstay of *AJP*, and the Peterswill Foundation, heir to most of the fortune of the company's founder, Peter Roundsmith, has long been a major supporter of ACFRP programs. But the Peterswill Corporation has gone through some difficult years recently. Sales of its mouthwash declined significantly after federally mandated changes were made in Peterswill's advertising claims, and the firm's share of the dentifrice market also slipped badly, chiefly because of the corporation's complacent attitude toward fluoride research. Now a new senior management group is in place, trying to turn things around by expanding Peterswill's markets, and a new senior researcher, hired away from a competitor, has developed Capwright. The firm's management believes that Peterswill's ability to survive now rides on the success of this product.

Capwright is an adhesive and seating compound for fixed prostheses. Its appeal lies in the fact that it is more than a cement. It will form itself to both surfaces, both the preparation and the prosthesis, and fill in any gaps which exist between the two without weakening the bond, thus making up for any errors in a dentist's preparation of the tooth or in the impressions that the dentist takes for the prosthesis. The copy from Peterswill's advertising agency doesn't make this point quite so explicitly, of course; it stresses Capwright's "ability to expand the general practitioner's ability to place caps and bridges, while giving even the most expert prosthodontist new confidence that his or her appliances will seat perfectly." But any dentist who reads the ad will understand what is being said.

The chief associate editor speaks first. "The first thing you have to ask yourself, Doctor, is what it means to say that we are professionals. We claim to be committed to quality treatment and to placing our patients' oral health ahead of our own desire for money and a flourishing practice. There isn't any doubt that quality treatment and the best care for our patients mean that teeth must be properly prepared for prostheses, and impressions and castings must be done with precision."

"What do we teach our students in the dental schools?" the associate editor continues. "Certainly not to just come close, and fill in the gaps that are left with a good cement. We teach them that an exact fit is expected between preparation and prosthesis, and we teach them the skills to carry this out in the routine case, and we teach them to send difficult cases to specialists because that is the standard of care.

"If that is true, then how can this journal publish an ad like this, which says to general practitioners and specialists alike: `Don't worry about your sloppy work; we'll cover your mistakes!' This journal has a reputation to protect; that's one thing, and I think it is important. But something more important than that is at stake. We are a profession. We hold a public trust, not just as individuals, but collectively through organizations like the College. If Capwright is a superior bonding agent, or if it is better at handling the microscopic imperfections that occur in even the highest quality prosthetic preparations and castings, let them say that and provide the research to prove it. But we would be guilty of a serious violation of our professional ethics if we were to publish an ad that encourages dentists to tolerate substandard preparations because they can cover up the results with Capwright!"

The managing editor responds. "Of course I respect the values that the associate editor refers to, but there are four additional facts that you need to take account of in your decision, Doctor. First of all, there is the financial issue. We rarely get a chance to run a full color four-pager, much less to have a chance to contract for one each month for the next two years. Besides, Peterswill has been one of our major advertisers. There is good reason to think that the firm's new management would pull their other advertising from the journal if we refused to run the copy for Capwright.

"You know as well as I do that if the only funding we had was the grant from ACFRP, this would be a quarterly journal of 40 or 50 pages, not a monthly that has room enough to serve our community in dozens of important ways on top of the first-rate research we publish. We can't ignore our advertisers and still serve the members of the College and the larger dental community. They are depending on us, too. That's the second point. In addition to our own bottom line considerations, we have an obligation to continue serving our readership because they need us and count on us for all that this journal does for them.

"Third, this product has been field tested by reputable laboratories. It has FDA approval. It won't decay anyone's teeth or compromise their health. The associate editor says he would be willing to advertise a product that claims to fill in microscopic imperfections. Well, we all know that there are many dentists out there who place prostheses with more than microscopic imperfections in the fit, and some patients eventually pay the price in pain and lost function. Why not encourage the general practitioner to use a product like this that will raise the quality of that dentist's prosthetic work? It is the G.P.s who are the most pressed right now, with the economics of dentistry changing so much. Don't we owe them some consideration? After all, this journal isn't published just for the members of the College. It tries to serve the whole dental community. It's the College's way of educating dentists generally about good prosthetic care. Here is a way that the care that ordinary dentists actually give their patients can be significantly improved. The standard of care in the dental schools is not the standard of care out in the offices, and it is *that* standard of care that we have a chance here to improve.

"Fourth, I want to ask whether the editors of this journal are the ones who ought to tell practicing dentists what is and what is not appropriate care. Dentists are professionals; that point has already be stressed by the associate editor. But that means they are the ones that have been entrusted with the decisions about the proper care of their patients. Each of them must make that decision about each particular patient; we cannot make those decisions for all of them. Our job is to inform them of the clinical techniques available to them, and you know as well as I do that our advertising is as important a vehicle for doing that job as our articles on current research. This product has FDA approval and is the result of extensive research in Peterswill's own labs and at several universities. So I submit that we would be going beyond our mandate, and doing a disservice to the dental community as well, if we refused to publish this ad, not to mention tightening the financial noose around the journal's neck instead of taking the opportunity to let it take a deep breath for the first time in years."

You are the editor, Doctor. What should you do?

THE OBLIGATIONS OF THE PROFESSION AS A WHOLE

To this point, this book has principally emphasized the obligations of individual dentists because of the commitments they have made in becoming professionals and because of the nature of the profession they have joined. But each profession as a whole also has obligations. This chapter will examine the obligations of the dental profession using the same eight categories of professional obligation that have guided the discussion of individual dentists' obligations in the preceding chapters.

First, however, the general idea that the dental profession as a whole can have obligations, and the implications of this fact for individual dentists and for dentistry's professional organizations, deserves some comment. The cultural bias mentioned in Chapter 4 that views all judgments and choices as the actions only of individual humans, rather than seeing some of them as the actions of groups of persons acting as a unit, hinders our understanding that a whole profession can and does have obligations. This idea is as contrary to that cultural assumption as the ideal proposed in Chapter 4, and reiterated often in these pages, that the relationship a dentist should be striving for with each patient involves shared judgments and a shared choice of treatment that the two parties make together as a single chooser.

It is beyond the scope of this book to carefully examine the arguments that philosophers and other social theorists have made for and against the idea that groups can perform actions and have obligations. As was stated in Chapter 4, human experience is filled with situations in which a group, sometimes small, sometimes large, makes judgments, makes choices, and acts in other ways as a single entity. Of course, groups of humans do these things only by virtue of and by means of the actions of the individuals who make them up. But this fact does not entail that a listing of all the individual actions involved will be sufficient to completely describe what is going on in such a situation, without anything missing. Instead, even after all the actions of the individual dentists and other persons involved have been thoroughly described, we propose, there will sometimes be still more to say about what the *group* as a whole judges, chooses, and does.

Because such a group acts only by virtue of and by means of the actions of individuals, however, it cannot act to fulfill its obligations unless the relevant individuals, playing various roles within it, act as they need to so that the group acts as it ought to. Thus every member of the dental profession has, by reason of that membership, an additional professional obligation not explicitly mentioned in the preceding chapters. This is the obligation, which principally falls into the category of *proper relationship to the larger community*, to do what is necessary so that the profession as a whole acts as it ought.

Exactly how an individual dentist can and ought to fulfill this obligation will depend on many factors in the dentist's professional and personal life. Some of the obligations of the dental profession as a whole are such that individual dentists work for their fulfillment day-in and day-out at chairside in what they do and what they communicate about the dental profession. Thus they routinely act in the name of the profession and play a role in some of its collective actions without noticing it (although their noticing it, and noticing that they have obligations about it, and reflecting on these, is one of the goals of this discussion).

For some of the other obligations of the dental profession that will be discussed below, individual dentists can work effectively for their fulfillment only by taking on additional roles within the dental community, especially through dentistry's professional organizations. As every dentist knows, the extra burden of being active in organized dentistry cannot be made to fit into every professional life in the same way. Most dentists find some times in their professional lives more suited to playing an active role in dentistry's professional organizations, and other times—for example, when their children are younger and their practices are not well established—less suited for the demands of such activity. But no dentist may ethically look upon the activities of dentistry's professional organizations simply as matters that "someone else" is responsible for. At some appropriate point, every dentist ought to be active in shaping the actions and policies and contributing in other ways to the activities of organized dentistry as an important element in the collective life of dentistry as a whole. For every dentist bears a share of the responsibility for the character of the dental profession as a whole, and must take seriously the obligation to shape that character from within and to participate actively in the dialogue with the larger community that shapes it also from without.

For analogous reasons, each of the dental organizations has obligations not only to fulfill its own narrower mission but also to contribute to the fulfillment of the obligations of the dental profession as a whole. A dental organization that saw the obligations of the dental profession as a whole as none of its distinctive business would be as myopic in understanding its obligations as the individual dentist who saw them as someone else's work. Thus as every member of a dental professional organization bears a share of the responsibility for that organization's actions and policies, so the members must routinely include the fulfillment of the obligations of the dental profession as a whole on its agenda. Moreover, since there are many professional organizations within dentistry, with many distinctive missions, each of them has an obligation to communicate effectively with the others to make certain that their individual activities advance, rather than hinder, the fulfillment of the obligations of the dental profession as a whole. For without such active, self-conscious collaboration on the part of dentistry's many organizations, it is very possible that important elements of the obligations of the dental profession as a whole will be overlooked.

Why differentiate the dental profession as a whole so carefully from the various professional organizations within dentistry? The reason, already alluded to in Chapter 2, is that none of the dental professional organizations can simply speak for or act in the name of the whole community of dental practitioners. One reason for this is that in the United States, for example, none of these organizations actually includes all present practitioners. A second, more important reason is that each of the dental professional organizations has, of necessity, a particular set of concerns, a particular mission. Even the most broad based of them, no matter how admirable its goals and its achievements, cannot actually attend to all that dental practice stands for and involves. So rich a reality as the professional practice of dentistry cannot be formalized into the aims or mission of a single formal organization, and it is doubtful that even a large number of formal organizations, either those that already exist or these and others that might exist, could encompass so complex a reality even through intense collaboration in some sort of federated "super-organization." It seems more accurate, then, to distinguish the formal organizations from the dental profession as a whole.

Nevertheless, when concrete acts are needed, it is far easier for a formal organization to perform them than for the profession as a whole. The profession as a whole, like any very large, informally constituted group, works much more slowly and subtly, for example, in its dialogue with the larger community about the contents of dentistry's professional norms. Therefore as events occur that require shorter-term responses than the whole profession can achieve, and as the direction of the whole profession's actions in some matter become clear but now need more concrete, formal actions to embody them, the concrete actions of the dental professional organizations are essential, just as the actions of individual dentists in their day-in, day-out practices are also essential. Therefore for most dentists, the fulfillment of their obligation to take responsibility for and become active in the name of the profession as a whole will ordinarily include service through one or more of the professional organizations.

Thus every dental organization must remember that its actions communicate to the larger community what dentistry as a whole stands for (and so are governed by the norm of integrity and education), and yet they do not simply represent the whole of dentistry because the dental profession as a whole is larger, richer, and more complex than any organization. The task of the dental organization parallels that of the individual dentist, who is obligated not to misrepresent dentistry to the larger community (under the norm of integrity and education), and yet is obligated to represent it with some measure of humility, because he or she does not represent all that it stands for.

A very good example of this point is the ADA's *Principles of Conduct and*

Code of Professional Ethics. As was noted earlier, this document, and the official statements of the ADA's Council on Ethics, Bylaws, and Judicial Affairs that interpret it, is both one of the most important statements of the contents of dentistry's professional obligations, and yet it is also *not* a complete statement of those obligations, nor the last word about their content on the matters covered in it. Its importance lies in its being a carefully constructed document whose key elements have been formulated through a process that is widely representative of the membership of the largest dental professional organization in the United States. But its limitations lie in that it is the work of a formal organization, that this organization does not include all dentists in the society, and most importantly that the larger community dialogues with the dental profession about the contents of the profession's obligations in many other forums, some of them extremely subtle and informal. So the contents of the *Principles* are not legislative of the contents of dentists' professional obligations, nor are they finally determinative of their content in any other way. Yet it remains one of the most important expressions of dental professional obligations in the dialogue between dentistry and the larger community, and also one of the most important educational documents for dentists themselves regarding these obligations.

All those who play a role in a dental organization or act in some way in the name of dentistry as a whole have a similar double task. They are to correctly represent dentistry (and not misrepresent it). Yet they are also to be clear themselves and make it clear to those with whom they speak that they do not simply represent the whole profession, do not act simply in the name of the whole by themselves, but are at most partial actors for the whole. It is only when organizations understand and carry out this subtle task that dentistry as a whole can act and can fulfill its collective obligations through its professional organizations.

In spite of its importance to the life of the dental profession and its members, neither the idea that the dental profession as a whole has obligations nor the roles of individual dentists and dental professional organizations in contributing to their fulfillment have been much examined. But it is beyond the scope of this chapter to examine these themes in any greater detail. With these brief comments as background, the next task is to survey the main categories of professional obligation of the dental profession as a whole.

CHIEF CLIENT, CENTRAL VALUES, AND COMPETENCE

One of the most important roles of the dental profession in our society is its contribution to the society's understanding of what is to count as oral health and what are instances of its absence, especially with a view to professional intervention. As will be explained, the profession's obligations in carrying out this role require consideration of three different categories of professional norms, namely, chief client, central values, and competence.

The most general meanings of the concepts of health and disease are probably consistent across cultures and eras. But as these meanings are specified more concretely and grounded on more and more concrete understandings of desirable human functioning, the distinctive values of a given society's culture and even of the accepted modes of practice of each particular health care profession become incorporated into them. Thus what counts as oral health in a given society like our own is not something timeless, though it is connected to or is a specification of something of lasting and general human value. Instead, its functional content has been determined in large part by cultural conceptions of acceptable versus unacceptable levels of pain/comfort and function/dysfunction, and these in turn are significantly affected by the interventions that are performed by those considered expert in the society in addressing and modifying people's oral pain/comfort and function/dysfunction.

These last are the society's dental professionals. The interventions they perform do not include all possible interventions that they might perform. Only certain classes of possible interventions are considered constructive for oral health by the dental community. So the dental community, to a significant degree, creates what counts as oral health, as well as proper oral function and oral dysfunction. Yet which classes of intervention are considered proper is also partly determined by the culture's values regarding oral pain/comfort and function/dysfunction. Thus these two groups—the society's dental professionals and the community at large that is the carrier and shaper of its culture— work together to shape the concepts of oral health and its absence that guide the practice of the one and the expectations of the other.

To take an absurd example, suppose a patient came to a dentist to request assistance in strengthening his or her teeth and bite so that the patient could routinely crack the shells of nuts as squirrels do. Today's dentists would refuse the request as being dangerous to the patient's oral health and would likely view the patient as a crackpot, and they would be easily supported in this judgment by the larger community. But suppose that the vast majority of people in the society routinely made this request of dentists, and they did so for nutritional or environmental reasons that had acquired considerable currency in the society. Long before such a scenario became commonplace, the dental community would have begun to address the issue, either looking for alternatives for those in such need or working to challenge the reasoning that made this appear a reasonable health request when it is really a very risky one from the point of the society's previously accepted understandings of oral health. If these efforts failed over a period of time—how long is difficult to say—eventually the society's views of oral function and dysfunction would have changed, and very likely, the dental community would come to the point of devising modes of assisting the society's people in performing this function in as safe a manner as possible, given the rest of what the society and the dental community understand as constituting oral health and its absence.

The point here is certainly not to recommend this strange scenario, but to illustrate the fact that the dental profession does not unilaterally determine the content of oral health in a society. Nevertheless, its contribution to this process is far greater than that of any other definable group in society and is perhaps even equal to that of the larger community as a whole because of the community's continuing respect for the dental profession's relevant expertise. Consequently, the dental profession has an obligation to contribute to the shaping of these important concepts carefully and conscientiously. The dental profession makes its contributions to this process in three ways, corresponding to the three categories of professional norms identified above, namely, by determining the classes of persons that will be considered the profession's chief clients, the central values that it will work to achieve for its patients, and the sorts of interventions that will be included within the range of its competence.

There are classes of persons whom dentistry rightly serves and there are classes of persons whom it does not serve, like the "nut-cracker" patient of the previous example. Those whom it serves are rightly served because their conditions are considered appropriate needs for dentists to address. Those whom it refuses to serve fall outside the classes of persons whose needs are appropriate for dentists to address. In identifying certain classes of persons as those rightly served by its members, namely as its chief clients, the dental profession contributes to the society's understanding of oral health, even as the society for its part contributes to this determination as well.

There are also, as has been stressed often in these pages, certain values that dentistry is rightly committed to achieving for its patients, and other values that dentistry has no particular commitment to serve. In determining what the former values are, namely, its central values, and especially how they are to be understood concretely as the specific goals of dental practice at a given time in a given society, to be pursued in a given ranked order or hierarchy, the dental profession contributes to the society's understanding of oral health, even as the society for its part contributes to this determination, too.

Finally, there are interventions that members of the dental profession rightly perform under particular clinical circumstances, and other interventions that no dentist could appropriately perform under those circumstances. At work here is the professional norm of competence. The guidance that the profession's determinations of competent practice offer dentists at chairside is minute and may at first appear to be solely determined by scientific and technological fact. But these determinations are also controlled by an understanding of health that is embedded in the criteria that identify some interventions as competent under the circumstances and others as not so. As the dental community teaches new dentists and judges practicing dentists by these criteria of competent practice, it shapes the culture's understanding of oral health in great detail.

The dental profession, as it engages in dialogue with the larger community about the contents of the profession's norms of chief client, central values, and competence, has an obligation to attend carefully to the ways in which this dialogue shapes the whole community's understanding of oral health. The larger community has an obligation to participate thoughtfully in this dialogue, too. But the concepts and professional norms it yields will be employed more self-consciously by members of the dental profession, and in any case, the larger community accords first place in this dialogue to the dental profession by reason of its expertise. Therefore the dental profession has a special obligation to guide this dialogue carefully and to shape the contents of these important concepts for the whole community thoughtfully, and each dentist and each of dentistry's professional organizations also has an obligation, insofar as he or she or it plays a role in this dialogue, to contribute conscientiously to the fulfillment of the dental profession's obligations in this regard.

MORE ON COMPETENCE

The most obvious obligation of the dental profession as a whole was discussed in Chapter 9. It concerns the profession's supervision of the application of dental expertise so it is used (and not misused) to benefit both individual patients and, in the case of public health measures, the community at large.

This obligation is fulfilled in a variety of ways. First, the profession maintains standards of practice through the dental schools, continuing educations programs, and the professional organizations. Many individual dentists contribute to the profession's fulfillment of this obligation by serving as dental school faculty, by mentoring young dentists formally or informally, by supporting continuing education programs of many sorts, and also by providing financial support for all of these activities.

Second, the profession supports continuing research and quality control regarding procedures, materials, and many other aspects of clinical practice. It also supports the systems of licensure and, especially through professional organizations, has an active voice in legislative and other public forums dealing with competent dental practice. These are the settings where the ongoing dialogue between the dental profession and the larger community regarding standards of practice, the contents of the society's concepts of oral health, and the contents of the dental profession's ethical norms is most visible.

Third, the profession supports the work of peer review structures and the activity of individual dentists discussed in Chapters 9 and 10 to provide one another—and where necessary, appropriate review bodies—with effective communications about bad outcomes and bad work, whether minor and occasional, or serious or continual. The pressures on individual dentists against doing their part for the fulfillment of this aspect of the dental profession's obligations were discussed in those chapters. But without a committed effort on the part of individual practitioners to contribute to the work of the profession in this way, the dental profession will not be able to fulfill this aspect of its obligations. It was for this reason that in Chapter 9 the idea was stressed that every patient of any dentist is, in this respect, a patient of every dentist. For every dentist is an agent of the dental profession as a whole in this matter, and has an obligation to assure every patient of the profession that dental expertise will be used competently and to his or her benefit rather than misused.

A fourth and more subtle way in which the dental profession fulfills its obligations of competence, through the actions and judgments of its individual members and through its professional organizations, concerns the theme of different philosophies of dental practice. The point was made in Chapter 5 that, within the range of acceptable dental practice, there are a variety of philosophies of dental practice that a dentist may legitimately incorporate into his or her habitual patterns of practice. Dentists are not automatons, and neither are patients. Both groups benefit, and the oral and general health of patients and also their autonomy are all better served, when the profession supports different preferred patterns of practice and especially different philosophies of dental practice within the range of what is acceptable as competent dental care.

In all four of these areas, individual dentists and dentistry's professional organizations have obligations to continue to assist the profession as a whole, and where necessary to help it improve, in its efforts to fulfill its obligations under the norm of competence.

MORE ON THE CENTRAL VALUES

Another obvious component of the obligations of the dental profession as a whole concerns its efforts to achieve the central values of oral and general health and support and enhance patients' autonomy in oral health care outside the dental office.

With regard to oral and general health, the profession fulfills this obligation above all through the activities of every individual dentist and the members of his or her professional and nonprofessional staff who educate individual patients for self-care. It also fulfills this obligation through the educational efforts of its professional organizations and through other public health initiatives like support for the fluoridation of water supplies. The American Dental Association's program for evaluating and approving over-the-counter dental health products is another important example of an organizational effort that contributes to the profession's fulfillment of this aspect of its obligations.

It is worth noting that these efforts, whether of individual dentists or dental organizations, also support patients' autonomy. For they provide patients with increased control over the challenges to oral health that can affect them and enable patients to exercise this control at their own convenience, in their own preferred manner, and in the exercise of their own understanding of what is involved rather than in dependence on another's expertise.

The sixth of dentistry's central values, "Efficiency in the Use of Resources," has barely been mentioned since it was first identified in Chapter 5. Because most dentists practice as individual entrepreneurs or in very small groups, and because most patients are concerned about the cost of their dental care, we have assumed that such efficiency would be an automatic concern of dentists and patients alike and did not need more careful attention in these pages. But when this central value is considered from the perspective of the whole profession, a concern arises that does deserve attention.

American society has become increasingly conscious in recent years that health care resources are not unlimited. Whether or not this concern will issue in a national plan for the distribution of health care resources, and whether or not such a plan will be responsive to the kinds of questions about ethical distribution raised in Chapter 13, these are still important questions that the dental profession ought to be asking. Such questions ought to be on the agendas of both individual dentists and dentistry's professional organizations, as should similar questions about the typical ways in which today's dental resources are actually distributed.

If the dental profession does not thoughtfully initiate this conversation, it is very likely that the initiative will be taken by others less knowledgeable about what dental interventions can and cannot do and about what is at stake in oral health. The obligation of the dental profession as a whole to work for the most effective and appropriate employment of our society's dental care resources can only be fulfilled if both individual dentists and dentistry's professional organizations take up this initiative.

RELATIONSHIP TO CO-PROFESSIONALS

The theme of collaboration among health professionals that was stressed in Chapter 10 applies at the level of the whole dental profession as well. America's health professions have a great deal in common (and will likely have more so if the larger community begins to make serious policy decisions regarding the limits of its resources for health care). But this society's health professions have unfortunately spent at least as much effort in political struggles for turf as they have in trying to learn from and support one another or in working to collaborate in achieving the elements of human health that are common among their goals and values.

Health is not neatly divisible into tidy, profession-specific components. Therefore the dental profession's commitment to patients' oral and general health requires that the profession as a collective entity, again through the efforts of both individual dentists and dentistry's professional organizations, work toward increasing levels of cooperation with other health professions for the sake of its patients.

It is difficult to predict what such collaboration might yield, and it is difficult to predict how each profession's understanding of itself might benefit from the health professions' trying to work together and learn from one another. Each can surely learn much that is valuable from the others about the institution of profession and about the pursuit of people's health. But to date this learning is almost completely untapped. Therefore the dental profession has an obligation to begin to make effective use of the resource of the other professions to carry out its social role more effectively.

INTEGRITY AND EDUCATION, AND THE PRIORITY OF THE PATIENT

The obligation of each dentist, under the rubric of *integrity and education*, to practice and possibly to live in other aspects of his or her life consistently with the values and commitments of dentistry was a central theme of Chapter 8 and has been stressed in other chapters as well. This obligation carries an automatic reference to the dental profession as a whole, since it is the profession's values and commitments, and not simply those of the dentist as a particular individual, to which the dentist is obligated to bear witness. But there is another implication of this category of professional norms that concerns the dental profession as a whole. For the profession as a whole can also bear witness—or fail to—to dentistry's principal commitments, in particular those concerned with the theme of the priority of the patient and professional sacrifice discussed in Chapter 6.

The obligations of individual dentists to represent the dental profession correctly specifically in their business affairs were discussed at length in Chapter 14. It is important that a dentist not communicate to the public that the principal determinant of dentists' treatment decisions and relations with their patients is economic gain, but rather the achievement of their patients' well-being, especially the central values and the ideal of an interactive relationship.

For the very same reasons, it is important that the dental profession as a collective entity both act and communicate to the public in a manner that does not misrepresent dentistry's commitments to place patients' well-being and the health of the community ahead of other goals. Statements by dental organizations and their officers, and other dentists identified by the media as spokespersons or representatives for whatever reason, ought therefore to represent the commitments of dentistry accurately rather than presenting a picture of the profession as committed to something else, and the collective actions of dentists and dental organizations should be judged by the same standard.

The operative assumption about many organizations in American society is that they exist principally to serve the interests of their members, which is routinely taken to mean the self-interests of their members. This is a correct assumption about many groups and organizations in our society, including many that look outwardly not very different from most dental organizations, for example, the many trade associations that abound in American life. It is therefore of special importance that dental organizations, as the most visible indicators of what the dental profession stands for, carefully act on and communicate dentistry's message of commitment and priority.

Chapter 2 articulated this message by claiming that dentists and the dental profession have obligations, as expressed in the Normative Picture of the dental profession and denied in the Commercial Picture. Chapter 6 articulated it by claiming that the ethical practice of dentistry requires some genuine measure of sacrifice on the part of dentists for the sake of their patients. It is worth asking whether this claim ought not also be true of the dental profession collectively, and of each of dentistry's professional organizations, if it is to be a plausible message to those who hear it. For this message will impress few of its listeners if the profession or its organizations are perceived to be more interested in protecting dentists' turf or economic position, or in protecting a particular organization's turf or voice within dentistry, than in the well-being of patients and the health of the larger community. Sacrifice is a difficult message to communicate without falling into bland rhetoric. Nevertheless, each individual dentist and each dental organization has a special obligation to assist the profession as a whole in not only correctly communicating the profession's commitment to sacrifice and to the priority of the patient, but also in acting collectively in accord with it.

THINKING ABOUT THE CASE

Since the issues in this chapter's introductory case focus chiefly on the topic of the preceding section and the themes of the two sections on competence in this chapter, we will begin with the obligations of the dental profession as a whole under the norm of competence.

The final decision in the case clearly depends on a number of important technical judgments, required to be carefully made by the norm of competence, about exactly what Capwright does and exactly how its use might change, for good or ill, the standard of practice for prosthetic preparations. The associate editor is correct in proposing that the adoption of this bonding material could change the standard of practice regarding preparations by gradually shifting the point at which general dentists would refer a case to a prosthodontist. This is an example of the point stressed previously in this chapter that determinations of competent practice by the dental profession affect what counts as oral health in the society. But the associate editor's suggestion that making such shifts is inappropriate simply because changes in standards of treatment are involved is incorrect. Rather the relevant question is whether patient health will be significantly affected for the worse, or, if there is some slight loss of benefit or increase in risk of complications, whether that negative outcome is possibly sufficiently outweighed by a gain in efficiency in the use of dental care resources (i.e., by making more kinds of care more accessible to patients in general dentists' offices). The case as presented does not offer enough detailed clinical information to decide this matter here.

On the other hand, the managing editor is surely incorrect to suggest that decisions about such matters belong solely in the hands of dentists at chairside. The obligation to play a role in the dental profession's acting properly to evaluate a new dental product is not only the obligation of chairside dentists. It is at least equally the obligation of those assigned relevant roles within organized dentistry, with researchers and the technical editors and staffs of research journals having a particularly important responsibility in such matters. The editor of *AJP* is surely not mandated to make these important technical judgments alone. But he or she is surely mandated to play an important role in them, often enough as final arbiter, at least from the point of view of publication, of whether the judgments of many different judges are taken to support presenting a new product to the dental community or declining to do so.

Thus this case suggests many difficult questions about competence or standards of care and about who ought to play what roles in the shaping of these standards within the dental community. Some of them cannot be resolved here because the case does not provide enough technical data about Capwright. But others depend not on details of the case, but on views about the proper interplay of various roles within the dental community in fulfilling the dental profession's obligations with regard to competence and about what is to count as oral health. This commentary cannot explore these questions further either, but they deserve careful reflection both by individual dentists and by the professional associations within which such special roles are ordinarily assigned.

The case also raises questions about the mission of the organization that publishes *AJP* and of the purpose of the journal itself, both capable of being viewed as activities of the dental profession as a whole. Does the association exist to further the work only of the prosthodontists that are its members so that reducing the number of referrals from general dentists to prosthodontists would be inappropriate? Neither editor suggests this view, with the managing editor explicitly proposing that the association and the journal exist to improve the quality of dental care wherever it is given. Is this view appropriate, or would a narrower view of this organization's mission be acceptable, or even preferable?

What about the financial security of the journal? Does the managing editor speak against dentistry's commitment to the priority of patients' well-being in proposing that this lucrative ad copy will enable the journal to survive and continue its tradition of services to its readership? May the editor ethically publish advertising copy that he or she judges to be borderline from the point of view of competent practice, at least by current standards, in order to preserve a journal that provides important services to dentists? Or must borderline advertising copy be rejected in the name of patients' oral and general health, even if these might actually suffer in time if the journal's research and other services are less available?

We do not propose that these are easy questions (although they might become easier if the final technical data about Capwright points in one direction rather than another). The point is rather to notice that such questions are, as much as chairside issues are, important questions of professional ethics in dentistry. Every dentist, not just those in special roles within organized dentistry, ought to reflect on these issues and offer the fruits of their reflections to the profession as a whole to help it guide its actions and its communications to the larger community.

RELATIONSHIP TO THE PATIENT AND TO THE LARGER COMMUNITY

Dentistry as a whole does not deal directly with the individual patient as the dentist at chairside does. In that respect, the obligations of the dental profession as a whole touch the relationship between patient and dentist only insofar as the dental profession supports proper dentist-patient relationships educationally and through the actions of dental organizations and the like. But the question of the ideal relationship, as well as the choice between the four models of relationship considered in Chapter 4, is relevant to the obligations of the dental profession as a whole in another way, namely, with regard to the relationship between the profession as a whole and the larger community as these two parties engage in dialogue and act in concert in many other ways: what is the ideal relationship here?

We have proposed that in contemporary U.S. society, the Interactive Model represents the ideal relationship between dentist and patient. This claim seems to have very wide support within the dental community as well. Many dentists today work hard to achieve as interactive a relationship with each patient as is possible. Very few dentists are not guided in their relationships with patients by at least the minimal standard of interaction, which is informed consent. But the question is now worth posing whether a comparable effort ought not be under way within dentistry for the profession as a whole to relate to the larger community according to the same ideal of relationship.

As of this writing, dental organizations have rarely sought the input of members of the lay community in their deliberations on any matter, including matters in which technical dental knowledge or practice experience are of little importance. For example, as was noted in Chapter 14, the deliberations of dental organizations regarding the proper limits of ethical advertising by dentists, though they require information specifically about how nondentists understand dental advertising copy, have rarely included nondentists in the conversation. The evidence, in other words, suggests that the Guild Model is still the operative model of the relationship between the dental profession as a whole and the larger community.

Yet, as has been stressed throughout this book, the authors of the contents of the professional obligations of both individual dentists and dentistry as a whole profession include the larger community as well as the dental community. The contents of dentists' and dentistry's professional obligations are of necessity the fruit of a dialogue if they are to be meaningful at all. Yet when formal conversations are convened by dentistry's formal organizations, one party to that dialogue—the larger community—ordinarily goes unrepresented. If the Interactive Model of relationship is indeed the ideal relationship between those with dental expertise and those without it, as the authors have claimed, then the dental profession, and the organizations and individuals who act as parts of it, ought to think seriously about applying it conscientiously to the profession's ongoing dialogue with the larger community.

This proposal does not claim to have resolved the many difficult questions that will immediately arise about how this obligation, if it is indeed an obligation of the dental profession, ought to be carried out. Clearly, simply working through the most obvious voices within the larger community, such as its legislative or elected officials, is unlikely to answer the need. Nevertheless, however the details are resolved, we propose that a serious initiative to bring representatives of the larger community into active dialogue with the dental profession is in order.

What will be the topics of this dialogue? There may be many. But the most important topics of this dialogue, from the point of view of this book, will be the contents of the professional obligations of dentists and the dental profession. This book has attempted to identify the contents of these obligations as they currently exist, that is, as they are currently delineated within the ongoing dialogue that ought to become much more explicit as being a dialogue and much more self-conscious on both sides. But discussing the obligations of dentists and of the dental profession as a whole, as these obligations currently exist, is only half the task. The other half is to inquire whether the content these obligations currently have matches the content they *ought* to have. This is a question that the dental community and the larger community in dialogue need to keep on asking as the circumstances of social and professional life keep changing.

The proposal that the dental profession and the larger community be interactively related in explicit dialogue is most important with regard to this last question, with determining whether what is the case about dental professional obligations is what ought to be the case about them. Chapter 2 and other chapters in this book have stressed the theme that professional obligations are "made" obligations, the fruit of a dialogue, obligatory because they are accepted and committed to by the parties involved. This means they can be changed by those parties, and staying abreast of changing circumstances, as well as amending and adapting the professional obligations of dentists and of the dental profession as a whole accordingly, will require that the explicit dialogue being proposed here continue actively.

Thus one of the most important obligations of the dental profession as a whole, we propose, is to initiate a much more explicit and active dialogue with the larger community, on the model of the Interactive Model of dentist-patient relationship. In such a relationship, the two parties view each other as equals, not in dental expertise, but in having important information and important values to contribute to their collective deliberations, and as being moral equals and co-choosers of the path they will follow together. Developing such a relationship with the larger community, we believe, would place the dental profession in the best possible position to address the challenges that dentists and the dental profession will face as social and professional life and the realities of health care and its delivery all undergo major changes in the years to come.

CONCLUSION

The purpose of this book has not been to offer the last word on anything, but rather to provide a detailed, concrete impetus to more thoughtful and more extensive conversation about one of the most essential features of dentistry, its professional ethics. Our aim above all has been the stimulate reflection and conversation about the contents and the grounds of the obligations of individual dentists and of the dental profession as a whole. At the same time, the authors have argued that our society has gone through an important change regarding dental care over the last several decades.

At many points in this book, we have noted the differences between professional life according to the Guild Model and professional life according to the Interactive Model, based on mutual respect and the moral equality of the two parties, who work together to achieve shared judgments about what to do and a shared choice to do it. We are convinced that the Interactive Model is now normative for dental professionals in this society. That is why we have proposed many times in these pages that it is a key element for dentists' professional ethical reflections now and into the next century.

If this book prompts more thoughtful conversations about professional-ethical matters in dentistry between individual dentists, that would be a fine outcome. If it prompts conversations within and between groups of dentists and dental organizations, especially if the conversation crosses geographic lines and specialty divisions, that would be wonderful. If it prompts conversation from every corner of the dental community, from the most powerful in organized dentistry and the most respected in academic dentistry and dental research, to the most experienced in chairside practice, that would be outstanding. But this would still not be all that dentistry needs.

Our hope is that this discussion of professional-ethical issues in dentistry will also stimulate conversations about dental ethics between dentists and their patients, between dental organizations and groups within the lay community, between the dental profession and the larger community. Then all parties to the dialogue will be actively involved. Then, too, there will be a broad enough base of relevant experience that the answers that are the fruit of that dialogue—about how men and women who are committed to caring for others' oral health ought and ought not to act—will likely be the best possible.

Appendix: Bibliographic Essay

The most complete bibliography of materials in dental ethics is *The PEDNET Bibliography: 1993*, published by the Professional Ethics in Dentistry Network (PEDNET) and available from that organization. In this Appendix, we will identify some items listed in that document and some additional sources that readers will find useful for further study of the issues discussed in this book.

CHAPTER 1

There are two other book-length discussions of ethical issues in dentistry. One is *Dental Ethics*, edited by Bruce D. Weinstein (Lea and Febiger, 1993). This is a collection of 13 essays in dental ethics by leading authors in the field and includes an earlier version of the PEDNET Bibliography. The other is *Ethical Questions in Dentistry* by James T. Rule and Robert M. Veatch (Quintessence, 1993). Part One of this book is an introductory essay about moral theory and its relation to practical ethical issues. Part Two describes 109 cases drawn from dental practice, along with a brief commentary about the ethical issues in each case.

The American Dental Association's *Principles of Ethics and Code of Professional Conduct* and the codes of ethics of other dental professional organizations are one of the most important resources for studying dental professional ethics, and they provide, each in its own way, useful surveys of important issues in the field.

Some shorter introductions to issues in dental ethics include "Ethical Issues in Dentistry" by Laurence B. McCullough, in *Clinical Dentistry*, edited by Jefferson Hardin (Philadelphia: Lippincott, 1983, 1993); "Ethics in Dentistry: Review and Critique of Principles of Ethics and Code of Professional Conduct" by David A. Nash, *J Am Dent Assoc* 109(10):597-603, Oct 1984; "Ethical Issues in Dental Care" by Anthony W. Jong in Jong's book, *Community Dental Health*, 2nd edition (Mosby, 1988); "The Normative Principles of Dental Ethics" by Courtney S. Campbell and Vincent C. Rogers, in *Dental Ethics* edited by Bruce D. Weinstein (Lea and Febiger, 1993); and "Dentistry" by David T. Ozar, in the *Encyclopedia of Bioethics*, revised edition, edited by Warren Reich (Macmillan, 1994).

More intensive examination of ethical issues in dentistry will also benefit greatly from study of the major philosophical approaches to moral reflection. There are many introductory surveys of moral philosophy. Among the most readable are James Rachels, *The Elements of Moral Philosophy* (Temple University Press, 1986); Robert L. Holmes, *Basic Moral Philosophy* (Wadsworth, 1993); and Lawrence Hinman, *Ethics: A Pluralistic Approach to Moral Theory* (Harcourt Brace Jovanovich, 1994).

CHAPTER 2

The best short introduction to the general topic of professional ethics is *Professional Ethics* by Michael D. Bayles, 2nd edition (Wadsworth, 1989). Two other thoughtful books on this general theme are *The Moral Foundations of Professional Ethics* by Alan Goldman (Rowan and Littlefield, 1980) and *Grounding Professional Ethics in a Pluralistic Society* by Paul F. Camenisch (Haven, 1983). There are also several good books of readings on professional ethics that include both cases and essays about a number of different professions. Unfortunately, dentistry is rarely represented in such surveys. Two of these are *Ethical Issues in Professional Life* edited by Joan C. Callahan (Oxford University Press, 1988) and *Ethical Issues in the Professions* edited by Peter Windt et al. (Prentice-Hall, 1989).

Dentistry's status as a profession and the appropriateness of the Normative Picture of the dental profession is a frequent topic of editorials and letters to the editor in dental journals and of keynote addresses at professional society meetings. But these forums rarely offer an opportunity for detailed moral reasoning and consideration of alternative viewpoints. One happy exception is "The Privilege of Practice" by R. H. Scholl, in *J Am Dent Assoc* 98(1):159-60, Jan 1979. See also David T. Ozar's "Three Models of Professionalism and Professional Obligations in Dentistry," in *J Am Dent Assoc* 110(2):173-7, Feb 1985.

CHAPTER 3

The eight categories of professional obligation that are offered here as a conceptual tool for identifying and analyzing a profession's obligations are original with this book. An earlier version of this approach appeared in "Ethics for the Practicing Dentist: A Framework For Studying Professional Ethics" by David T. Ozar, *J Am Coll Dent* 58(1):4, 6-9, Spr 1991; but only the first seven categories were considered in that essay, and only very briefly. Obviously, many of the authors cited elsewhere in this bibliography also offer sets of key questions or themes to use in identifying and analyzing ethical issues and dentists' professional obligations.

CHAPTER 4

The relationship between the health care professional and the patient is probably the most discussed topic in the literature of contemporary health care ethics. Numerous articles have been written on the health care provider's obligation to respect the capable patient's autonomous decisions about treatment, and to provide patients with sufficient information that their decisions can be autonomous, and on the many other ways in which the patient-professional relationship can become ethically complex.

Several standard works about these topics are written with all the health professions in mind, not just dentistry: *Making Health Care Decisions: The Ethical and Legal Implications of Informed Consent in the Patient-Practitioner Relationship*, Volume One (U.S. Government Printing Office, 1983), which is the report on this topic from the President's Commission for the Study of Ethical Problems in Medicine and Biomedical and Behavioral Research; *A History and Theory of Informed Consent* by Ruth Faden and Thomas Beauchamp (Oxford University Press, 1986); and *Informed Consent: Legal*

Theory and Clinical Practice by P. Appelbaum, C. Lidz, and A. Meisel (Oxford University Press, 1987). The most thorough study of autonomy currently available is *The Theory and Practice of Autonomy* by Gerald Dworkin (Cambridge University Press, 1988).

There have been a number of valuable articles and one brief book on ethical issues related to informed consent in dental practice: "Informed Consent in Dentistry" by Herman Segal and Richard Warner, *J Am Dent Assoc* 99(6):957-958, Dec 1979; "Ethics in Dental Practice" by A. C. Hirsch and Bernard Gert, *J Am Dent Assoc* 113(4):599-603, Oct 1986; and "Ethical, Moral, and Legal Dilemmas in Dentistry: The Process of Informed Decision Making" by Burton R. Pollack and R. D. Marinelli, *J Law Ethics Dent* 1(1):27-36, 1988. See also Herman Segal and Richard Warner, *Ethical Issues of Informed Consent in Dentistry* (Quintessence, 1980); "Endodontic Intervention—Is It Paternalism?" by David J. Sokol, *J Am Dent Assoc* 117(1):5, July 1988; "Informed Consent in Dentistry" by David J. Sokol, *J Dent Pract Adm* 6(4):157-61, Oct/Dec 1989; "Can a Rational Patient Make an Irrational Choice? The Dental Amalgam Controversy," *Gen Dent* 40(3):184-7, 1992, by Gary T. Chiodo and Susan W. Tolle; "Informed Consent and Refusal" by John G. Odom and Donald F. Bowers, in *Dental Ethics*, edited by Bruce D. Weinstein (Lea and Febiger, 1993); and "The Dentist-Patient Relationship" by Jeffrey P. Kahn and Thomas K. Hasegawa, which also appears in *Dental Ethics*.

Our proposal that the Interactive Model identifies the ideal relationship between dentist and patient was first made in "Three Models of Professionalism and Professional Obligations in Dentistry" by David T. Ozar, *J Am Dent Assoc* 110(2):173-7, Feb 1985. Robert Veatch contrasts several models of patient-practitioner relationships, but with an emphasis on medical practice, in "Models for Ethical Medicine in a Revolutionary Age," *Hastings Center Report*, 2:5-7, June 1972, and develops his own preferred "triple contract" model in detail in his book *A Theory of Medical Ethics* (Basic Books, 1981). Another important model of the professional-patient relationship has been developed by Sally Gadow, this one in the context of nursing practice: "Existential Advocacy: Philosophical Foundation of Nursing," in *Nursing: Images and Ideals*, edited by Sally Gadow and Stuart Spicker (Springer, 1980). See also "Three Models of the Nurse-Patient Relationship" by Sheri Smith, published in the same collection. The obstacles to attaining the ideal of shared decision-making in the context of medical practice are eloquently discussed by Jay Katz in *The Silent World of Doctor and Patient* (The Free Press, 1984).

CHAPTER 5

An earlier version of the proposed hierarchy of central values appeared as "Value Categories in Clinical Dental Ethics" by David T. Ozar, David L. Schiedermayer, and Mark Siegler, *J Am Dent Assoc* 116(3):365-8, Mar 1988. The idea for the hierarchy came initially from efforts by Mark Siegler, Albert Jonsen, and William Winslade to identify the hierarchy of goals for medical practice in their book, *Clinical Ethics: A Practical Approach to Ethical Decisions in Clinical Medicine* (Macmillan, 1982). The hierarchy of central values proposed in Chapter 5 also functions as a fundamental principle of the 1991 revision of the Canadian Dental Association's *Code of Ethics*.

Of course, professional ethics in dentistry and in the other health professions has been discussed in terms of serving the patient's interest, *beneficence*, and doing no harm, *non-maleficence*, for as long as these professions have existed, and every effort to identify relevant interests or harms will involve considerations of the same sort that have been discussed in this book in the language of values. So it is not specifically the emphasis on values, whether worded as such or as interests to be furthered or harms to be avoided, or articulated in some other way, that is original with this book. The original contribution is rather in the particular hierarchy of values proposed in Chapter 5 and in the way this hierarchy is employed to assist moral reflection in the rest of the book.

The literature on the themes of beneficence and non-malevolence in health care ethics is very large. One especially thoughtful study of these traditional themes is Edmund Pellegrino and David Thomasma's recent book, *For the Patient's Good: The Restoration of Beneficence in Health Care* (Oxford University Press, 1988).

One particular central value receiving special attention in contemporary dental practice is esthetic values. Recent discussions of this topic include "Professional Ethics and Esthetic Dentistry" by David A. Nash, *J Am Dent Assoc* 117(4):7E-9E, Sept 1988; "Ethics and Esthetics," by John A. Gilbert, *J Am Dent Assoc* 117(3):490, Sept 1988; and "Esthetic Dentistry: A Case and Commentary" by John A. Gilbert and Mary Ellen Waithe, in *Dental Ethics*, edited by Bruce D. Weinstein (Lea and Febiger, 1993).

CHAPTER 6

Keynote speakers and professional journal editors frequently refer to dental professionals' obligations to accept some measure of sacrifice for the sake of their patients. But, as Chapter 6 indicates, until the advent of HIV and AIDS there had been little careful discussion in the literature of the extent of or the limits of this obligation. The ethics literature related specifically to HIV and AIDS will be discussed below in connection with Chapters 11 and 12.

CHAPTER 7

A standard, very thorough discussion of health care decisions for patients who are incapable of participating is Allan E. Buchanan and Dan W. Brock's *Deciding for Others: The Ethics of Surrogate Decision Making* (Cambridge University Press, 1989). Bruce L. Miller's essay, "Autonomy and the Refusal of Lifesaving Treatment," *Hastings Center Report* 11(4):22-28, Aug 1981, provides valuable guidelines for determining the extent of a patient's capacity for autonomous judgment and choice. Two other well-known discussions of that topic are "Tests of Competency to Consent to Treatment," *Am J Psychiatry* 134(3):279-284, 1977, by L. Roth, A. Meisel, and C. Lidz, and "Assessing Patients' Capacities to Consent to Treatment," *N Engl J Med* 319(25):625-638, 1988, by P. Appelbaum and T. Grisso.

There is far less literature on decision-making with patients with partial capacity. Two useful articles are "The Many Faces of Competency" by James F. Drane, *Hastings Center Report* 15(2):17-21, 1985 and "Paternalism and the Mildly Retarded" by Dan Wikler, in *Paternalism*, edited by Rolf Sartorius (University of Minnesota Press, 1983). Mary Mahowald's *Woman and Chil-*

dren in Health Care: An Unequal Majority (Oxford University Press, 1993), contains a discussion of children's decision-making. Another useful book is *Children and Health Care: Moral and Social Issues*, edited by John Moskop and Loretta Kopelman (Reidel, 1989).

Articles addressing these themes specifically in connection with dental professional ethics include "Ethical Issues in Pediatric Dentistry" by David T. Ozar, *Pediatr Dent* 13:374 1991; "Ethical Issues in Dental Care for the Compromised Patient" by David T. Ozar, *Spec Care Dent* 16:6, 1990; "Diminished Autonomy: Can a Demented Patient Consent to Dental Treatment?" *Gen Dent* 56(9):372-3, Sept/Oct 1992, by Gary T. Chiodo and Susan W. Tolle; "Ethics and the Patient with Dementia" by S. K. Shuman, *J Am Dent Assoc* 119(6):747-8, Dec 1989; and "Dental Care for the Cognitively Impaired: An Ethical Dilemma" by Anthony W. Jong, *Gerodontics* 4(4):172-3, Aug 1988.

CHAPTER 8

Many practice management consultants strongly advise the collaborative picture of practitioner-patient relationship proposed in this chapter. This is also the theme of some of the authors mentioned above in connection with the discussion of the ideal dentist-patient relationship in Chapter 5. But there is not much literature that focuses directly on the professional-ethical significance of integrity and education.

Several articles that touch on this theme are David T. Ozar's "Ethics of Management Techniques and Therapeutic Approaches" in *Behavior Management for the Pediatric Dental Patient*, edited by John A. Bogert and Robert L. Creedon (American Academy of Pediatric Dentistry, 1989); David J. Sokol and Carol K. Sokol, "A Review of Non-intrusive Therapies Used to Deal with Anxiety and Pain in the Dental Office," *J Am Dent Assoc* 110(2),217-222, 1985; Carol K. Sokol, Scott M. Sokol, and David J. Sokol, "Attitude Change Through Affective Dentistry: The Initial Assessment," *Internat J Psychomat* 33(1):88-91, 1986; and Patricia Marshall, "Reducing Emotional Distress Associated with Childhood Illness," *Compr Ther* 15:3-7, 1989.

CHAPTER 9

There is some literature on the legal aspects of malpractice and on the strategies that dentists can use to minimize their risk of and in malpractice suits. But there has been very little systematic discussion of the ethical aspects of bad outcomes, much less careful analysis of the important distinction between occasional, minor bad work and gross or continual bad work that is stressed in this chapter.

David J. Sokol's "Some Aspects of the Emerging Dental Malpractice Crisis," *J Law Eth Dent* 1(1):22-26, 1988, identifies several clear ethical challenges for dentists because of the malpractice crisis. See also the essay by Lisa S. Parker and Jeffrey Holloway mentioned below in connection with Chapter 10. "Am I My Brother's Warden? Responding to the Unethical or Incompetent Colleague" by Haavi Morreim, *Hastings Center Report* 23(3):19-27, 1993, distinguishes levels of adverse outcomes to assist health professionals in assessing one another's conduct and forming an ethical judgment about it. Though her examples are drawn from medical practice, many parts of her analysis apply equally well to dentistry. "Whistle-Blowing in Dentistry: What Are the Ethical Issues" by David A. Baab and David T. Ozar, *J Am Dent Assoc* 125(2):199-205, 1994, addresses some of the same questions in the context of dental practice. David T. Ozar's "Malpractice and the Presuppositions of Medical Practice," *Ann Health Law* 3, 1994, tries to picture what medical practice and health care generally would look like if the myths of infallible technologies and infallible practitioners were rejected by our society.

CHAPTER 10

The idea of building strong, positive relationships within one's referral network, within one's office, and with others who care for the same patients is not only a matter of common sense, but a common theme for many practice management consultants. Chapter 10 proposes that it is also a significant component of a dentist's ethical commitments as a professional. We know of very few systematic discussions of this topic from the perspective of professional ethics, either in the dental literature or in the health care literature generally. Four recent essays on various aspects of this topic all appear in *Dental Ethics* edited by Bruce D. Weinstein (Lea and Febiger, 1993): "Professional Responsibilities Towards Incompetent or Chemically Dependent Colleagues" by Lisa S. Parker and Jeffrey Holloway; "Relationships with Dental Hygienists and Dental Assistants" by Mary Alice Gaston and Marcia A. Gladwin; "Race, Gender, and Class: What Can the Profession Do to Promote Justice?" by Teresa A. Dolan, Linda C. Niessen, and Mary B. Mahowald; and "When the Dentist Tells the Hygienist, 'Just Do It!'" by Beverly Bizup Hawkins.

CHAPTER 11

HIV and AIDS have been discussed extensively in the health care literature since the mid-1980s. Of particular importance for dental ethics is the ADA's *AIDS Policy Statement, J Am Dent Assoc* 115(6):833, 1987. Among the articles discussing the dentist's professional obligation to treat HIV-positive patients, and the limits of that obligation, are the following: "Dentistry and AIDS: Ethical and Legal Obligations in Provision of Care" by Vincent C. Roger, *Med Law* 7(1):57-63, June 1988; "AIDS, Risk, and the Obligations of Health Professionals" by David T. Ozar in *AIDS and Ethics: Biomedical Ethics Reviews-1988*, edited by James M. Humber and Robert F. Almeder (Humana Press, 1989); "AIDS and Dentistry: Conflicting Right and the Public's Health" by Mary Ellen Waithe in the same volume; "Are You Willing to Treat AIDS Patients?" by Donald Sadowsky and Carol Kunzel, *J Am Dent Assoc* 122(1):29-32, 1991; "AIDS, Ethics, and Dental Care" by David T. Ozar in *Clark's Clinical Dentistry*, edited by Jefferson Hardin (Lippincott, 1993); and "HIV-Infection in Dentistry: Ethical and Legal Issues" by Mary Ellen Waithe and Gordon G. Keyes in *Dental Ethics*, edited by Bruce D. Weinstein (Lea and Febiger, 1993).

Two thoughtful articles on the special confidentiality issues that can arise when a dentist is caring for an HIV-positive patient are "Doctor-Patient Confidentiality and the Potentially HIV-positive Patient" by Gary T. Chiodo and Susan W. Tolle, *J Am Dent Assoc* 119(5):652-4, Nov 1989 and "A Challenge to Doctor-Patient Confidentiality: When HIV-positive Patients Refuse Disclosure to Spouses" by the same authors, *Gen Dent* 40(4):257-7, 1992.

CHAPTER 12

The citations in the text from Glantz et al. are taken from "Risky Business: Setting Public Health Policy for HIV-Infected Health Care Professionals" by Leonard H. Glantz, Wendy K. Mariner, and George J. Annas, *The Milbank Quarterly*, 70(1):43-79, 1992. See also "HIV-Infected Surgeons and Dentists: Public Threat or Public Sacrifice?" by Norman Daniels in the same issue of *The Milbank Quarterly*. Another valuable discussion of public policy regarding HIV-infected health care providers will be found in the *Michigan Recommendations on HIV-Infected Health Care Workers* by the Ad Hoc Committee on HIV-Infected Health Care Workers (Michigan Department of Public Health, October 1, 1991).

Additional discussion of the professional ethical issues that arise when a dentist is HIV-positive will be found in "AIDS, Ethics, and Dental Care" by David T. Ozar in *Clark's Clinical Dentistry*, edited by Jefferson Hardin (Lippincott, 1993) and in "An Analysis of the Ethics of Health Care Providers with HIV" by Gary T. Chiodo and Susan W. Tolle, *Gen Dent* 40(6): 460-6, Nov/Dec, 1992. See also the "Report and Advisory Opinion Concerning the Advertising of Negative Results of HIV Tests" by the American Dental Association Council on Ethics, Bylaws, and Judicial Affairs (American Dental Association, October, 1992); "The HIV-Infected Dental Professional: A Challenge to Law, Ethics, and the Dental Profession" by Mary K. Logan, *J Dent Pract Adm* 6(4):162-8, Oct/Dec 1989; and "HIV-Positive Health Care Professionals: Should They Still Provide Patient Care?" by James J. Koelbl, *J Law Eth Dent* 4:63-72, 1991.

CHAPTER 13

Many philosophers and political theorists have proposed accounts of the fundamental principles of distributive justice for human societies, some in very great detail and with considerable sophistication of reasoning. A useful survey of the approaches that are most often discussed today is *Justice: Alternative Political Perspectives* edited by James Sterba (Wadsworth, 1991). Joel Feinberg's brief survey of principles of distributive justice in "Social Justice," Chapter 7 of his book, *Social Philosophy* (Prentice-Hall, 1973), is also very useful.

A number of health care ethicists have applied these more general theories of justice specifically to the distribution of health care resources in American society. A standard resource on this topic is *Securing Access to Health Care: The Ethical Implications of Differences in the Availability of Health Care* by the President's Commission for the Study of Ethical Problems in Medicine and Biomedical and Behavioral Research (U.S. Government Printing Office, 1983). Charles J. Dougherty also provides a good survey of these approaches in his book *American Health Care: Realities, Rights, and Reforms* (Oxford University Press, 1988).

Four theorists who have carefully developed positions on the ethical distribution of health care resources are Larry R. Churchill, *Rationing Health Care in America: Perceptions and Principles of Justice* (Notre Dame University Press, 1987); H. Tristram Engelhardt, Jr., *The Foundations of Bioethics* (Oxford University Press, 1986); Norman Daniels, *Just Health Care* (Cambridge University Press, 1985); and Erich Loewy, *Suffering and the Beneficent Community* (State University of New York Press, 1991).

Unfortunately, none of these authors pays specific attention to *dental* care resources. We know of no previous systematic study of the application of the ethical criteria of social justice to dental care resources. A strong polemic against the idea that members of our society have any sort of rights regarding health care resources will be found in "Health Care, Human Rights, and Government Intervention" by G. F. Kuskey, *Ca Dent Ass J* 1(1):10-3, Jl 1973.

CHAPTER 14

Much has been written and spoken to encourage dentists to address the ethical challenges to which both the changing social environment for health care and the business aspects of dental practice unavoidably give rise. There is also a lot of conversation among dentists and within dental organizations about the ethics of dental advertising. But systematic efforts to examine these issues against the background of a detailed understanding of dentists' professional obligations are few and far between. The dental community would benefit greatly if more of its members undertook the task of carefully formulating their views on these matters.

A number of the articles mentioned elsewhere in this bibliography do address the issues of Chapter 14, at least by implication. In addition, on the topic of ethical advertising in dentistry, there are a number of significant articles: Federal Trade Commission's "Final Order on Ethical Restrictions Against Advertising by Dentistry," *J Am Dent Assoc* 99(12):927-93, Nov 1979; "Dental Advertising: A Help or a Hindrance? New Patients Use Advertising to Find Dental Care" by Anthony W. Jong, *Dentistry* 7(2):9-12, Apr 1987; "The Process of Professionalization: Getting Down to Business in Dentistry: The Effect of Advertising on a Profession." by David L. Schiedermayer, *J Am Coll Dent* 55(1):10-16, Spr 1988; "Dentists' Advertising—Patient Welfare or *Caveat Emptor*" by Thomas H. Boerschinger, *Dent Prac Adm* 9(4):5-9, Dec 1989; "Professional or Commercial Enterprise? An Ethical Analysis of Dental Advertising" by Linda S. Scheirton, *Tx Dent J* 190(9):19-27, Sept 1992; and "Advertising" by Linda S. Scheirton and Thomas H. Boerschinger, *Dental Ethics*, edited by Bruce D. Weinstein (Lea and Febiger, 1993).

Finally, on the ethical issues involved in capitation and similar insurance arrangements, see "Informed Consent in Dentistry: The Impact of `Who Pays the Bills'," by David J. Sokol, *J Law Eth Dent* 2(2):64-8, Apr/June 1989.

CHAPTER 15

Although the officers, committees, and councils of dentistry's many professional organizations undoubtedly discuss the proper ethical role of their organizations and of dentistry as a single profession on a daily basis, the literature of dental ethics includes few examples of systematic ethical reflection on these matters. Many a journal editor has also called readers' attention to such issues as well. But editorial writers rarely have the opportunity to work out the ethical issues in careful detail. Nor does this chapter's brief survey of the ethical obligations of the dental profession as a whole and of its professional organizations fill this need sufficiently. This is a task that deserves the serious attention of both individual dentists and the various dental organizations.

Index